NURSING CARE OF THE ELDERLY

4th Edition

Edited By
John Lantz, RN, Phd

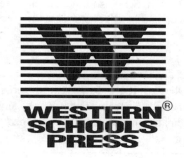

WESTERN®
SCHOOLS
PRESS

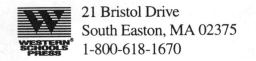

21 Bristol Drive
South Easton, MA 02375
1-800-618-1670

ABOUT THE EDITOR

John Lantz, RN, PhD, is currently a professor and program chair in Community Health Nursing, School of Nursing, San Diego State University. He is a 1990-1991 postdoctoral fellow in Applied Gerontology, The Gerontological Society of America.

FOURTH EDITION REVISED BY

Joan Cagley-Knight, MSN, ARNP, is a registered nurse specialist in field operations with Health Quality Assurance, Agency for Health Care Administration, Area 8, Fort Myers, FL. She holds a Master of Science in Nursing from the University of South Florida, Tampa, FL and a Master of Arts in Counseling from the University of Northern Iowa in Cedar Falls, IA. For 10 years Ms. Cagley-Knight was a nursing instructor at Hawkeye Community College in Waterloo, IA. She is also a certified federal/state survey-or for long term care facilities and the former director of educational services at a national educational video company where she wrote and/or produced 50 educational video tapes for long term care and home health staff use.

ABOUT THE AUTHORS

Doris Bower, RN, ANP, C, is a nurse practitioner at the University of California, San Diego, Alzheimer's Disease Research Center.

Kimberly Butrum, RN, MS, is at the University of California, San Diego, G.N.P. Alzheimer's Disease Diagnostic and Disease Program. Her master's degree is in gerontological nursing.

Ann Harbord, MS, RD, is a consultant providing clinical and administrative dietary services to seven convalescent hospitals and skilled nursing facilities in the San Diego area.

Susan Johnson, RN, CNA, MS, is a geriatric nurse practitioner with the Division of Family Medicine at the University of California, San Diego.

Marcie Lepkowsky, Pharm D, is an assistant clinical professor for the University of California, San Francisco, San Diego Program. She is also staff pharmacist at the University of California, San Diego Medical Center.

Deborah Lubow, MS, RN, C, is an adult nurse practitioner in Hospital Based Home Care at the Veteran's Administration Medical Center, Baltimore, Maryland.

Barbara Santamaria, MPH, RN, C, is an adult nurse practitioner in Hospital Based Home Care at the Veteran's Administration Medical Center, Baltimore, Maryland.

Angela Staab, RN, MN, CGNP, is currently chairperson of the nursing department at Rockingham Community College in North Carolina. She is also an adjunct assistant professor at both University of North Carolina-Greensboro and University of North Carolina-Chapel Hill schools of nursing.

Revision by: Joan Cagley-Knight, MSN, A.R.N.P.

Subject Matter Expert: Suzanne Doyle Friedman, MS, RN

Indexer: Sylvia Coates

Typesetter: Kathy Johnson

Western Schools' courses are designed to provide nursing professionals with the educational information they need to enhance their career development. The information provided within these course materials is the result of research and consultation with prominent nursing and medical authorities and is, to the best of our knowledge, current and accurate. However, the courses and course materials are provided with the understanding that Western Schools is not engaged in offering legal, nursing, medical, or other professional advice.

Western Schools' courses and course materials are not meant to act as a substitute for seeking out professional advice or conducting individual research. When the information provided in the courses and course materials is applied to individual circumstances, all recommendations must be considered in light of the uniqueness pertaining to each situation.

Western Schools' course materials are intended solely for *your* use and *not* for the benefit of providing advice or recommendations to third parties. Western Schools devoids itself of any responsibility for adverse consequences resulting from the failure to seek nursing, medical, or other professional advice. Western Schools further devoids itself of any responsibility for updating or revising any programs or publications presented, published, distributed, or sponsored by Western Schools unless otherwise agreed to as part of an individual purchase contract.

ISBN: 1-57801-031-4

IMPORTANT: Read these instructions *BEFORE* proceeding!

Enclosed with your course book you will find the FasTrax® answer sheet. Use this form to answer all the final exam questions that appear in this course book. If you are completing more than one course, be sure to write your answers on the appropriate answer sheet. Full instructions and complete grading details are printed on the FasTrax instruction sheet, also enclosed with your order. Please review them before starting. *If you are mailing your answer sheet(s) to Western Schools, we recommend you make a copy as a backup.*

ABOUT THIS COURSE

A "Pretest" is provided with each course to test your current knowledge base regarding the subject matter contained within this course. Your "Final Exam" is a multiple choice examination. **You will find the exam questions at the end of each chapter.** Some smaller hour courses include the exam at the end of the book.

In the event the course has less than 100 questions, mark your answers to the questions in the course book and leave the remaining answer boxes on the FasTrax answer sheet blank. **Use a <u>black pen</u> to fill in your answer sheet.**

A PASSING SCORE

You must score 70% or better in order to pass this course and receive your Certificate of Completion. Should you fail to achieve the required score, we will send you an additional FasTrax answer sheet so that you may make a second attempt to pass the course. Western Schools will allow you three chances to pass the same course...*at no extra charge!* After three failed attempts to pass the same course, your file will be closed.

RECORDING YOUR HOURS

Please monitor the time it takes to complete this course using the handy log sheet on the other side of this page. See below for transferring study hours to the course evaluation.

COURSE EVALUATIONS

In this course book you will find a short evaluation about the course you are soon to complete. This information is vital to providing the school with feedback on this course. The course evaluation answer section is in the lower right hand corner of the FasTrax answer sheet marked "Evaluation" with answers marked 1–25. Your answers are important to us, please take five minutes to complete the evaluation.

On the back of the FasTrax instruction sheet there is additional space to make any comments about the course, the school, and suggested new curriculum. Please mail the FasTrax instruction sheet, with your comments, back to Western Schools in the envelope provided with your course order.

TRANSFERRING STUDY TIME

Upon completion of the course, transfer the total study time from your log sheet to question #25 in the Course Evaluation. The answers will be in ranges, please choose the proper hour range that best represents your study time. You MUST log your study time under question #25 on the course evaluation.

EXTENSIONS

You have 2 years from the date of enrollment to complete this course. A six (6) month extension may be purchased. If after 30 months from the original enrollment date you do not complete the course, *your file will be closed and no certificate can be issued.*

CHANGE OF ADDRESS?

In the event you have moved during the completion of this course please call our student services department at 1-800-618-1670 and we will update your file.

A GUARANTEE YOU'LL GIVE HIGH HONORS TO

If any continuing education course fails to meet your expectations or if you are not satisfied in any manner, for any reason, you may return it for an exchange or a refund (less shipping and handling) within 30 days. Software, video and audio courses must be returned unopened.

Thank you for enrolling at Western Schools!

WESTERN SCHOOLS
P.O. Box 1930
Brockton MA 02303
(800) 618-1670

NURSING CARE
OF THE ELDERLY

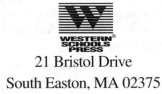

21 Bristol Drive

South Easton, MA 02375

Please use this log to total the number of hours you spend reading the text and taking the final examination (use 50-min hours).

Date	Hours Spent
_____	_____
_____	_____
_____	_____
_____	_____
_____	_____
_____	_____
_____	_____
_____	_____
_____	_____
_____	_____
_____	_____
_____	_____

TOTAL

Please log your study hours with submission of your final exam. To log your study time, fill in the appropriate circle under question 25 of the FasTrax® answer sheet under the "Evaluation" section.

PLEASE LOG YOUR STUDY HOURS WITH SUBMISSION OF YOUR FINAL EXAM. Please choose which best represents the total study hours it took to complete this 30 hour course.

A. less than 25 hours   C. 29–32 hours

B. 25–28 hours   D. greater than 32 hours

NURSING CARE OF THE ELDERLY

WESTERN SCHOOLS' NURSING
CONTINUING EDUCATION EVALUATION

Instructions: Mark your answers to the following questions with a black pen on the "Evaluation" section of your FasTrax® answer sheet provided with this course. You should not return this sheet. Please use the scale below to rate the following statements:

A Agree Strongly	**C Disagree Somewhat**
B Agree Somewhat	**D Disagree Strongly**

The course content met the following education objectives:

1. Described the areas which are important in gerontological nursing.

2. Discussed the major causes of mental and emotional changes in the geriatric populace.

3. Discussed normal aging changes occurring to the senses of vision, hearing, taste, and smell, and described nursing caregiving strategies to cope with the problems these changes present to the older adult.

4. Discussed normal physiological changes that occur with aging and discussed risk factors that these normal physiological changes may present in activities of daily living for an elderly person.

5. Discussed the manifestations of coronary artery disease/myocardial infraction, congestive heart failure, hypertension, cerebrovascular accident (stroke), osteoarthritis, osteoporosis, and gout in the older adult.

6. Discussed physiological changes that affect drug disposition and how different drugs are used for geriatric patients.

7. Identified the nutritional problems that are prevalent in geriatric patients.

8. Delineated that dementia is a disease process and not a part of normal aging. Discussed the development of a comprehensive care plan for the patient with Alzheimer's disease.

9. Discussed death and dying, and the legal and ethical issues involved.

10. Identified needs of the elderly in a variety of settings and strategies to promote healthy aging.

11. The content of this course was relevant to the objectives.

12. This offering met my professional education needs.

13. The information in this offering is relevant to my professional work setting.

14. The course was generally well written and the subject matter explained thoroughly? (If no please explain on the back of the FasTrax instruction sheet.)

15. The content of this course was appropriate for home study.

16. The final examination was well written and at an appropriate level for the content of the course.

Please complete the following research questions in order to help us better meet your educational needs. Pick the ONE answer which is most appropriate.

17. What is your work status?

    A. Full-time employment

    B. Part-time employment

    C. Per diem/Temporary employment

    D. Inactive/Retired

18. For your LAST renewal did you take more Continuing Education contact hours than required by your state, if so, how many?

    A. 1–15 hours

    B. 16–30 hours

    C. 31 or more hours

    D. No, I only take the state required minimum

19. Do you usually exceed the contact hours required for your state license renewal, if so, why?

    A. Yes, I have more than one state license

    B. Yes, to meet additional special association Continuing Education requirements

    C. Yes, for professional self-interest/cross-training

    D. No, I only take the state required minimum

20. What nursing shift do you most commonly work?

    A. Morning Shift (Any shift starting after 3:00am or before 11:00am)

    B. Day/Afternoon Shift (Any shift starting after 11:00am or before 7:00pm)

    C. Night Shift (Any shift starting after 7:00pm or before 3:00am)

    D. I work rotating shifts

21. What was the SINGLE most important reason you chose this course?

    A. Low Price

    B. New or Newly revised course

    C. High interest/Required course topic

    D. Number of Contact Hours Needed

22. Where do you work? (If your place of employment is not listed below, please leave this question blank.)

    A. Hospital

    B. Medical Clinic/Group Practice/ HMO/Office setting

    C. Long Term Care/Rehabilitation Facility/Nursing Home

    D. Home Health Care Agency

23. Which field do you specialize in?

    A. Medical/Surgical

    B. Geriatrics

    C. Pediatrics/Neonatal

    D. Other

24. For your last renewal, how many months BEFORE your license expiration date did you order your course materials?

    A. 1–3 months

    B. 4–6 months

    C. 7–12 months

    D. Greater than 12 months

25. **PLEASE LOG YOUR STUDY HOURS WITH SUBMISSION OF YOUR FINAL EXAM.** Please choose which best represents the total study hours it took to complete this 30 hour course.

    A. less than 25 hours

    B. 25–28 hours

    C. 29–32 hours

    D. greater than 32 hours

CONTENTS

PRETEST

Begin by taking the pretest. Compare your answers on the pretest to the answer key (located in the back of the book). Circle those test items that you missed. The pretest answer key indicates the course chapters where the content of that question is discussed.

Next, read each chapter. Focus special attention on the chapters where you made incorrect answer choices. Exam questions are provided at the end of each chapter so that you can assess your progress and understanding of the material.

1. A major factor contributing to an older person's ability to recover from illness is

   a. hospitalization.
   b. medicare reimbursement.
   c. caregivers' attitude.
   d. number of medications prescribed.

2. Which of the following healthcare maintenance activities is recommended for the elderly?

   a. Annual pneumonia immunization
   b. Annual influenza immunization
   c. Never take more than three medicines at a time
   d. Exercise is a safety hazard

3. A nurse is most likely to help an older patient recover by doing which of the following?

   a. Being sure to teach the patient everything in the care plan.
   b. Proving he or she has a positive attitude by doing everything he or she can for the patient.
   c. Communicating understanding and a belief that improvement is possible.
   d. Setting limits so the patient will learn independence.

4. Alcoholism can have the same signs and symptoms as what other condition?

   a. Liver disease
   b. Unexplained injuries
   c. Hallucinations
   d. All of the above

5. Delirium is characterized by

   a. rapid onset.
   b. fluctuating course.
   c. impaired attention.
   d. all of the above.

6. A major cause of conductive hearing loss in older adults is

   a. accumulated cerumen.
   b. noise damage.
   c. presbycusis.
   d. tinnitus.

7. Decreased pupil size results in

   a. presbyopia.
   b. less light reaching the retina.
   c. night blindness.
   d. less color in the iris.

8. The risk factor for the development of cataracts other than age is

    a. obesity.

    b. alcoholism.

    c. night driving.

    d. poor nutrition.

9. Overall physiological changes of aging can be traced to

    a. basic cellular changes.

    b. heredity.

    c. body system changes.

    d. alterations in the integrated whole.

10. It is estimated that by age 80 cardiac output has decreased as much as

    a. 5%.

    b. 10%.

    c. 25%.

    d. 50%.

11. Which of the following is true regarding sleep and elderly persons?

    a. It's hard to awaken them once they have fallen asleep.

    b. They have fewer sleep-stage changes.

    c. They need less sleep.

    d. They awaken more often during the night.

12. The preferred treatment for osteoporosis includes:

    a. Skeletal traction for 3–4 weeks.

    b. Calcium, vitamin D, and estrogen replacement.

    c. Bed rest for a week at a time before ambulating again.

    d. Calcium, vitamin A, and vitamin E supplementation.

13. What is gout?

    a. Osteophyte formation and degeneration that limits usual range of motion.

    b. An acute infection of the great toe.

    c. An acute inflammation of synovial tissue caused by the deposit of urate crystals.

    d. Degeneration or rheumatoid condition of hyaline articular surfaces, which causes pain.

14. Enzymatic biotransformation of drugs is an example of which type of pharmakinetic activity?

    a. Elimination

    b. Distribution

    c. Metabolism

    d. Absorption

15. Which of the following is among the guidelines for medication use specified by Title 22 in the chapter Health Facilities and Referral Agencies?

    a. Prn orders are no longer allowed.

    b. Prn orders must be accompanied by appropriate indications for drug use.

    c. Drugs may be used as chemical restraints as long as they are ordered by a physician.

    d. Drugs may be used as chemical restraints if there is limited staff available to care for that patient.

16. Which drugs most often cause adverse reactions serious enough to lead to hospitalization of elderly patients?

    a. Antimetabolites

    b. Diuretics

    c. Antibiotics

    d. Laxatives

17. Which of the following is the best way to prevent osteoporosis?

    a. Ensure adequate fluid intake.

    b. Engage in moderate, routine endurance exercise throughout one's lifetime.

    c. Eat a variety of foods.

    d. Maintain normal weight for height and age.

18. What is the most frequently used enteral feeding product in the elderly?

    a. Hyperosmolar formula

    b. Isotonic, lactose-free formula

    c. Blenderized food

    d. Carnation Instant Breakfast

19. The best treatment for prevention of further infarcts in multi-infarct dementia is

    a. control of hypothyroidism.

    b. control of hypertension.

    c. control of symptoms of depression.

    d. limited use of anticholinergic drugs.

20. Which of the following conditions could cause delirium in a demented elderly patient?

    a. Impaction, urinary tract infection

    b. Dehydration, noisy environment

    c. Hunger, change in routine

    d. Thirst, emotional upset

21. Which of the following activities is appropriate for a nurse to offer demented patients as a response to their wandering when the wandering is viewed as agenda behavior?

    a. Asking them to assist with setting out craft supplies.

    b. Letting them pace in the hallway undisturbed.

    c. Having them watch television in the dayroom.

    d. Orienting them to reality every hour.

22. Which of the following is a key factor in determining the dosage of pain medications for a cancer patient?

    a. Risk of addiction

    b. The patient's weight

    c. The needs of the family or caregiver

    d. Whether the medication relieves the pain

23. Which of the following statements about ethics is true?

    a. Ethical decisions are legally correct.

    b. Withdrawing a treatment is more serious than withholding it.

    c. Ethical principles will enable caregivers to make a single correct decision.

    d. Ethics apply to everyone equally.

24. Regular physical exercise and activity aid in which of the following?

    a. Preparing one for marathon running

    b. Reducing obesity, blood pressure, and blood lipids

    c. Increased risk of falls

    d. Increasing osteoporosis

25. What is the most common psychosocial disorder in American men 18–65 years old?

    a. Depression

    b. Alcoholism

    c. Heart disease

    d. Stress

CHAPTER 1

INTRODUCTION

by
Susan Johnson, RN, CNA, MS

CHAPTER OBJECTIVE

After studying this chapter, the reader will be able to recognize the areas that are important in gerontological nursing.

LEARNING OBJECTIVES

After studying this chapter, the reader will be able to:

1. Recognize the potential for improvement in the health of an older person.

2. Differentiate between the process of aging and the disease process.

3. Select nursing characteristics that enhance the health of older clients.

4. Specify that the population over 65 is expected to almost double between 1985 and 2030, with the over-85 population growing fastest of all.

5. Select lifestyle characteristics that tend to maximize successful aging.

6. Recognize that aging probably has a multiple causation, involving biological, psychological, and social causes.

Gerontology is the study of older adults. It includes the contributions of many disciplines, including sociology, psychology, biology, medicine, and nursing. The term "geriatrics" was created in approximately 1905 to describe the field of applied gerontology, which involves the medical care of the elderly. Geriatrics has come to mean applied gerontology in any discipline. Another term, "gerontic nursing," was coined to describe the field of nursing care of older people, but it has not yet achieved wide acceptance.

AGING AND DISEASE

There are two truths to be kept in mind by those attempting to provide healthcare for the elderly. Although these truths may seem to be contradictory, understanding both of them will give nurses and other healthcare personnel a clearer vision of the work needed. The first truth is:

Being old is not the same as being ill.

Robert Butler, a leading gerontologist, tells a story that illustrates this point: A 120-year-old man goes to his doctor complaining of a pain in his right knee. The doctor looks at the knee, palpates it, and takes radiographs of it, but can not come up with a diagnosis. He sits down with the patient and tells him, "You're 120. You've got to expect some aches and pains at your age." The elderly man looks back at the doctor and replies, "But Doc, my left knee is 120 too, and it feels fine!" As diagnostic techniques become more sophisticated, and as research looks more carefully at the distinction between aging and disease, physical changes once considered a part of aging are often found to be the result of disease or deconditioning.

Nurses and other caregivers need to look with a critical eye and with a mind-set of prevention and rehabilitation at the discomforts and functional losses that often accompany aging. Only if caregivers believe there may be a way to correct a problem will they be motivated to try. And *communicating* this belief in improvement is the only way to encourage patients to believe in their own recovery and be willing to put forth the effort required to achieve it.

The second truth is related to the fact that aging is often accompanied by disease. More than 80% of people over 65 have at least one chronic health problem, and the number increases with advancing age. Health and the ability to function decline with age. The most common chronic conditions among the elderly are, in order of prevalence, arthritis, hypertension, hearing impairment, heart conditions, chronic sinusitis, visual impairments, orthopedic problems, diabetes, varicose veins, and hemorrhoids (Eliopoulis, 1995). The nine leading causes of death for the population over age 65 are: heart disease, malignant neoplasms, cerebrovascular accidents, chronic obstructive pulmonary disease, pneumonia/influenza, diabetes mellitus, accidents and adverse effects, chronic liver disease (cirrhosis), and suicide. Admissions to the hospital are three times more frequent in older adults than in younger persons, hospital stay is 50% longer, and twice as many prescription drugs are used (DeMaagd, 1995). Acute episodes of one or more chronic illnesses account for most hospitalizations of persons more than 65 years old. The most frequent findings are of the circulatory problems (31%), digestive diseases (12%), respiratory diseases (11%), and neoplasms (10%). The elderly have about 4 diagnoses per hospital discharge, compared with only 2.5 for younger patients. This information accounts for the disproportionate use of acute care facilities in the elderly. The annual rate of hospitalization for persons over age 65 is 365 per 1000 or twice that of younger persons. For those over age 75 the rate is over 50% (Jahnigen, 1997).

While hospitalized, the elderly individual is vulnerable to a number of unfavorable events. These may include: side effects of medications, falls, adverse effects from the diagnostic studies, nosocomial infections, and surgical complications. The term "hospital deconditioning syndrome" has been adopted to acknowledge the rapid decline in functional status brought on by bed rest. Changes include joint stiffness, decreased muscle mass, bone demineralization and lost aerobic capacity. This association between aging and disease and the difficulty in knowing what is the result of aging itself and what is the result of disease bring us to the second truth:

To draw a distinction between disease and normal aging is to attempt to separate the undefined from the undefinable.

Both of these truths are valuable in guiding our practice, despite the seeming contradiction. And the contradiction can be resolved by realizing that both are part of a larger truth. In the 1960s, a conflict raged in the field of child development concerning whether development was determined by inherent nature or by the "nurture" or upbringing a child received. It was resolved through understanding that nature and nurture are interacting elements, each influencing the other. So, too, in gerontology, aging and disease are interacting elements of later life. The work for nurses and for other healthcare workers can then focus on what to do about any decrease in function or comfort. Instead of asking, "Is this problem due to aging or to disease?" caregivers can ask instead, "Can this problem be prevented or remedied?" And the job for healthcare workers becomes providing care that fosters prevention and remediation for everyone, no matter what age.

EFFECTIVE NURSING CARE IN HEALTH AND ILLNESS

Nurses are involved in all phases of health-care for older people preventing illness and promoting health, helping people cope with disease and maintain an existing level of health, and caring for people unable to care for themselves. Nurses provide care at three levels of prevention. **Primary prevention** is aimed at detecting and reducing risk factors that predispose people to disease. Immunization and counseling on smoking cessation are examples of primary prevention. **Secondary prevention** involves early detection of a disease before the disease becomes dangerous or disabling. Early detection of hypertension or elevated blood sugar is an example of secondary prevention. **Tertiary prevention** consists of detecting a disease that is symptomatic and taking action to maximize recovery. Teaching a diabetic patient to self-administer insulin or providing fluid to a dehydrated patient in a nursing home are examples of tertiary prevention.

In all phases of prevention, nurses assess patient needs, plan the care needed, and implement the plan. Implementing the care plan includes hands-on caregiving and coordinating with others to get the necessary care. Usually, the care plan also involves teaching the patient or the patient's family about the problem and about ongoing care. Frequently, care includes counseling in some form to help patients and family members cope with illness. These caregiving and counseling functions can only be successful if the nurse understands the patient's perspectives and priorities. This understanding is called empathy. It is also important that the patient believe in the competence and caring of the nurse. This belief is called trust.

Empathy involves understanding. To have empathy for a patient, a nurse must act from a desire to understand the patient as much as from a desire to help. One model of human interaction that explains this need to act from a desire to understand is that all human interaction is directed either by a desire to protect oneself or by a desire to understand the other person. Whenever people act out of a desire to protect themselves—and most human interaction is of this type—they increase the barriers between themselves and the people with whom they are communicating. Only when separation and isolation become painful do people switch to a desire to understand. Behavior motivated by the desire to understand another person increases sharing and respect between people. Nurses need to nurture the ability to approach clients not with a protective attitude but with a desire to understand the clients' problems from *the clients'* point of view. Since nurses usually work in settings where they are responsible for accomplishing a specific set of tasks, the need to protect oneself by "completing" the assigned work may become the main motivating force. But providing care that does not fit the patient's own perception of his or her needs will not contribute to the well-being of that patient in the long run. All the care that nurses provide should be given with an underlying desire to understand that patient—in other words, with empathy.

Most basic nursing texts describe communication techniques that contribute to the development of a therapeutic relationship. Although specific techniques such as reflecting the person's words, asking open-ended questions, or waiting in silence can contribute to effective communication, any of them used in a mechanistic fashion will fail to convey a sincere desire to understand.

Establishing and maintaining a relationship or counseling another does not involve putting on a facade of behavior to match a list of characteristics. Rather both you and the client will change and continue to mature. As the helper, you are present as a total person while assisting the senior client to come to grips with needs, conflicts, and self (Murray, Huelskoetter, & O'Driscoll, 1980).

Reece and Faryna (1990) describe the qualities of active listening that will be most helpful in developing an empathic and trusting relationship:

- Quiet attention to the patient's responses.

- Body language that communicates interest.

- Using phrases such as "what else" or "go on."

- Repeating or paraphrasing key words of the patient.

A HEALTHY PERSPECTIVE FOR NURSES

Often barriers exist between people that are based on a lack of understanding or fear of understanding. By making special efforts to retain our desire to understand the client, nurses can sometimes overcome these barriers and develop an empathic and trusting relationship. In caring for older patients, one major source of barriers is the caregiver's own unexamined fears about aging and loss. An older person who is exhibiting agitated or regressive behavior is doing so because that is the best way he or she can cope at that time. Nurses who have unexamined assumptions and fears about aging find it very difficult to accept such a patient as a full human being and very difficult to retain the motivation to understand. Protective actions such as avoiding the patient, or even intimidation, may make the nurse feel safer, but such actions are hurtful to the patient and inconsistent with quality nursing care. Similarly, when a compliant patient expresses dependence and tells a nurse that the nurse is the only one who cares, a nurse with unexamined fear of loss or isolation may react with an inappropriate self-protective action, such as encouraging the patient's dependency.

As more and more of America's population enters the "geriatric" category, more and more nurses will be involved in caring for the elderly. These nurses need to be aware of their own feelings about aging and be willing to attempt to understand their clients. One way to examine your feelings about older people is to look at how you characterize specific older people and determine whether those characterizations are more positive or more negative.

DEMOGRAPHICS

Although demographic trends may be uncertain given current birth and death rates, the proportion of the United States population over 65 will grow dramatically in the next 60 years. One way to describe this trend is to look at absolute numbers, and these numbers are increasing. In 1900, there were 3.1 million persons over 65 in the United States. By 1990, that number increased to 31.1 million. It is projected that by the year 2050, the number of persons over age 65 will be nearly 69 million, well over twice as many as there are today. The elderly population increased 11-fold from 1990 to 1994, compared to only a 3-fold increase for those under 65. In July, 1994 there were 33.2 million elderly (one-eighth of the total population) (U.S. Bureau of Census, 1996).

Another way of looking at the growth of the older population is to calculate the percentage of persons over 65. This is a significant measurement in our society, because people over 65 tend to be retired from the work force. In 1986, 12.1% of the U.S. population was over 65. It is estimated that by the year 2000, 13% will be over 65, and by the year 2030, this may rise to 21.1%. Surely the problems associated with aging will become greater and greater in the foreseeable future.

Not every area within the United States has the same percentage of elderly persons. Although seniors are less likely to move than their younger neighbors, in the 5 years between 1980 and 1985, 880,000 people over 65 moved, and more than a third of that number shifted from the Northeast and Midwest to the South or West. *Figure 1-1* shows the projected distribution of the over-65 population by area from 1993 to 2020.

One of the demographic trends facing our society is that not all of the elderly are in one group. There are those who are still functionally independent and often lead vigorous lives. Others are more likely to be frail, having more illnesses, less functional independence, and fewer reserves with which to cope with illness or accidents. This second group is increasing in relative size even faster than the whole group of the elderly. It is probable that even more healthcare will be needed in the decades to come. It is also apparent that some of the care of the elderly will be provided by their aging children.

SUCCESSFUL AGING

Our society will be able to cope better with the increasing numbers of older citizens if there is better health and less disability in the older population. Also, we all would like to be fully alive and functionally independent for as long as we live, without prolonged illness or disability. Advances in medical care have extended the life span of people today, but medical care has not yet been able to ensure that morbidity will be decreased. Now that many people live well into their seventh or eighth decade, we must turn our attention to decreasing morbidity and the loss of health and function that can result from disease.

Many baby boomers, who have received better medical care and had better work environments than their predecessors, will enter old age healthier than previous generations. They also will strive for wellness and will expect the health care system to assist them in healthy aging, not just in providing care when they become ill (Beck & Chumbler, 1997).

RESEARCH ON AGING

By looking at examples of successful aging, caregivers can develop guidelines for preventive practices that will minimize the health problems of older people and maximize health, functional ability, and independence in the elderly. Nursing's role in this process begins with a thorough knowledge of the entire aging process, both physical and psychosocial. Assessment skills that are age-appropriate and the ability to identify and plan for risk factor reduction on primary, secondary and tertiary levels are essential (Stanley & Beare, 1995). Nurses play a critical role in all practice areas for developing and implementing nursing research in aging. Nurses have common sense about the clinical issues and concerns and can implement research findings.

The most accurate data about the effects of aging come from longitudinal studies of groups of people, which examine how the group changes over time. These studies are conducted over a period of several years, some of them over several decades. They are very expensive to do, and so there are not very many of them. A more common method of studying older people is to look at differences between age groups, or cohorts, at the time of the study which is cross-sectional. These studies can make an error of attributing a change to age that is actually the result of differences in life history. An example is the study of dental care for the elderly. The older people are, the less dental care they seek. But this is a cohort difference rather than the result of aging. By looking at the pattern over time, it becomes apparent that the 60-year-olds of 10 years ago sought the same amount of dental care as the 70-year-olds of today. And the amount of dental care today's 50-year-olds received 10 and 20 years ago is the same as those same people get today. It is extremely common for an elderly person not to have sought dental care for years (Berkey & Valdez, 1997). Most of the health

FIGURE 1-1 *(1 of 2)*
Population 65 Years and Over and 85 Years and Over for States: 1993, 2000, 2010, and 2020

Region, division, and State	Persons 65 years and over					Persons 85 years and over				
	Number				Percent change, 1993 to 2020	Number				Percent change, 1993 to 2020
	1993[1]	2000	2010	2020		1993[1]	2000	2010	2020	
United States	**32,791**	**35,322**	**40,104**	**53,348**	**62.7**	**3,369**	**4,333**	**5,969**	**6,959**	**106.5**
Northeast	7,199	7,304	7,600	9,348	29.9	753	923	1,198	1,295	72.0
New England	1,832	1,853	1,979	2,537	38.5	207	257	338	369	78.6
Middle Atlantic	5,366	5,451	5,622	6,811	26.9	546	665	861	926	69.4
Midwest	8,060	8,367	8,912	11,206	39.0	906	1,099	1,407	1,549	71.0
East North Central	5,533	5,754	6,097	7,578	37.0	583	719	941	1,032	77.1
West North Central	2,527	2,613	2,815	3,627	43.6	323	380	466	517	60.0
South	11,360	12,724	15,058	20,513	80.6	1,115	1,512	2,158	2,613	134.4
South Atlantic	6,228	7,132	8,560	11,644	86.9	587	840	1,264	1,549	163.9
East South Central	2,007	2,167	2,461	3,247	61.8	207	260	335	391	89.3
West South Central	3,125	3,425	4,037	5,622	79.9	321	412	559	673	109.6
West	6,173	6,927	8,534	12,281	99.0	595	800	1,206	1,501	152.1
Mountain	1,677	1,925	2,361	3,374	101.2	155	222	338	417	169.9
Pacific	4,496	5,002	6,174	8,906	98.1	441	578	868	1,084	145.9
New England	1,832	1,853	1,979	2,537	38.5	207	257	338	369	78.6
Maine	170	176	192	256	50.4	19	23	30	34	79.5
New Hampshire	134	141	166	237	76.8	15	19	25	29	98.1
Vermont	69	72	82	110	59.1	8	9	12	14	66.6
Massachusetts	842	842	881	1,109	31.7	97	120	155	168	73.6
Rhode Island	155	151	153	195	26.2	17	21	27	28	66.2
Connecticut	462	471	504	630	36.3	51	65	88	96	88.3
Middle Atlantic	5,366	5,451	5,622	6,811	26.9	546	665	861	926	69.4
New York	2,388	2,426	2,526	3,028	26.8	257	301	379	418	62.7
New Jersey	1,071	1,112	1,192	1,480	38.2	102	128	171	187	83.3
Pennsylvania	1,908	1,913	1,904	2,303	20.7	187	236	310	320	71.1
East North Central	5,533	5,754	6,097	7,578	37.0	583	719	941	1,032	77.1
Ohio	1,480	1,547	1,619	1,986	34.2	151	186	252	276	82.4
Indiana	728	772	836	1,048	44.0	77	95	125	139	80.1
Illinois	1,479	1,513	1,588	1,952	32.0	157	193	243	262	66.2
Michigan	1,171	1,211	1,277	1,579	34.9	116	148	200	219	88.4
Wisconsin	676	711	776	1,013	50.0	80	97	121	136	69.2
West North Central	2,527	2,613	2,815	3,627	43.6	323	380	466	517	60.0
Minnesota	568	602	683	918	61.5	73	88	110	126	73.3
Iowa	436	439	449	546	25.1	58	67	80	85	46.5
Missouri	741	769	837	1,072	44.6	89	104	129	143	61.1
North Dakota	94	93	93	117	23.9	13	16	18	20	55.7
South Dakota	105	108	111	142	34.3	14	16	20	22	55.6
Nebraska	229	236	248	317	38.5	31	35	42	46	47.6
Kansas	353	366	395	517	46.5	46	54	67	75	64.3

See footnotes at end of table.

Source: Bureau of the Census. Current Population Reports, Special Studies, P23-190, *65+ in the United States.* U.S. Government Printing Office, Washington, DC, 1996.

promotion and disease prevention measures that have been identified as decreasing mortality and morbidity are actually lifestyle changes rather than the direct result of medical care. And the lifestyle patterns that are recommended need to begin long before a person enters the geriatric category. So, we can consider that one job for people concerned with the health of older people is to address the issue of healthful and preventive lifestyles for younger people as well as for seniors.

PRIMARY PREVENTION

Primary prevention of illness and disability for older people includes several measures that should ideally be a part of their lives

FIGURE 1-1 *(2 of 2)*

Population 65 Years and Over and 85 Years and Over for States: 1993, 2000, 2010, and 2020

Region, division, and State	Persons 65 years and over					Persons 85 years and over				
	Number				Percent change, 1993 to 2020	Number				Percent change, 1993 to 2020
	1993[1]	2000	2010	2020		1993[1]	2000	2010	2020	
South Atlantic	6,228	7,132	8,560	11,644	86.9	587	840	1,264	1,549	163.9
Delaware	87	100	113	146	67.2	8	10	16	19	134.6
Maryland	549	602	701	929	69.2	52	66	95	111	115.1
District of Columbia	77	73	72	87	13.2	8	10	12	12	47.3
Virginia	712	803	967	1,319	85.3	67	91	134	162	143.7
West Virginia	278	277	280	342	23.1	28	35	44	46	67.3
North Carolina	865	998	1,200	1,633	88.7	80	114	170	213	166.3
South Carolina	426	482	575	738	84.9	35	52	79	96	171.8
Georgia	695	798	998	1,419	104.0	65	89	125	156	138.2
Florida	2,539	2,999	3,654	4,982	96.2	245	372	589	735	200.4
East South Central	2,007	2,167	2,461	3,247	61.8	207	260	335	391	89.3
Kentucky	482	509	563	729	51.3	52	62	77	88	70.1
Tennessee	651	717	839	1,129	73.5	66	84	112	133	102.9
Alabama	545	591	668	874	60.4	54	69	90	106	95.4
Mississippi	329	350	391	514	56.3	35	45	55	64	82.4
West South Central	3,125	3,425	4,037	5,622	79.9	321	412	559	673	109.6
Arkansas	362	383	436	580	60.1	39	49	62	72	86.5
Louisiana	487	514	565	741	52.0	47	60	77	88	88.0
Oklahoma	440	454	501	661	50.4	50	60	75	85	70.6
Texas	1,835	2,074	2,534	3,640	98.4	186	244	344	428	130.3
Mountain	1,677	1,925	2,361	3,374	101.2	155	222	338	417	169.9
Montana	113	118	130	174	54.2	12	16	22	24	102.9
Idaho	130	144	172	246	89.4	13	18	25	29	121.7
Wyoming	51	51	54	74	43.4	5	6	8	8	69.5
Colorado	357	416	514	743	108.0	37	48	72	89	143.8
New Mexico	178	204	247	350	97.3	16	24	35	44	166.6
Arizona	529	623	783	1,121	111.9	46	72	117	146	221.2
Utah	165	187	230	334	102.4	16	23	34	42	161.1
Nevada	155	183	231	333	115.6	10	15	27	34	245.3
Pacific	4,496	5,002	6,174	8,906	98.1	441	578	868	1,084	145.9
Washington	612	676	836	1,245	103.5	62	84	123	146	135.5
Oregon	418	434	505	724	73.2	43	56	76	84	95.2
California	3,303	3,704	4,605	6,622	100.5	323	418	636	809	151.0
Alaska	26	31	38	54	103.3	2	2	3	4	197.0
Hawaii	137	158	190	262	91.6	12	18	30	40	241.8

Note: Totals may not add due to independent rounding and percents are computed on unrounded numbers.

[1]These estimates are consistent with the population as enumerated in the 1990 census, and have not been adjusted for census coverage errors. Includes Armed Forces residing in each State.

Source: U.S. Bureau of the Census, 1993 data consistent with 1994 Census Advisory, *Updated National/State Population Esimates*, CB94-43; 2000, 2010, and 2020 from *Population Projections for States, by Age, Sex, Race, and Hispanic Origin: 1993 to 2020*, Current Population Reports, P25-1111, U.S. Government Printing Office, Washington, DC, 1994, Series A - preferred series.

Source: Bureau of the Census. Current Population Reports, Special Studies, P23-190, *65+ in the United States*. U.S. Government Printing Office, Washington, DC, 1996.

well before they become senior citizens. These measures include the following:

Smoking Cessation

Older smokers respond as well as younger ones to smoking cessation. Within 1–5 years, after stopping smoking, older people can expect a reduction in risk of coronary heart disease to the level of non-smokers. Risk of other diseases also decrease, leading to an increased life expectancy. While "lecturing" patients is probably not helpful, being willing to discuss the issue and convey a caring and optimistic attitude may help significantly. Referral to smoking cessation programs and support groups can increase the success of smoking cessation efforts.

Alcohol Limitation

Alcoholism is a problem for many older people; estimated prevalence is between 5% and 25%. Not only does alcoholism lead to liver disease and esophageal varices, it is also implicated in malnutrition, increased smoking, accidental falls, and adverse drug interactions. Nurses are often in an ideal position to detect inappropriate alcohol use and can encourage patients and family members to seek appropriate treatment.

Safety Precautions

Seat-belt use significantly decreases injury and disability from automobile accidents. Safe sex—either through monogamous relationships or through condom use—is as important for sexually active older people as for younger ones. In assessing these safety practices, nurses can communicate to older people who matured before such safety habits were considered routine the importance of such precautions. Falls are also a source of injury to the elderly. Nurses can examine the environment around the older person and recommend changes to decrease the chances of a fall. Some specific suggestions for the home include removing loose rugs and cords that cross pathways, installing grab bars and nonskid surfaces in the tub or shower, and making supplies and equipment (such as cooking tools) easily reachable to prevent the temptation to climb unsafely. In the nursing home or hospital, nurses can prevent fall injuries by leaving call bells, water pitchers, and other needed items within reach of older patients who are bed-bound.

Adequate Nutrition

Although caloric needs may diminish with decreasing activity levels, adequate protein, vitamins, and minerals are still needed for the body to be able to resist or recover from injury or infection. Adequate fiber and fluid are essential components to prevent constipation, which has been linked to cancer of the bowel. Although fats generally should

make up only 20% of the diet, it is important to be willing to compromise on that measure when a person is having difficulty getting sufficient calories and is underweight. Weight control is a preventive measure for many ills, from heart disease and hypertension to degenerative joint disease. Nurses often evaluate food intake and counsel patients about appropriate diets or refer the patients to nutritionists. In evaluating nutritional intake, nurses should be aware of the problems created by poverty, cultural food preferences, and poor nutritional habits of some older people. An example of the failure to do this is the case of a 78-year-old woman on a hospital medical ward whose records indicated that she chose her own meals. However, further investigation revealed that the diet she had been receiving consisted mostly of desserts with very little nutritional value. This patient's eating habits were the result of many years of indulging her preference for sweets. A person who has insufficient income, or no transportation, or no facilities for cooking, can be at high risk for malnutrition.

Immunizations

Although not a lifestyle measure, immunizations are also a part of primary prevention. One-time immunization against pneumonia is generally recommended, but it may be more effective if done at about age 55, when the immune system is more effective than in later years. Influenza vaccine, given at the start of every flu season, can reduce the prevalence of influenza by about 70% with very little risk. Tetanus immunization should be repeated every 10 years. Although tetanus is not a common disease, it is much more likely to be fatal for an elderly person.

Exercise

Many geriatricians recommend exercise, even in old age, as a method of improving well being (Hall, 1997). Benefits of exercise can include improved cardiovascular functioning, decreased bone loss, buildup of lean body mass and muscle strength, increased flexibility, and improvements in glucose tolerance and cholesterol levels (Rubenstein, 1998). *(See Table 1-1, Benefits of Exercise).* Recommendations include starting slowly; using low-impact, unstressed exercise vs. non-stressful; and progressing gradually with such activities as swimming and stationary bicycling. Not only vigorous physical exercise but also less intensive exercise has benefits.

SECONDARY PREVENTION

Cancer Screening

Early detection of many types of cancer, although not preventing disease, leads to dramatically improved survival rates. Breast cancer and colon cancer are two relatively common diseases for which annual screening is effective in achieving a cure. The American Cancer Society also recommends that women continue to get Pap smears every third year after three negative annual tests. Physicians usually include an examination of the prostate in their regular screening for older men. The American Cancer Society (1998) recommends that both the PSA (prostate-specific antigen) blood test and the digital rectal exam be completed annually for all men over age 50. Nurses can reinforce teaching about cancer screening, encourage patients to do it, and discuss the fears that may cause a client to avoid recommended testing.

TERTIARY PREVENTION

One preventive measure that commonly involves nurses is teaching patients about appropriate medication use. Older people use more medicines, and as a person takes more medicines, the chance of an adverse drug reaction increases. Nurses are often in the position to review medication use, especially when more than one

physician is involved and prescriptions may be duplicated or conflicting. Teaching patients about proper drug use is also frequently a nursing task. Seniors who take their own medicine should know not only what it is for and when and how to take it, but also what side effects should be reported to their doctor, whether it can have any effect on their lifestyle (such as a sedating drug affecting ability to drive), and whether it will interact with over-the-counter drugs, food, or alcohol.

SUCCESSFUL AGING: A CASE STUDY

In the 1960s, Sula Benet (1971) investigated the lifestyle and health practices of the Abkhasians of Soviet Georgia. Through a series of yogurt commercials, these people had become notable in the United States for their long lives. Although some question whether the Abkhasians exaggerate their ages, there is little doubt that these Georgians routinely live well past their eighties and retain functional abilities until the very end of their lives. A description of their way of living can be seen as a prescription for a healthy old age. Cultural factors enter into their successful aging and include increased prestige given to older people. They have lived in the same area for centuries, and originally herdsmen, by the 1960s they were primarily farmers living in small villages. Abkhasians do not have a word for calling people "old." Instead, people over 80 are called "long-lived." Death is seen as an unnatural occurrence, and grief is often very strong. Abkhasians themselves attribute their longevity to lifestyle practices in sex, work, and diet.

Although modesty is an important social norm, sexual activity is not seen as a source of guilt (with the exception that a double standard exists; women are expected to be virgins at their first marriage). Sexual activity is considered "a pleasure to be regulated for the sake of one's health, like a good

---

TABLE 1-1
Functional Benefits of Exercise with Aging

MENTAL

Improved memory especially logical.

EMOTIONAL

Reduced stress and loneliness.

Improved sleep.

Enhanced feelings of well-being.

MUSCULOSKELETAL

Improved muscle strength.

Improved absorption of calcium.

Increased agility.

Improved range of motion.

Enhanced equilibrium (fall prevention.)

CARDIOPULMONARY

Improved lung expansion.

Increased endurance.

Improved peripheral circulation..

Lowering of cholesterol level.

Decreased blood pressure, if needed.

GASTROINTESTINAL

Improved elimination and digestion.

Decrease in body fat percent and weight.

---

wine". Sexual activity is postponed until the twenties or even the thirties, but continues to the eighties and beyond.

In their work, Abkhasians never retire, but there is little stress, because everyone works at his or her own pace. Everyone continues to work in whatever way he or she can. People tend to do less strenuous work as they reach their eighties and nineties, but they remain active contributors to the community. Farmers will switch from plowing to weeding; housewives will do less heavy housework but will continue to cook, raise chickens, and knit. Abkhasians maintain an attitude that work is an integral part of living.

The diet of Abkhasians is stable and does not change significantly with age or economic status. They eat slowly, taking small bites, chewing slowly. Their calorie intake is 23% less than that of their industrialized neighbors. They eat three meals a day. Meat is eaten only once or twice a week and is fresh and lightly cooked. They rarely eat fish. The staple is a cornmeal mash, boiled without salt. They eat cheese and buttermilk daily (not yogurt) and occasionally eat eggs. Fruit and vegetables are eaten daily, providing a high vitamin content. A hot sauce and garlic are served at every meal. Honey is used, but not sugar. They do not drink coffee or tea, but do drink small quantities of a low-alcohol red wine at lunch and dinner. Interestingly, they never eat leftovers, using them instead to feed farm animals. Few Abkhasians smoke.

Aside from diet, work, and sex, Abkhasian culture is notable for its strong sense of community. Extended families are very strong, and kinship is a major factor regulating interpersonal relationships. Each person is a valued and needed member of the group. There was no written language before the Russian revolution, and the older members of the group are greatly valued as historians and storytellers. The lifestyle of these long- lived people can be seen as a prescription for successful aging:

* Keep fit with regular exercise.

* Eat a high-fiber, low-fat diet with many fruits and vegetables.

* Avoid promiscuous sexual contact.

* Do not smoke.

* Stay active in the life of your community.

* Pace yourself, and relax.

It would be interesting to see how the lifestyle of Abkhasians has changed over the last 30 years, and how these changes have affected their health and longevity.

THEORIES OF AGING

Most individual theories about the causes of aging, like early theories about child development, seem to center on a particular environmental or hereditary factor. There is growing opinion, however, that many factors happening together cause aging, with increasing probability that the changes of aging will occur as we get older. Some of the biological and environmental theories of aging are summarized here, including a discussion of how some of them are interrelated *(see Figure 1-2)*.

At the level of the cell, human aging shows the buildup of biological and chemical waste materials, which reduce the efficiency of the cell until it loses ability to function. Cellular degeneration can result from environmental influences, such as damage caused by free radicals, radiation, viral cross-linking, or lipofuscin or it can come from an intrinsic genetic influence, such as the inability to eliminate waste products (Eliopoulis, 1995). Free radicals are highly charged ions that damage many cellular structures, including DNA. Environmental radiation, which includes the solar radiation that everyone is exposed to every day, also can damage cells and their DNA. Viral cross-linking occurs when viruses borrow DNA strands from host cells and scramble the strands before giving them back. The scrambled DNA cannot work properly in making the cellular components it made before. As one ages, lipofuscin, a by-product of metabolism, accumulates, especially in the liver, heart, ovaries and neurons. The function of lipofuscin is unknown.

An intrinsic limit to aging was proposed by Hayflick, which is now called the *Hayflick limit* or *Hayflick phenomenon*. His proposal was that cells lose the ability to reproduce themselves after approximately 50 divisions. This limit may parallel the gradual accumulation of nonfunctional cells that is also considered a part of aging. Interestingly, cancer cells do not have this limit and instead continue to grow indefinitely. However, if an old cell is combined genetically with a cancer cell, the new cells will no longer be able to divide indefinitely. In the interactions between cells, both environmental stress and genetics have an effect. For instance, environmental stress causes activation of the sympathetic nervous system, known as the fight-or-flight response, which in time causes the calcification of cells. But genetic factors also influence both the severity of the stress reaction and the amount of cellular change it causes. Environmental factors such as poor diet, inadequate exercise, and smoking can decrease respiratory and circulatory function, leading to many kinds of chronic disease. Intrinsically, the immune system looses its specificity as we age. We simultaneously lose our immunity to foreign antigens, called *isoimmunity,* and acquire an increasing immunity to our own changing cells, called *autoimmunity*. Involution of the thymus occurs with age and causes a diminished number of newly formed T lymphocytes and a decreased capability of T lymphocytes to proliferate. It is apparent that a cell can change quite a bit before it loses its ability to function, but a very small change can result in a cell's being seen as an intruder to be attacked by our own immune system. This immune response may cause many of the problems that occur in people as they get older, such as arthritis, diabetes, heart disease, cancer, and even tooth loss. There is also a theory that an intrinsic aging hormone begins to be produced at adolescence and increases over time, causing many of the changes of aging.

In evolutionary terms, there is no pressure for a species to evolve individuals who continue to live beyond their reproductive life. Since humans have a long developmental period, there may have been natural selection for people who lived long enough to raise and protect their children, but once the chil-

FIGURE 1-2
Theories of Aging

Factor	*Extrinsic*	*Intrinsic*
Genetic	Free radicals Radiation Viral cross-linking	Hayflick limit
Cellular	Buildup of toxic substances	Buildup of nonfunctional components
Intercellular	Cell calcification caused by stress response	Immune changes Isoimmunity lost Iutoimmunity increased
Physiological	Circulatory decrease (diet, activity, smoking)	Aging hormone
Theoretical	No resources for future generations if no senescence and death	No evolutionary pressure to create a species that continues to survive past reproductive age

dren were able to take care of themselves, the parents were biologically redundant. At the same time, the increased mutation rate in children of older women can explain why humans have not evolved to have a longer reproductive life. These theories of biological aging may help us to understand the physical process of aging, but they do not begin to explain the interpersonal behavior that occurs as a person ages. In order to understand interpersonal interactions, several social theories of aging have been proposed.

SOCIAL THEORIES OF AGING

Several theories have evolved to explain the social interaction of people as they age, and each increased in complexity as it became unable to meet the test of experience. The old theory of **disengagement** was that the elderly and society withdraw from each other in a mutually sought and mutually satisfying separation. This theory has not been able to explain why seniors who are not withdrawn are generally healthier and happier. The activity theory proposes that there is a connection between activity and life satisfaction. Both interpersonal activity and physical activity contribute to a persons sense of well-being as he or she becomes older. A **socioenvironmental theory** was developed that proposed that senior citizens living with others of their own age would have increased social interaction and therefore have increased life satisfaction. This theory fit in with surveys that indicated that, on the average, the elderly would rather live with others of their own age and *near,* but not *with,* their children. But the social interaction theory could not explain why many satisfied elderly lived in age-integrated communities, or why many elderly living in age-segregated communities were not happy or healthy.

An exchange theory, adapted from political science, explained that people tend to maximize rewards of social interaction while minimizing costs:

PROFIT = REWARD - COST

Therefore, two people will continue to interact if it is to the social profit of each. When one person receives more social profit from an interaction, that person gains power over the person who receives less profit. In our society, in which youth and modernization are valued, the elderly may lose more and more power as they become more dependent on the young. Seniors can restore this power through three mechanisms: They can (1) withdraw, which decreases their cost; (2) develop alternative skills that will be valued by others and increase the others' reward; or (3) form social and political coalitions that increase the seniors' power directly.

MODELS THAT EXPLAIN HEALTH BEHAVIOR

Two other models have been developed to try to explain why older people behave as they do, especially regarding their health. These are the **health belief model** and the **locus of control model.**

The **health belief model** proposes that people will take action to prevent or cope with a problem only if they believe themselves at significant risk of harm and that the proposed action will reduce the harm at less personal cost than the problem itself. Unfortunately, people often do not believe they are at risk of something until it happens to them, and frequently do not believe that a prescribed preventive action will help. A clinical example of how the health belief model can affect health status is given in the following story:

> A 72-year-old woman living alone did not believe that a loose rug was a safety hazard, and so she did not get it fixed. She tripped over it and broke her hip. While she was hospitalized, she did not believe that she could recover, and so she became despondent and stopped eating and drink-

ing. She got weaker, and a fever developed because of dehydration, which kept her from going home as scheduled. Eventually the strong belief of her caregivers that she could recover changed her own health belief, and as she developed a trust that recovery was possible, she drank more fluids, began to participate more actively in therapy, and began to eat better. Her body temperature went down, her strength increased, and she went home able to function and eagerly participating in physical therapy—and she fixed her carpet. The outcome could have been different at many points of this story if the health beliefs had been different. It is especially easy to see how a health belief by the caregivers that assumed she would not recover because of her advanced age could have had a disastrous effect on her recovery.

The **locus of control model** proposes that people who believe they can control what happens to them will do better in systems where they maintain that control, whereas people who feel controlled by outside forces will manage better in systems where they are not forced to make decisions. This model can help explain why some people show increased satisfaction and health with increased independence. One factor that can significantly change someone's locus of control is serious illness, leading the ill person to feel that he or she cannot control his or her own life. And so people who are admitted to hospitals and nursing homes may become increasingly dependent and unwilling to make decisions on their own. Nurses and other caregivers need to work to counter this influence. By helping them maximize their feelings of control, nurses maximize patients' ability to function independently.

SUMMARY

Although aging is accompanied by biological and psychosocial changes, it is important to keep in mind that the majority of older people have the ability to remain functionally independent throughout their lives. When a person becomes unable to accomplish activities that he or she had previously done, caregivers need to realize that this is an indication of illness and not just getting old. With the identification of an illness, remedies can be sought that can restore health and function. Prevention of illness includes teaching and counseling patients about healthy lifestyle and specific preventive practices such as immunization and cancer screening. Health promotion and disease prevention will become ever more important as a greater percentage of the population reaches older age.

EXAM QUESTIONS

CHAPTER 1
Questions 1–10

1. A major factor contributing to an older person's ability to recover from illness is

   a. hospitalization.

   b. medicare reimbursement.

   c. caregiver attitude.

   d. number of medications prescribed.

2. The notion of disengagement reflects a

   a. cellular theory of aging.

   b. physiological theory of aging.

   c. genetic theory of aging.

   d. social theory of aging.

3. Which of the following is predicted demographically?

   a. The population over 85 will increase to more than 20% by 2030.

   b. The population over 65 will increase to more than 20% by 2030.

   c. The percentage of older people will double in the next decade.

   d. The percentage of the population over 65 will more than double by the year 2030.

4. Which of the following contributes most to healthy aging?

   a. Not smoking

   b. An annual physical examination

   c. Not eating leftovers

   d. Eating a high-protein diet

5. Which of the following healthcare maintenance activities is recommended for the elderly?

   a. Annual pneumonia immunization

   b. Annual influenza immunization

   c. Never take more than three medicines at a time

   d. Exercise is a safety hazard

6. Which of the following is true about theories of aging?

   a. Genetic changes are solely responsible for the aging process.

   b. Environment is stronger than heredity.

   c. Disengagement explains the isolation of older people.

   d. Aging is probably caused by multiple factors.

7. Which theories explain aging best?

   a. Biological theories

   b. A combination of theories

   c. Social interaction theories

   d. Psychological theories

8. Which of the following is true of the over-85 population?

   a. They will experience more disability in the future than they do now.

   b. They are the fastest growing segment of our population.

   c. Most of them will end their lives in a nursing home.

   d. Most live in the Northeast and Midwest.

9. A nurse is most likely to help an older patient recover by doing which of the following?

   a. Being sure to teach the patient everything in the care plan.

   b. Proving he or she has a positive attitude by doing everything he or she can for the patient.

   c. Communicating understanding and a belief that improvement is possible.

   d. Setting limits so the patient will learn independence.

10. Which of the following statements about aging and disease is correct?

   a. Both can contribute to functional losses.

   b. They are not related to each other.

   c. They are always directly related.

   d. They are both inevitable.

CHAPTER 2

MENTAL AND EMOTIONAL CHANGES: COPING AND CAREGIVING STRATEGIES

by
Susan Johnson, RN, CNA, MS

CHAPTER OBJECTIVE

After studying this chapter, the reader will be able to discuss the major causes of mental and emotional changes in the geriatric population.

LEARNING OBJECTIVES

After studying this chapter, the reader will be able to:

1. Specify two psychological tasks that occur for the majority of older people.

2. Differentiate between descriptions of dementia and other mental and emotional problems.

3. Recognize that rapid onset of mental changes is a component of delirium and requires immediate intervention.

4. Specify two emotional, two cognitive, and two physical symptoms that are indicators of depression.

5. Recognize exemplars of personality disorder, paranoia, phobia, and psychosis.

6. Select two reasons for decreasing medications that affect the mental abilities of older people.

7. Specify alternatives to drug therapy in the treatment of mental and emotional problems.

8. Select indicators that point to excessive alcohol use.

INTRODUCTION

Many myths are associated with aging. Many of these deal with the mental and emotional condition of older people. This chapter begins by describing elements of mental and emotional functioning, and the interaction of mind and body. Next comes a description of aspects of interpersonal interaction that are an inevitable part of our experience as social beings. A discussion of common life events and successful and unsuccessful coping patterns follows. Then nursing assessment of mental and emotional health is discussed. Last, some specific psychological problems are covered, including delirium, depression, anxiety, abuse, personality disorders, psychosis, and substance abuse. Dementia of the Alzheimer's type is discussed in a separate chapter.

THE MIND-BODY INTERACTION

The division of mind, or *psyche,* and body, or *soma,* is an artificial one that we use to attempt to analyze and understand ourselves better. But our thoughts are dependent on what our sensory system perceives, and can only occur if the physical mechanisms of our nervous system are working properly. In turn, our thoughts can affect how we perceive the world around us, and how we react physically to that world. One very graphic example of how our minds and bodies are connected comes from a small 1990 study of depression, which found that all patients who were rated as depressed both according to an objective test and by nursing staff were either at a higher level of care or were dead within 6 months (Keane & Sells, 1990). Another small study in 1989 found a significant relationship between physical impairment and higher levels of mental distress in a group of subjects 60–80 years old, and this result was stable over time. The more severely disabled of these older adults experienced higher levels of anxiety, suicidal ideation, and overall distress than did the participants who had a moderate disability (Zatura, Maxwell, & Reich, 1989). The Framingham Study, which is one of the larger and more well-known longitudinal studies, has shown that cognitive impairment, or memory deficit, is associated with a reduced ability to follow a prescribed drug regimen for control of hypertension (Farmer et al., 1990). With these examples, it is easy to see that our minds and bodies are inevitably interrelated. We use the categories of mind and body, however, to help us examine and learn about how these systems work, just as we create a division between heart and lung in order to study them, always keeping in mind that these organs are intimately interrelated.

INDIVIDUAL-SOCIAL INTERDEPENDENCE

Our minds not only interact with the internal system of our bodies, they are also in constant interaction with the outside world, perceiving, interpreting, and reacting. One of the major external influences on our mental health is the social support we receive from family, friends, neighbors, and other caregivers. A 9-year study found that physical health and social support were the major coping resources in preventing decline in mental health. Interestingly, although poor mental health and decreased cognitive ability were predictors of mortality, they were less significant than the availability of social resources (Haug, Breslaw, & Folmar, 1989). Another study found that social support can buffer the effect of stressful situations on the coping ability of older people. Also, people who had better mental health in turn had better social support systems (Cutrona, Russell, & Rose, 1986).

A person's social support system tends to remain stable with aging. Someone who is close to family and friends tends to maintain these relationships and makes new ones as needed. People who are isolated tend to remain isolated. The 14-year Berkeley Older Generation Study found that family relationships were especially stable. Also, women tended to retain beyond-family relationships more than men. With "very-old" age, over 85 years, friendships tended to decrease, but while involvement with friends declined in very-old age, satisfaction with children tended to increase (Field & Minkler, 1988). Though it is common for people as they age to experience the loss of family members and friends, people who have had a good social support system tend to find new friends, or become close to younger members of their family.

THE DEVELOPMENTAL TASKS OF AGING

Erik Erikson (1963) described eight developmental stages of mankind, ending with the task in later life of achieving ego integrity rather than surrendering to despair. Ego integrity is the development of a sense of wholeness and satisfaction with one's life. It can also be seen as emotional maturity. Several lesser developmental tasks go into the achievement of emotional maturity, and different authors describe different elements, including the following:

- Flexibility in adapting to the environment, and the ability to solve problems

- Acceptance of personal strengths and limitations—a good sense of identity

- The ability to balance conflicting influences

- Autonomy, independence

- Social sensitivity, treating others as worthy of concern

- Striving to live up to one's highest potential

Although no one ever becomes perfectly "mature" in all aspects of emotional and social life, a person who functions adequately in society, maintains appropriate life roles and relationships, and evaluates his or her own life as a positive experience is generally considered emotionally mature. The ability to reach emotional maturity, to develop ego integrity, depends on many factors. Erikson suggests that each developmental task depends on the successful completion of previous developmental tasks. At each developmental stage, a person is dependent on the resources available, on the people who serve as role models, and on experience in coping with life. It is possible to continue to develop throughout the life span, improving one's adaptation to life and moving toward the achievement of ego integrity.

COMMON LIFE EVENTS AND COPING STRATEGIES

One universal fact of life is change. As people get older, sometimes these changes are more and more often characterized by loss. Losses can be grouped into three broad categories: loss of relationship or of people; loss of ability or roles one has held; and loss of objects, or possessions. An example of loss of ability is the development of chronic disease. In coping with this loss, a person can focus on remaining abilities and specific skills that can improve function. Or a person can focus on negative aspects, focus on the loss itself, with self-blame or wishful thinking or avoidance, all of which tend to decrease the ability to adapt to the illness (Bombardier, D'Amico, & Jordan, 1990).

Coping with loss becomes a major task for older people. Losses can be obvious and large, such as the loss of a spouse or confidant, or they can be smaller, such as the loss of a neighbor or a personal possession. The extent to which a loss is felt by an older person can only be determined by that person and depends on the meanings the person associates with the loss. The death of a distant relative can mean little ("After all, I hardly knew her"), or it could be severe ("We were the same age, and lived through the Depression together"). A person's ability to cope with loss is a major factor in determining whether old age will be a satisfying experience or a catastrophic one.

The use of coping mechanisms tends to remain stable throughout adult life, according to an analysis of data from the Baltimore Longitudinal Study on Aging (McCrae, 1989). Coping abilities are developed by experiencing stress and learning useful ways to react. Unfortunately, sometimes we learn a coping mechanism in one area only to find that it does not work in another area. An example of this situation is when an older person who has coped by being independent is admitted to a hospital where the staff expect a patient to be dependent. The older patient, trying to retain control over his or her own life, is seen as uncooperative by the staff, and conflict or withdrawal occurs. The ideal situation would be for everyone to develop flexible coping skills that enable a person to cope with different situations in different ways. Unfortunately, this is not easily done. Coping strategies tend to be fairly stable over time and seem to be part of the enduring characteristics of each individual.

McCrae (1989) analyzed 28 specific coping mechanisms and found that aging has little effect on the use of coping behaviors, and that coping behavior is independent of personality. The following are some coping behaviors:

- Hostile reaction

- Rational action

- Seeking help

- Perseverance

- Isolation of affect (feelings)

- Fatalism

- Expression of feeling

- Positive thinking

- Distraction

- Escapist fantasy

- Intellectual denial

- Self-blame

- Taking one step at a time

- Social comparison

- Sedation

- Substitution

- Restraint

- Drawing strength from adversity

- Avoidance

- Withdrawal

- Self-adaptation

- Wishful thinking

- Active forgetting

- Humor

- Passivity

- Indecisiveness

- Assessing blame

- Faith

Humor and laughter have become recognized as effective ways to cope with changes that occur as we age. Humor serves as a means of relieving tension, coping with stressful situations, and setting up bonds with others (Wooten, 1996). There are several theories that suggest how and why humor is effective. These theories range from "relief," in which laughing is seen as a release of nervous energy and from focusing on disagreeable aspects of a situation, to a theory of incongruity in which things are put together in a surprising way that brings humor to the situation. All of these theories try to help us understand the role of humor in life situations particularly as we age. It seems that humor may have a physiological effect on the aging process. Research has shown a physical response to laughter distinguished by a pattern of stimulation followed by relaxation. Studies have shown similar responses by the cardiovascular and respiratory systems. As a coping mechanism, humor can break down communication barriers between age groups and between nurses and individuals as they age.

Although most people can probably think of situations in which they might use most of these coping mechanisms, it is easy to realize that some of them would be more effective than others in reaching a desirable outcome or in achieving what might be called emotional maturity.

PERSONALITY

Personality is the combination of characteristics that make people different from each other and lead them to behave in an individual way. Research on personality changes with aging has not been particularly successful, partly because there is no universally accepted theory of what personality is.

One model of personality proposes three dimensions of personality (Costa & McCrae, 1988):

Neuroticism: anxiety, hostility, depression, self-consciousness, impulsiveness, vulnerability

Extroversion: warmth, gregariousness, assertiveness, activity, excitement seeking, positive emotion

Openness: fantasy, aesthetics, feelings, actions, ideas, values, curiosity, agreeableness, conscientiousness

Neugarten (1973) reviewed the literature of personality changes and concluded that three traits have been consistently observed to change with age. First, there is an increase in introversion, or focusing on the inner world. Second, there is a shift in active mastery of the environment or adaptation. Third, there is increased cautiousness. A more recent study, however, using a sample of more than 10,000 people (the National Health and Nutrition Examination Survey; Costa et al., 1986) found that although older people were slightly lower in scores for extroversion, openness, and neuroticism, these trends were not consistent. The authors came to the conclusion that personality tends to be stable in adulthood.

In summary, a person seems to become "more of the same" with increasing age, retaining and possibly strengthening many of the traits that were developed at a younger age. With this increasing development of a "unique" personality, there is at least as much variation among older people as there is among younger ones.

ASSESSMENT OF MENTAL HEALTH

Mental health depends on a wide variety of factors. The ability to adapt to the outside world and cope with the stresses of life is a central component of mental health. Another essential component is the ability to maintain interpersonal relationships, to interact appropriately with the people in one's life. Nurses can evaluate the mental and emotional health of older people by asking questions about these two areas of life. Questions about coping can include the following:

• How are you feeling today?

• What are the sources of stress in your life?

• What have you done in the past when you were under stress?

• What do you do in a typical day?

• What do you do to have fun?

• What do you do when you are angry? sad?

• What are your strengths?

• What do you like about yourself?

• How did you get through the tough times in the past?

Questions about social and interpersonal interaction can include the following

• Whom in your family do you feel close to?

• Do you have close friends?

• Can you talk about your feelings to anyone?

• Do you belong to any groups?

• Who helps you when you are in trouble?

While asking such questions, nurses can also be evaluating other aspects of a person's mental health. To evaluate speech, determine whether the speech is at a normal, fast, or slow rate. Is the tone normal? Is the amount of speech appropriate, or does the person answer with monosyllables or talk continuously? **Thoughts** should be expressed logically. Are thoughts expressed disjointedly, with the client jumping from topic to topic? Are thoughts constructive? Are they self-destructive, or do they indicate an obsession with fears or delusions? Do the thoughts indicate an obsession with bodily concerns? **Nonverbal behavior** or "body language" can give important clues about a person's mental state. Does the person make eye contact? Is motor activity depressed or excessive? Is posture relaxed, tense, or blocking, as with crossed arms and legs?

Mood or affect can also be evaluated by using observation. Does the patient seem happy, sad, angry, fearful, up, down, high, and so on? Is a range of emotions expressed? Do facial expressions and nonverbal behavior match the person's expressed mood?

The nurse's assessment of these aspects of mental status can be strengthened by validating observations with the patient. This is done by stating the observation and asking the patient if he or she is aware of the behavior and if it is normal. An example would be to observe that a person is fidgeting during the interview and ask, "You seem to be moving a lot. Is this normal for you, or do you think it's because of how you're feeling?" To a patient who speaks slowly in a low tone of voice, answers in monosyllables, and sits slumped in a chair, the nurse could say, "You seem sad to me. Are you feeling sad?" Either a yes or a no answer could then be further explored.

One factor nurses need to consider when evaluating someone's behavior is the cultural norm for that person. People of different cultures may express their mental state in very different behaviors. If you are unsure of a patient's ethnic background, it is appropriate to ask the patient what that background is. Another factor to consider is how distressed a person is. When you are confronted with someone who is talking incessantly in a loud, high-pitched voice, with disjointed thoughts and delusions that someone is trying to hurt him, it would obviously not be a good time to try to validate your observations; this person is simply in too much distress to hear what another person is saying.

Two additional components of mental health include **perception** and **cognitive function.** Perception includes what the person sees, hears, feels, smells, and tastes. Perception of the outside world depends both on how our sensory system receives data from that world and how our minds interpret that data. When our sensory system is not functioning well, it is more difficult for our minds to process the data and more difficult for us to react appropriately. The chapter on sensory abilities deals more fully with this topic.

Cognitive function is the ability to process and remember data. In addition to memory, cognitive function includes the ability to pay attention, to reason and calculate, to use judgment, and to use language skills appropriately. The chapter on dementia goes into more detail on cognitive function. One example of change in cognitive function is delirium, which is a short-term, acute change and is a nursing and medical emergency.

DELIRIUM

Delirium is an acute disorder characterized by sudden onset of changes in cognition. Nurses need to understand delirium and be able to identify it separately from dementia, which is a long-term, progressive disorder of attention and cognition. The reason nurses need to be able to identify delirium is that it is almost always caused by an underlying condition that can be treated. Infections of the bladder, lungs, or brain can cause delirium, as can systemic infections such as influenza, septicemia, and AIDS. Oxygen deficiency; dehydration; hypoglycemia; electrolyte imbalances; thyroid, pituitary, or adrenal hormone abnormalities; vitamin deficiencies; and pain can all cause delirium. Medications, especially sedatives and tranquilizers, and alcohol as well as withdrawal from these substances can cause delirium. Diseases such as cardiac or vascular insufficiency, head trauma, brain tumors, and multiple sclerosis can cause delirium. This partial list illustrates both the variety of possible causes of delirium and the treatable nature of many of them.

Nurses and physicians often overlook delirium, thinking the signs and symptoms are the result of dementia, psychosis, or depression. One study found that 32% of cases of delirium went unrecognized by physicians (Francis et al., 1988). A nurse who notices that a patient is suddenly more agitated and calls a physician for an order for a tranquilizer might be ignoring the real possibility that a delirium exists and may fail to obtain appropriate treatment for the underlying condition(s). Inouye et al. (1990) have proposed a simple and elegant method for detecting delirium called the confusion assessment method (CAM). To evaluate whether an abnormality of attention and cognition is a delirium, ask the following four questions:

1. Does the abnormal behavior have an **acute onset** and **fluctuating course?**

2. Is the person characterized by **inattention,** having difficulty concentrating or keeping track of what is being said?

3. Is the person showing **disorganized thinking,** with rambling or incoherent speech, irrelevant or incoherent ideas, jumping from subject to subject?

4. Does the person demonstrate an **altered level of consciousness,** such as hypervigilance, lethargy, stupor, or coma?

To arrive at a diagnosis of delirium, the patient needs to demonstrate both 1 and 2 as well as either 3 or 4.

DEPRESSION

It is the common misconception that to be old is to be depressed. In actuality, depression in the elderly appears to be less frequent than in younger adults. In the Epidemiologic Catchment Area study, 15% of community residents older than 65 were found to have depressive symptoms (Buffum & Buffum, 1997). Many rigorous studies indicate that significant symptoms of depression affect about 10 to 15 percent of all community-living individuals over age 65 (Buckwalter, 1995). Depression in elders can be related to bereavement or adjustment disorder, or can be atypical or dysthymic. Rates of depression increase dramatically among the institutionalized elderly, with as many as 50 to 75 percent of long term care residents suffering from mild to moderate depressive symptoms. A significant number of these noncognitively impaired elderly (10 to 20 percent) experience severe symptoms making depression a critical public health problem. Luckily, about 80 percent of all people with serious depression respond positively to treatment and return to health. Depression is more common in older women, but this may merely be a result of survivability (American Psychiatric Association, 1994).

Depression is a serious problem for older people, not only because it causes psychological and spiritual distress but also because it contributes to loss of functional independence, self-neglect, and failure to thrive. Also, older people who have difficulty accepting that they may have a psychological disorder will often have physical signs and symptoms related to their distress. This process of expressing emotional problems as physical ones is called somatization. The medical costs of attempting to diagnose and treat these somatic complaints can be enormously high. Sometimes depression can be such a serious problem and a person becomes so dependent that admission to a nursing home is sought, and then the increased dependency of that setting can lead to further depression. Altogether, the emotional and economic costs of depression can be enormous, especially if it is not recognized and treated.

The Development of Depression

Historically, depression has been described as being either *reactive,* that is a short-term reaction to a life stress, or *endogenous,* a chronic disease without a specific precipitating event. This separation into distinct categories may be more of an artifact of how we assess people, the setting they are in, and how self-aware they are about their own emotional reactions than an absolute distinction between two types of illness. Depression can be characterized along a continuum of duration—recent onset vs. chronic—but there is no clear evidence that either the physiological process or emotional experiences are different for endogenous and reactive depression (Chaisson-Stewart, 1985). It is important to note, however, that transient sadness and normal grieving do not constitute depression. When sadness and grieving are prolonged or are more severe than expected, or are accompanied by ongoing physical signs and symptoms as well as feelings of worthlessness (low self-esteem), then a diagnosis of depression may be made.

Depression is probably caused by an interaction between an emotional response to a stress and a physiological change in chemical neurotransmitters. Normally our nerve cells release chemical substances called neurotransmitters, which carry impulses from one nerve cell to the next. Norepinephrine and serotonin are the two neurotransmitters most commonly implicated in mood disorders. With increasing age, these transmitters decrease, resulting in a slower neurological response. Although there is still usually a more than adequate supply of neurotransmitters to keep people moving, eating, breathing, thinking, and so on, the reduction of neurotransmitters may be partially responsible for several mental and emotional problems, including depression.

Depression can be assessed by nurses by using the Geriatric Depression Scale (GDS) created specifically for assessing depression in elders (Yesavage & Brink, 1983). The 30-item scale is easy to administer or can be self-administered by a patient. Scoring ranges describe the depression: 0-10 = normal; 11-20 = mild depression; 21-30 = severe depression. This is a screening tool only but is widely used in cognitively intact elders and is important because it eliminates physical signs and symptoms so often seen in the elderly as a result of chronic disease.

Assessment of Depression

Depression usually is characterized by an awareness of sad feelings by the depressed person and general feelings of hopelessness and helpless-

ness. Sad feelings can be experienced in different ways, including the following:

- Being blue, discouraged, downhearted
- Being frequently irritated
- Feelings of failure
- Lack of satisfaction
- Inability to enjoy activities that used to be fun (this is called *anhedonia*)
- Feeling unattractive to others
- Feeling that others would be better off if the depressed person did not exist

Associated feelings of guilt or anxiety can also be present and can contribute to the depression. Sometimes older persons will either be unaware of their feelings or be unable to express them to health professionals or even family members. In this instance, depression may not be manifested as a problem with sad feelings but through other signs and symptoms that are not always easy to recognize as depression. Nurses need to be alert for behavioral and physical expressions of depression as well as emotional ones. Depression tends to be characterized by a "slowing down." Activity levels may decrease, and the person may cut down on all activities, especially social ones. The decreased social and sensory stimulation may in turn contribute to deepening depression. Thought processes may slow down also, with memory difficulties sometimes severe enough to mimic dementia. The depressed person may have difficulty making decisions.

Physical signs and symptoms can include sleep disturbances, especially early awakening, and feelings of fatigue even after resting or sleeping. Appetite disturbances can be characterized either by increased appetite or loss of appetite. Physical "slowing down" can include slowed gastrointestinal peristalsis, which results in constipation. A depressed person may put less effort into taking care of herself or himself, which can have such consequences as not seeking health care as needed, not taking medications that are needed to control chronic illness, not taking basic safety precautions, looking disheveled, and just not "taking care" of oneself. The prevalence of depression in nursing home residents is high and, according to studies, underdiagnosed and undertreated (Ryden et al., 1998). These authors developed a two-step protocol for assessing all newly admitted residents to nursing homes. The initial screening is recommended for all residents upon admission to aid early detection and treatment. The focus is, also, on educating staff to recognize symptoms and respond aggressively.

In differentiating depression from normal bereavement, nurses can assess both the duration and the acuity, or seriousness, of the signs and symptoms. Even a short-term grief reaction may need referral for psychological evaluation if the "slowing down" is severe enough to threaten a person's life. Although grief for the loss of a significant other may last well over a year, if it is still preventing the patient from participating actively in life, a referral is a good idea. Sometimes grief will be difficult to cope with because previous losses still carry a heavy emotional burden. Whenever a depression continues for many months after a loss, a psychological assessment is indicated to evaluate the person's ability to recover independently. The physician or psychiatrist may decide that antidepressants should be used. Regardless of age, all people deserve to feel better.

Drug Treatment

The use of antidepressant drugs for depression is a popular form of therapy. Tricyclic antidepressants have been most frequently used, and the newer heterocyclic drugs are gaining rapidly in popularity. These drugs have a similar effect on depression, so the choice is based on side effects. One major type of side effect is called *anticholinergic,* and causes drying of secretions, constipation, urinary hesitancy, and blurred vision. These side effects can impair cognitive function and can worsen a dementia or delirium. Consequently, drugs with high anticholinergic effects are not recommended for older people. Some examples of tricyclic and heterocyclic drugs and their advantages and disadvantages are as follows (Buffum & Buffum, 1997):

Tricyclic Antidepressants

- **Amitriptyline HCl (Elavil):** high anticholinergic effect, highly sedating, orthostatic hypotension, tachycardia.

- **Imipramine HCl (Tofranil):** low anticholinergic effect, moderately sedating, orthostatic hypotension.

- **Doxepin HCl (Sinequan, Adapin):** low anticholinergic effect, highly sedating.

- **Desipramine HCl:** very low anticholinergic effect, low sedative effect.

- **Protriptyline HCl:** low anticholinergic effect, low sedative effect.

- **Nortriptyline HCl:** low anticholinergic effect, moderately sedating, develop cardiac arrhythmias.

Heterocyclic Antidepressants

- **Amoxapine (Asendin):** low anticholinergic effect, moderately sedating, extrapyramidal side effects and seizures reported.

- **Maprotiline HCl (Ludiomil):** low anticholinergic, moderate sedative effect, seizures reported, skin rash in 10% of users.

- **Trazodone HCl (Desyrel):** no anticholinergic effect, high sedative effect (useful for sleep problems), rare reports of priapism in men, increased libido in women, no life-threatening consequences of overdose, interacts with digoxin (decrease digoxin dose), higher dose needed: 400mg equivalant to 150mg imipramine.

Serotonin Reuptake Inhibitors & Serotonin/
Norepinephrine Reuptake Inhibitor

- **Fluoxetine (Prozac):** no anticholinergic effect, not sedating, given in a.m. to prevent insomnia, dosage range 20-80mg.

- **Paroxetine (Paxil):** little anticholinergic effect, may be more sedating than others in this class (Small, 1997).

- **Sertraline (Zoloft):** no sedating effect; little or no anticholinergic, orthostatic, or cardiac effects, may suppress appetite.

- **Bupropion (Wellbutrin):** little or no sedating, anticholinergic, orthostatic, or cardiac effects.

- **Nefazodine (Serzone):** safe and effective for elderly.

- **Venlafaxine (Effexor):** caution when used in patients with hypertension (Yoshikawa, Cobbs & Brummel-Smith, 1998).

Monoamine oxidase (MAO) inhibitors are less frequently used because of adverse interactions with other drugs and with many foods, but they are sometimes effective when tricyclic antidepressants do not work. Patients need to be closely watched for orthostatic changes and for changes in liver function.

In summary, many drugs can be very effective in helping elders cope with severe depression. However, care must be taken that side effects of the medications do not cause a worsened cognitive state; excessive sedation; or intolerable anticholinergic drying of mucous membranes, urinary retention, or constipation. "Start low and go slow" is the best practice for the use of antidepressants in the elderly. They must realize that relief of symptoms takes up to 6 weeks.

Nondrug Therapy

Psychotherapy for older patients has not been widely used, probably because of a combination of factors that include lack of reimbursement for such therapy and a disinclination on the part of the current cohort of elderly to seek therapy for emotional problems. Some therapists believe that modified, goal-directed forms of therapy, such as cognitive therapy, can be effective in treating depression in older people. Cognitive therapy focuses on concrete behavioral change, with the therapist and patient in an active partnership to develop self-help problem-solving techniques. Studies yield conflicting results for the use of cognitive therapy to treat depression in nursing home residents (Ebersole & Hess, 1998). Group therapy is also a mechanism used to provide more affordable therapy. Being with other people is very important in the process of successfully dealing with depression. Several types of psychosocial group intervention are recommended (Buckwalter, 1995). These include: Reminiscence and Life Review Methods, Music Therapy, Movement Therapy, Sensory Stimulation, Pet Therapy, and Remotivation Therapy. The method is much less important than the process of what happens between the individual and others in the group.

Electroconvulsive therapy (ECT) is used by geropsychiatrists to treat depression. It has the advantage of not having drug side effects. ECT can have the side effect of a transient memory impairment, which is usually limited to a few hours but in some cases can be more prolonged. ECT is very safe, but as it takes specialized equipment, specially trained staff, and requires several treatments, it is an expensive form of therapy. ECT appears to be as effective in geriatric patients with severe or psychotic major depressive disorder as in nongeriatric groups of patients (AHCPR, 1993). Stereotypes of ECT as a frightening or inhumane experience are outdated, but many people are still influenced by them sufficiently to be unwilling to consider this type of therapy.

Nutrition and exercise both play a part in treating depression. Malnutrition can contribute to a depression, and the depression in turn can result in inadequate dietary intake. Overeating during a depression can also present a problem of lessened self-esteem and feelings of loss of control. Evaluating diet and providing nutritional counseling can help correct these problems. Exercise is known to cause increased physical well-being. It also causes the release of endorphins in the brain, which act to improve emotional well-being. Although many older people have physical limitations that prevent participation in exercise programs designed for younger people, most can participate in some kind of regular physical exercise.

Suicide Associated With Depression

The incidence of suicide increases with age, especially for white men more than 65 years old. Persons in this cohort tend to use extremely lethal means and have more "success" than any other age group (Mellick, Buckwalter, & Stolley, 1992). It is sometimes very difficult to determine whether such deaths are the result of carefully thought-out, rational decisions in the face of loss of independence or anticipated pain or the result of a reversible depression. Suicides in the over age 75 white male increased during the period from 1981 to 1986 from about 46 to 60 percent while statistics for men in the 65 to 74 year-old group increased only from 30 to 38 percent (Buckwalter, 1995). Suicide is seldom a cry for help in the elderly, but reflects a serious desire to kill themselves. As dramatic as the increases in suicide statistics are for elderly individuals, they most likely hugely underestimate the true enormity of the problem. Two reasons for this are, not listing suicide as the actual cause of death on death certificates and, second, not recognizing passive suicide, such as abusing alcohol and mixing deadly combinations of medications or accidental overdoses of medications.

While much controversy exists over the right of individuals to end their lives, most people would agree that suicide resulting from a depression is an unfortunate tragedy. Nurses can encourage people who seem depressed to seek treatment from physicians or therapists. By conveying a belief in the reversibility of depression, nurses can help older clients look for affirmative choices rather than succumb to feelings of hopelessness and helplessness. The issue of suicide is further discussed in the chapter on death and ethical issues.

ANXIETY

Although some anxiety is a normal human experience, abnormal levels of anxiety can cause severe distress to older people. Women tend to be affected more often than men. Total anxiety rates for the elderly vary across studies from less than 1 percent to almost 20 percent (Small, 1997). Anxiety can be combined with dementia, psychosis, or depression and change the therapeutic approach from what would be needed for any of these problems individually. Anxiety-induced disorders in later years include **panic disorder, phobic disorder, generalized anxiety, agoraphobia, obsessive-compulsive disorder,** and **posttraumatic stress disorder.**

Panic disorder is characterized by acute panic attacks unrelated to actual physical danger. Panic attacks are periods of intense fear accompanied by physical signs and symptoms such as choking, dyspnea, dizziness, tachycardia and chest pain, trembling, sweating, nausea, numbness or tingling of extremities, flushing or chills, and fear of losing control or of dying. Phobic disorders occur when exposure to a certain identifiable stimulus provokes an anxiety attack. Phobic disorder is the most common anxiety disorder for persons of all ages, including elderly persons, and the male-to-female ratio is 1:2. In fact, phobia is the second most common psychiatric disorder next to cognitive impairment in individuals 65 years and older (Small, 1997).

Generalized anxiety is similar to panic disorder except that the anxiety tends to focus on specific life circumstances, such as health, finances, and children. Indications include increased motor tension; increased vigilance; and signs and symptoms of a fight-or-flight response, such as dyspnea, tachycardia, dry mouth, or dizziness.

Agoraphobia is the fear of being in public places such as standing in line or sitting in a bus. It can be severe enough that the person is unable to leave home or go to the hospital.

Obsessive-compulsive neurosis is more acute than an obsessive-compulsive personality disorder and is characterized by repetitive thoughts that are not wanted by the person experiencing them and may be suppressed and by repetitive, ritualistic behavior that is performed excessively in an attempt to neutralize the obsessive thoughts. The behaviors include **checking** rituals, such as confirming that the stove is turned off numerous times, and **cleaning** rituals, such as washing the hands repeatedly after they become "contaminated."

Posttraumatic stress disorder (PTSD) can result when a person has experienced a trauma outside the range of normal human experience. It is characterized by recurrent unwanted recollections of the event, unrealistic anxiety about one's current safety, and/or "flashbacks." Symbolic events, such as anniversaries, can be greatly anxiety provoking. In the effort to avoid thoughts connected with the trauma, a person may start to avoid stimuli and people that are only remotely or symbolically connected with it and live in a detached, low-emotion, protective cocoon. Alternatively, the person may demonstrate increased vigilance and arousal, as if to prevent the trauma from recurring. People who have lived through wars and natural disasters can retain anxiety from PTSD indefinitely. Nurses providing care to refugees, veterans, and other "sur-

vivors" need to be aware of the long-lasting effects that such experiences can have.

Drug Treatment

Drug treatment of anxiety has changed significantly over the years. Bromide was replaced in the 1950s with phenobarbital and other barbiturates and in the 1960s with benzodiazepine antianxiety medications. After several years of enthusiastic use of benzodiazepines, however, long-term effects of addiction emerged. For the elderly, the side effects include sedation with increased prevalence of falls and injury and impaired memory. Whereas these drugs can work well to reduce anxiety, their long-term use can create dependency and severe withdrawal effects. Research demonstrating benzodiazepine safety for younger people is not applicable to older patients because of the longer half-life of these medications in older persons. Nurses need to evaluate the efficacy of antianxiety medications: are they working? Nurses also need to watch for unwanted side effects such as sedation, confusion, impaired coordination, dizziness, and blurred vision. Abrupt withdrawal should be avoided, because it can result in severe signs and symptoms which are anxiety, irritability, insomnia, fatigue, muscle twitching and sweating. Buspirone (Buspar) has been found to be clinically effective for anxiety and well-tolerated by the elderly (Schneider, 1996; Small, 1997). Buspirone is unrelated to the benzodiazepines and has little sedation and no anticonvulsant or musculoskeletal side effects. Further studies need to be done, but its' usefulness is apparent.

Sedative-hypnotic antianxiety medications can exacerbate an underlying depression, or disinhibit demented patients and cause more inappropriate behavior. A depressed patient will respond to antidepressants.

Nondrug Therapy

Non-drug treatment of anxiety includes having the patient discuss and ventilate anxieties in a safe and reassuring environment. Since elderly persons may be reluctant to discuss psychological problems, education about the biological basis of anxiety may increase compliance. Sometimes the environment can be changed to reduce or eliminate factors that precipitate anxiety. Another technique that is used for phobias (such as agoraphobia) is progressively greater exposure to the phobic item, which can result in desensitization. There are self-help groups for agoraphobics that involve support and desensitization by people who are recovered agoraphobics themselves. Minimizing polypharmacy may improve or even remove symptoms (Small, 1997). Nurses are in a critical spot and role to help identify and amend the adverse effects of polypharmacy. Nurses should not hesitate to refer a patient for psychiatric evaluation if the patient continues to have distressing signs and symptoms of anxiety.

BIPOLAR DISORDER

A bipolar affective disorder, referring to characteristic emotional mood swings between mania and depression, may also be referred to as Manic Depressive Disorder. This disorder usually begins between 30 and 50 years of age almost never after age 60. The disease that begins earlier usually lasts into old age, however, so geriatric nurses may see patients who have this problem. The treatment for the disorder is the drug lithium carbonate, which prevents manic episodes and improves the intermittent depression. It is important for the patient to receive a thorough evaluation before starting lithium so that reversible causes of mania such as drugs (steroids, isoniazid, procarbazine, levodopa, bromide), metabolic disturbances (hemodialysis, postoperative state), infection, neoplasm, or epilepsy can be ruled out. In order to assure the safety of lithium treatment in elderly patients, kidney function, thyroid function, and ECG should be monitored. Lithium may have

many side effects, even at therapeutic levels. Patients may be tempted to discontinue the drug when they are feeling good but should be encouraged to continue taking it. Lithium doses are titrated by measuring lithium levels in blood serum. As with most drugs, the elderly are more easily and more severely affected by the toxic effects of lithium than younger persons are (Master, 1996).

Side effects of lithium at therapeutic levels are

* tremor, urinary frequency, mild nausea

Early indications of toxic levels are

* increasing tremor, ataxic gait, weakness, slurred speech, blurred vision, tinnitus, drowsiness or excitement

Severe toxic effects include

* increased deep tendon reflexes, nystagmus, confusion, lethargy that may progress to stupor, seizures, coma

When lithium is not tolerated or is ineffective, anticonvulsants and calcium channel blockers may be a better option (Master, 1996). Medications for the elderly individual with mania must be carefully monitored and titrated slowly.

PERSONALITY DISORDERS

W hen people with a predominant character type become ill, the physical and psychological stress can result in inappropriate coping patterns. Several of these personality types are described (Geringer and Stern, 1986).

Oral Personality. Coping tends to be dependent and demanding. Patients with this personality type may act is if the caregiver has unlimited time and may become angry and reproachful when their unreasonable demands are not met. Depression and addictive tendencies often accompany this character pattern. Nurse management involves setting firm limits while communicating a positive regard. Short, frequent contact may be more effective than infrequent, longer visits.

Compulsive Personality. Behavior is very controlled, reserved, and rational, often focusing on detail without being able to see the larger context of a situation. These patients tend to have a rigid moral system. They are self-controlled and conscientious and usually have great difficulty in situations where they cannot be in control. Nurses can help most by explaining carefully what they are doing, by encouraging the patient to participate in his or her care, and by accepting the patient's desire to be in control.

Hysterical Personality. These patients tend to be charming and imaginative, and they try to form close personal relationships, often inappropriately so. They attach great importance to their attractiveness and may feel this is threatened by their illness. Nurses can be most helpful by providing reassurance, allowing ventilation of feelings. Since these patients can feel overwhelmed by details, nurses need to be alert to cues that the patients do *not* want thorough explanations.

Masochistic Personality. These patients are characterized by having a history of repeated suffering combined with an exhibitionistic display of suffering. They tend to be self-sacrificing. Illness may be either a proof of their lack of self-worth or the only way to justify being cared for by others. They may get a sufficient secondary gain from their illness that makes them resist therapies that may improve their health. The best nursing approach is to acknowledge their suffering and their self-sacrifice while continuing to have a positive expectation that they will help themselves.

Schizoid Personality. Behavior tends to be remote, reserved, and isolated. When these patients become ill, they must interact with others, which can be so threatening that they may refuse to acknowledge they are ill. Nursing care should include accepting the person's high need for privacy and refraining from intruding whenever possible. It is unlikely that these patients will respond well to attempts to "get to know them," and the truly empathic response is to give them the privacy that helps them feel more secure.

Paranoid Personality. Behavior is fearful and suspicious, oversensitive to criticism. They expect the worst in others and may act in a manner that brings out the worst in others, creating a self-fulfilling prophecy. Often when older people start to forget things, they explain their memory lapse by attributing evil intent to someone else, either real or imaginary. The woman who cannot find the dishes she wants accuses her daughter of stealing. The woman who moved into her son's house, losing most of her personal possessions, repeatedly accuses an imaginary intruder of taking her things. Nursing management of paranoid reactions can focus on the patient's underlying feeling of threat or loss, acknowledging the validity of the feeling without participating in the paranoid delusions.

Narcissistic Personality. To protect a fragile self-esteem, these patients react by acting grandiose, arrogant, and vain. Illness is a threat to their imagined self-perfection. They may react to caregivers with idealization—"my nurse is the best"—or with denigration—"I'm better than you." Nurses need to realize the fragile foundation of such people and communicate acceptance of the individual and support autonomy whenever possible.

Many patients may have more than one of these character patterns. Evidence for nurses that they are dealing with a personality disorder is when the nurse has a strong emotional reaction to the patient, often out of proportion to the situation at hand. When a nurse notices such a reaction, he or she can pause and analyze what is going on, why the patient feels the need for self-protection and what the nurse can best do to provide a therapeutic environment. Needless to say, this requires patience and takes practice.

PSYCHOTIC DISTURBANCES OF THOUGHT AND BEHAVIOR

Besides severe depression and manic-depressive illness, a major psychotic illness is schizophrenia. Psychotic behavior is characterized by agitation, delusions, hallucinations, a poor sense of self with resulting self-neglect, poor insight, and incoherent thought patterns. Psychotic people can live to old age. With the closing of many state mental institutions, elderly psychotic people often live in nursing homes, in single-room occupancy hotels, or as homeless street people.

Schizophrenia is a psychotic disorder that is neither manic-depressive nor depressive. It is a fluctuating disease, with prodromal, active, and residual phases. The prodromal phase in the elderly may be difficult to differentiate from organic diseases such as senile dementia of the Alzheimer's type, Huntington's disease, or drug side effects. The active phase is characterized by increased delusions and hallucinations and increased incoherence and/or catatonic behavior. The residual phase is a time of blunted emotional reactions when even hallucinations do not evoke much of a response from the patient. Magical thinking, peculiar behavior, and an inability to maintain functional roles can characterize both the prodromal and residual phases, making it difficult for schizophrenics to deal effectively with their society even when not in an active phase of the disease.

Drug Therapy for Schizophrenia

The major treatment for schizophrenia is drug therapy with a class of drugs called neuroleptics. These drugs all block dopamine, which is a neurotransmitter. Because a lack of dopamine is the cause of Parkinson's disease, one effect of neuroleptics is to cause parkinsonian signs and symptoms, and this side effect is related to the strength of the dose of neuroleptic. Other side effects include sedation and the anticholinergic effects of dry mouth, constipation, and urinary retention. A life-threatening complication of antipsychotic use is Neuroleptic Malignant Syndrome. Symptoms include muscular rigidity and dystonia. Autonomic symptoms are fever (up to 107°F), increased pulse and blood pressure. The treatment is to immediately discuntinue the antipsychotic and aggressively treat the symptoms. Low-potency neuroleptics such as chlorpromazine HCl (Thorazine) and thioridazine HCl (Mellaril) are given in higher doses and therefore have stronger sedating and anticholinergic effects. For elderly patients, high-potency neuroleptics such as haloperidol (Haldol) and thiothixene HCl (Navane), and risperidone (Risperdal) are given in very low doses to maximize the antipsychotic effect while minimizing sedation and anticholinergic effects. Unfortunately, along with maximizing the antipsychotic effect, these doses cause the maximum parkinsonian side effects except when given with Cogentin (benztrapine). Other drugs that seem to reduce episodes of agitated or aggressive behavior include carbamazepine (Tegretol) and lithium carbonate.

Nursing Intervention for Schizophrenia

Although the prognosis for cure of chronic schizophrenia is poor, many of those with the disease can be treated as outpatients for much of their lives. In the healthcare setting, appropriate nursing intervention can minimize the nurse's stress in caring for such patients and maximize the patient's ability to cope. First, nurses need to be aware of their own feelings. Discouragement and frustration are common. Besides administering drugs and monitoring their effect, nurses can help create a therapeutic environment that minimizes anxiety. Consistent care from all members of the healthcare team will help establish trust, as will small efforts at meeting the patient's immediate needs, such as lighting a cigarette or listening to his or her fears. Establishing a relationship is difficult, because the patients tend to remain withdrawn even while expressing dependency needs. With a trusting relationship beginning, nurses can encourage the withdrawn person to become more involved with others. This process can be very slow, with repeated false starts and regressions. It is important to give the patient sufficient distance; pushing will only increase anxieties and distrust. Throughout the process, the nurse needs to remain open to involvement and caring toward the patient.

SUBSTANCE ABUSE: ALCOHOL AND DRUGS

Alcohol and other substances may be used as a form of self-medication by elders who are troubled by emotional problems such as depression. Some older people have a primary alcoholism or drug addiction problem. The consumption of three to five drinks per day over a prolonged period has been linked to increased mortality. Higher levels of use lead to even higher rates of illness and death. The use of multiple medications and frequent co-existing dementia or depression further complicate the issue. Alcohol can cause behavioral and mood changes that mimic conditions such as dementia or depression and/or drug side effects (Zimberg, 1996). Alcohol is the most common substance abused, with sedatives and antianxiety drugs accounting for most of the rest. It is difficult to estimate accurately the prevalence of substance abuse in the elderly, partly because it is apparently an underdiagnosed problem.

The clinical manifestations of alcoholism may be nonspecific, with patients appearing to have dementia, depression, or physical illness. Nonspecific signs and symptoms such as falls, injuries, unusual behavior, malnutrition, self-neglect, incontinence, diarrhea, and hypothermia can all be indications of an underlying problem with alcoholism. Accurate diagnosis of alcoholism in the elderly becomes even more difficult when a misdiagnosis of dementia is made. Several screening tools exist that can help health workers recognize patients who have difficulty dealing with alcohol. One is the CAGE questionnaire:

1. Have you ever tried to **Cut** down on your drinking?

2. Are you **Annoyed** when people ask you about your drinking?

3. Do you ever feel **Guilty** about your drinking?

4. Do you ever take a morning **Eye-opener?**

A yes answer to even one of these questions means that a more careful evaluation of the person's alcohol consumption is indicated (Zimberg, 1996). Positive responses to the first and third questions are most common.

Alcohol can cause a wide range of problems, including intoxication with increased potential for injury and evidence of withdrawal, including delirium and hallucinations. Chronic alcohol abuse can also cause illnesses such as liver disease, ulcers, esophageal varices, damage to heart muscle, arrhythmias, and central nervous system (CNS) damage, such as memory loss and loss of coordination. Sedatives and anxiolytics, particularly the benzodiazepine tranquilizers, can cause problems of intoxication as well as withdrawal signs and symptoms ranging from malaise and insomnia to tachycardia, orthostatic hypotension, and delirium.

One of the major consequences of alcohol abuse is the development of liver disease. For the elderly with liver damage, many of the drugs used are metabolized at different rates. When alcohol is taken with other sedating drugs, a dangerous CNS depression can develop. For those with memory problems and loss of motivation for self-care, medications are often not taken as directed. For elderly alcoholic patients all these mechanisms combine to cause difficulties with prescribed drugs and the management of concurrent illness.

Another category of substance abuse in the elderly population is the overuse of over-the-counter (OTC) drugs. One third of all money spent on medicine by the elderly was spent on OTC drugs such as analgesics, laxatives, sedatives, cold and allergy remedies, alcohol-based cough medicine, and caffeine (Yee, Williams & O'Hara, 1990). These OTC medicines can become a problem when they are used excessively. Daily laxative use, for instance, can cause a dependence, with loss of normal bowel tone as well as electrolyte disturbances. Some of these drugs can interact in unhelpful ways with prescribed medications. When taking a nursing history, nurses should ask about OTC medications and how often the drugs are used.

Recent studies of middle to old age drinking has shown researchers that, there may be some potential positive effects from moderate drinking of alcohol (Thun, 1997; Doll, 1997). The benefits of drinking small amounts of alcohol when you are middle-aged and older include prolonging your life and helping to fight off the following: Heart disease, diabetes, certain cancers, age-related vision loss, ulcers of the duodenum, strokes, mental deterioration and some types of infections. The risks remain, so that if an individual doesn't drink, it is not advisable to start at any age to promote health. However, there may prove to be some health benefit from small to moderate drinking as one ages (daily, up to 4–5 ounces of wine for women, and for men no more than double that amount).

By being aware of the potential for substance abuse in the elderly, nurses can help identify people with this problem and support these patients in seeking treatment for the disease. Again, nurses need to be aware of their own attitudes toward alcohol and other substance abuse in order to help their patients effectively.

SUMMARY

Two categories of mental and emotional problems exist in geriatric populations: those that develop in older age, and those that develop earlier and have become "chronic" by later years. Although nurses may have more success in their efforts to affect less chronic problems, Jenicke (1989) outlines four principles that form the basis for nurses' approach to elderly people with any type of mental or emotional problems:

1. Fostering a sense of control, self-efficacy, and hope

2. Establishing a relationship

3. Providing or elucidating a sense of meaning

4. Establishing constructive contingencies in the environment

One technique that can help to accomplish much of this approach is the **life review.** Even in short patient-nurse interactions, reminiscing and life review can help the patient feel known, respected, and cared about. Therapeutic reminiscing is not just idle conversation; it involves a review of all the varied elements that contribute to the development of that individual. Life review is a way of looking back that allows comforting memories to be reexamined, and sharing with others the commonality of experiences while recognizing the individual's uniqueness. Exploring the memories of the past with a group of elderly or an individual can help the person reconstruct their reality today through the examination of the past.

Finally, in dealing with patients with emotional and psychological problems, nurses need to remain constantly aware of their own emotional well-being. It is essential not to get drawn into emotional reactions that may be countertherapeutic. It can be very challenging for a nurse to remain caring, involved, and therapeutic. If a nurse is unaware of feelings in reaction to a patient, it is difficult to focus on meeting the patient's need. For instance, nurses who have unexamined needs for control will have difficulty fostering a sense of autonomy in their patients. A nurse who holds negative beliefs about substance abusers will be unlikely to deal objectively with a person with a history of substance abuse. But a nurse who knows the limits of his or her own compassion and empathy will be much more likely to provide care according to patients' varied needs.

EXAM QUESTIONS

CHAPTER 2
Questions 11–20

11. The major influence on mental health in later years depends on

    a. marital status.

    b. personality type.

    c. income or financial security.

    d. social support systems.

12. A short screening test for alcoholism is:

    a. Testing the person's breath.

    b. A blood alcohol test.

    c. The CAGE questionnaire.

    d. A urine test.

13. Which of the following is the major physical consequence of chronic alcohol abuse?

    a. Withdrawal

    b. Diarrhea

    c. Arrhythmias

    d. Liver disease

14. Mr. K has a bedtime ritual of putting cushions on the floor in an exact pattern so that he will not get hurt if he falls out of bed. This is an example of

    a. paranoid psychosis.

    b. obsessive-compulsive behavior.

    c. realistic coping with the danger of falling.

    d. confabulation to deal with memory loss.

15. Depression in the elderly is which of the following?

    a. A normal part of aging.

    b. Usually a chronic illness.

    c. Not a significant problem.

    d. A common contribution to loss of independence.

16. One indicator of excess alcohol use is:

    a. Increased appetite.

    b. Getting angry when people ask you about alcohol use.

    c. Improved sleep patterns.

    d. Daily intake of one or two drinks.

17. Delirium is characterized by

    a. slow onset.

    b. progressive course.

    c. increased concentration.

    d. incoherent ideas.

18. Which of the following is true about substance abuse?

    a. Nurses can depend on physicians to diagnose it.

    b. Sedatives are the most frequently abused substance.

    c. It is frequently a hidden problem.

    d. It is not linked to higher mortality.

19. The development of ego-integrity means

    a. becoming honest.

    b. developing confidence.

    c. achieving a sense that one's life has been worthwhile.

    d. believing that one's ego is more important than other people's.

20. It is a good idea to use the lowest dose possible of medications that depress the central nervous system because they can cause

    a. increased prevalence of falls.

    b. dangerous interactions with other drugs.

    c. daytime sedation.

    d. All of the above.

CHAPTER 3

SENSORY CHANGES: COPING AND CAREGIVING STRATEGIES

by
Angela Simon Staab, RN, MN, CGNP

CHAPTER OBJECTIVE

After reading this chapter, the reader will be able to recognize normal aging changes that occur in vision, hearing, taste, and smell and describe nursing caregiving strategies to cope with the problems these changes present to older adults.

LEARNING OBJECTIVES

After reading this chapter the reader will be able to:

1. Describe the normal physiological changes that may occur with aging in the senses, including hearing, vision, taste, and smell.

2. Discuss the pathological processes frequently associated with sensory deficits in older adults.

3. Identify coping and caregiving implications for nursing care of older adults with sensory deficits.

4. Identify strategies for increasing communication in older adults with sensory deficits.

INTRODUCTION

The rapidly expanding body of gerontological knowledge will continue to change what is known about normal aging versus pathological aging. Nurses who work with the elderly population must make a special effort to keep abreast of new knowledge so they can deliver and promote the highest possible level of care to older adults. Alterations in the senses that occur with aging can have a profound effect on older adults' communication abilities and perception of the environment. Sensory impairment is a deficit that can influence perception, behavior, and personality. As the changes become more pronounced, they can affect communications, activities of daily living, and lifestyle.

As the senses diminish, older people become more vulnerable to accidents, injuries and falls, social isolation, disorientation, and cognitive decline, sometimes resulting in death.

Interactions with the environment may be altered as a result of decreased vision, hearing, taste, and smell. Professional nursing interventions can alter positively the outcome of these problems and assist older adults in developing skills needed to cope with a changing environment. The purpose of this chapter is to identify the changes that occur in the senses with normal aging, describe the pathological processes frequently associated with sensory deficits, and present nursing interventions and caregiving and coping strategies useful in the care of older adults.

LOSS OF HEARING

Physiological Changes of Aging

Hearing loss is one of the most prevalent sensory deficits in the elderly, increasing with each decade and affecting health and lifestyle. In addition to the impairment of sound conduction, the ability to understand speech may be hampered by background noises and speech distortions. In adults with normal hearing, hearing occurs through the combined action of the external ear (trapping sounds), tympanic membrane vibrations, bony joint vibrations, and the function of the eighth cranial nerve (auditory nerve). Impairment in any of these areas will cause a hearing deficit.

There is a loss of elasticity in the cartilaginous portion of the pinna (or auricle) of the ear. The skin of the auricles may become dry and lax with increased wrinkling. In the external auditory canals, itching and dryness can occur; the small hairs become longer, coarser, and more noticeable in older men. The term *conductive hearing loss* is used to describe alterations in sound wave transmission from outside the ears through the canals and tympanic membrane. Cerumen impaction represents the most common external cause of conductive hearing loss and is frequently overlooked as a cause of hearing impairment in the elderly (Heath & Waters, 1998). Cerumen (ear wax) becomes drier because of the decreased number and activity of ceruminal glands. Cerumen impaction of the external canal can block sound wave transmission, resulting in diminished vibration of the tympanic membrane. In older men, the larger hairs become imbedded in the accumulated wax, preventing the natural dislodging of cerumen. With aging, the tympanic membrane becomes thinner, paler, and more fibrotic, further reducing the transmission of sounds. Thickening and scarring of the membrane may be present as a result of infections and injury over the years.

In the middle and inner ear, degeneration of the bony joints, vestibular structures, cochlea, and organ of Corti occurs, affecting sensitivity to sound, understanding of speech, and maintenance of equilibrium. The bones of the ossicular chain become calcified and hardened, interfering with the transfer of sound vibrations from the tympanic membrane to the oval window. The gradual atrophy and degeneration of hair cells (cilia) and blood supply in the cochlea lead to decreased sound discrimination ability. To complicate matters further, older adults require more time than younger ones to process information in the higher auditory centers (Martin & Barkan, 1989). Sensorineural loss or perceptive deafness is related to degenerative changes in the ossicle and cochlea of the inner ear. Auditory nerve (eighth cranial nerve) neurons and the brainstem are cortical auditory pathways. The degenerative alterations to these include changes in vascular supply and biochemical and electrical changes.

Age-related Conditions

The physiological changes result in three major types of hearing deficits: conductive, sensorineural, and mixed. Conductive hearing loss occurs when there is interference with the normal movement of sound vibrations transmitted outside the external ear through the canal and tympanic membrane to the middle ear. Causes of conductive hearing loss include accumulation of cerumen impacted within the auditory canals, otosclerosis, otitis external, and scarring of the tympanic membranes from eardrum perforation or chronic otitis.

Presbycusis is the term associated with sensorineural hearing loss in old age that involves neural, sensory, metabolic, and mechanical structures of the inner ear. It is characterized by a gradual, progressive, symmetrical loss of hearing of high-pitched frequencies. It begins in midlife and continues on a progressive course into the older years and generally does not lead to total deafness

(Christian, Dluby, and O'Neill, 1989). Men are affected more often than women.

Presbycusis is characterized by a diminished ability to hear consonants. This high-frequency hearing loss causes poor discrimination for consonants such as *s, t, z, f,* and *g.* Even in a quiet environment, discrimination and comprehension are poor, especially with background noise or the presence of tinnitus (ringing in the ears). Hearing of vowels, or low-frequency sounds, generally remains intact (Staab & Lyles, 1990). Sounds become distorted, words jumbled, and sentences incoherent. These changes in hearing for consonants and vowels result in an inability to hear as a result of an impaired clarity of speech, as opposed to loss of volume (loudness). The speech of others becomes unintelligible and, therefore, a normal conversation becomes difficult to follow. For the person to hear, the speaker does not have to shout but only alter words or phrases to increase comprehension and hearing.

A mixed hearing loss involves a conductive loss superimposed on a sensorineural loss. It can be associated with otosclerosis, tumors, toxic effects due to drugs (especially aspirin or streptomycin). Tinnitus, a ringing or buzzing in the ear, is one example of mixed loss. Another is otosclerosis, a loss of compliance of the three bones of the ossicular chain. This fixation of the bones impedes the action of the stapes and interferes with transmission of sound vibrations from the external to internal ear.

Nursing Assessment

Nursing assessment of any hearing loss should begin with a complete history and an assessment of the level of hearing loss. The patient's ability to hear directions can be determined by simply asking if he or she can hear conversational-level speech or by estimating how close a speaker must stand to the patient in order to be heard and understood with the patient's back to the speaker. If there is a hear-

ing deficit, position yourself in easy view of the patient to enhance lipreading. Speak directly toward the patient slowly, with exaggerated speech (Staab & Lyles, 1990). Keep questions short and their wording simple. If a patient wears a hearing aid, be certain it is being worn and is turned on and that the battery is functional. If there is a language barrier, be certain an interpreter is present (Stanley & Beare, 1995). Ask the patient if he or she has ever had hearing loss, dizziness, vertigo, pain, or tinnitus, with special attention to onset. Evaluation of conductive hearing loss can include examining the external ear for abnormalities and lesions and inspecting the external ear canal for the presence of cerumen and the condition of the eardrum. Testing with a tuning fork can help assess hearing by detecting hearing impairments and differentiating between conductive and sensorineural loss. The Rinne test demonstrates the ability to hear through air and bone conduction. In the Weber test, if hearing is normal or if there is equal bilateral deafness, the tone will be heard equally in both ears. Unless the loss is bilateral, the Weber test will lateralize sound to the affected ear (Winters, 1989). The patient should have audiometric testing with precision equipment, either by a nurse trained to conduct the test or by an audiologist.

Nursing Caregiving Strategies

Impaired ability to hear may lead to a loss of independence and social isolation. Hearing loss may place older adults at greater risk for loss of independence and reduce motivation to adapt to the impairment or experience new learning. Hearing loss may be perceived as dementia, because diminished hearing can promote confusion and impairment of language comprehension. The ability to test reality may also be impaired. Persons who hear only parts of a conversation may often think that the conversation is about them. This can lead to suspiciousness, persecution delusions, and paranoia. *Table 3-1* presents nursing coping and care-

TABLE 3-1 *(1 of 2)*

Nursing Coping and Caregiving Interventions for Patients with a Hearing Deficit

ISSUE	INTERVENTIONS
Improving communication skills	1. Assess the level of hearing loss.
	2. Maximize hearing with visual cues and body language.
	3. Be aware that older adults will often try to hide their inability to hear.
	4. Facilitate communication with the patient:
	a. Place yourself in easy view of the patient.
	b. Speak directly toward the patient.
	c. Speak slowly, in a low and varied tone.
	d. Use short, simple sentences with hand and facial gestures.
	e. Rephrase rather than repeat.
	f. Talk toward the patient's best ear.
	5. Keep extraneous noise to a minimum: turn off televisions and radios, and quiet noisy roommates.
	6. Make certain the room is well lighted so all can see.
	7. Remove impacted cerumen from canals.
	8. Write out important communications.
Coping with sensorineural hearing loss	1. Investigate all causes of hearing loss.
	2. Review all drugs to eliminate any that may be ototoxic (aspirin, streptomycin).
	3. Be aware of any social isolation and acquire assistance from family, clergy, or social services to evaluate.
	4. Be certain the person can use and clean a hearing aid if it is available.
	5. Refer families and patients to local support groups and organizations for education, advice, and support.
	6. Install "home helpers" such as chimes, lights, and special TV captioning.
Coping with tinnitus	1. Relate to the patient that this condition is nonprogressive and may disappear in time or may increase with fatigue or stress.
	2. Encourage the patient to keep a bedside radio on at night as a source of ambient noise to mask the tinnitus.
	3. Discuss with the patient that tinnitus can interfere with communication, because it decreases listening ability.
General goals of care	1. Increase communication with others.

TABLE 3-1 *(2 of 2)*

Nursing Coping and Caregiving Interventions for Patients with a Hearing Deficit

ISSUE	INTERVENTIONS
General goals of care	2. Acquire a hearing aid if it can decrease hearing loss.
	3. Comprehension of patient and family regarding treatment.
	4. Assist patient with socialization rather than allowing isolation.
	5. Patient and family support therapeutic approach.
	6. Prevention of hazards in the environment.
	7. Provide an environment that is functionally adapted to the patient's hearing deficit.
Remedies for impacted cerumen	1. Use applications of over-the-counter products (Debrox or Cerumenex) to soften wax.
	2. Soften and remove cerumen by placing 2-3 drops of mineral oil in the auditory canal.
	3. Lavage the external ear canal with 25% hydrogen peroxide solution (one part hydrogen peroxide to three parts water).
	4. Avoid using cotton-tipped applicators to clean ears; frequently cerumen will be impacted instead of removed.
	5. Use tepid installations, *never* hot or cold to avoid complications such as pain or tympanic membrane perforation.

giving interventions that may help nurses detect and treat hearing loss in adults.

Caregiver interventions. Once the patient's actual deficits and capabilities are determined, the goal is to maximize strengths by using such strategies as visual cues, body language, and a hearing aid. Give the patient every opportunity to read your body language; do not cover your mouth with your hands or turn your face away when speaking. Talk toward the best ear of the listener and stay in a lighted area to allow the patient to see your face and lips clearly. Secure the attention of the patient with a gentle touch by facing him or her or speaking his or her name before you begin talking. Write down any important communication or directions that need to be followed specifically or in sequence. Deafness is a form of sensory deprivation that affects the patient and the patient's

family both physically and psychologically. Listening and talking can be reassuring for older adults with a hearing deficit; it can also be very frustrating and depressing. Nurses can make a difference with these people. Families need teaching and counseling about how to make listening situations optimal and improve lifestyle and self-esteem for the hearing-impaired older adult. It can make the difference between optimal functioning and loneliness and isolation.

Technological aids. Sound amplification is generally achieved through the use of hearing aids or assistive devices. The need for a hearing aid should be evaluated and avenues for financial reimbursement pursued as soon as the patient's need and consent are established.

A hearing aid should be individually fitted. It amplifies sounds but generally does not correct the distortion. Be certain that the patient and family realize that hearing aids do reverse the ability to communicate but do not restore hearing to normal quality. Encourage the family to obtain initial information from consumer and professional organizations rather than from hearing aid dealers. Older adults should have periodic audiometric examinations and prompt treatment of cerumen impaction and ear conditions, particularly infections, to minimize further hearing deficits. Assistive hearing devices are not personalized and amplify sound for individual or group communication. Hand-held voice amplifiers should be considered when only increased volume of sound is needed. It is better to use soft chimes or lights rather than loud buzzers or alarms to signal doorbells, telephones, and mealtimes. The family or long-term care facility may want to consider the purchase of low-cost captioning for the television or an induction apparatus for the radio and television.

Community referrals. Acquire community support for the patient from groups such as the National Hearing Aid Society, the American Speech and Hearing Association, and the National Association for the Deaf. Referrals to these agencies can be made directly by a nurse. Phone numbers for these organizations can be found in the telephone book or through a social worker.

LOSS OF VISION

Physiological Changes of Aging

It is now realized that loss of vision in late life is not an inevitable consequence of aging (Oberlink et al, 1997). The Framingham Heart Study revealed that corrected vision of at least 20/25 in the better eye is retained by 98% of persons age 52 to 64 years, 92% of those age 65 to 74,

and 70% of those age 75 to 85. Although visual acuity may remain sharp for many older persons, the quality of an individual's vision generally is not what it was in younger years. Vision is altered in older adults by four major physiological changes: an elevation of the minimal threshold for light perception, decreased visual acuity and peripheral fields, decreased ability to adjust to changing amounts of dark and light, and a loss of accommodative power. The eyelids lose their elasticity, and there is a loss of subcutaneous fat in the orbit of the eye which can limit upward gaze.

The eyebrows and eyelashes gray and decrease in fullness. The conjunctiva becomes pale and appears slightly yellow. Corneal sensitivity lessens, causing a decreased corneal reflex. An age-related deposition of a lipid (called *arcus senilis* or corneal rings) produces a whitish-gray ring just outside the limbus of the eye. The iris of the eye gradually loses its pigment.

Loss of elasticity in the lens and atrophy of the ciliary muscle decrease the ability to focus on fine details. The lens increases both in thickness and size throughout life because of the continual proliferation of new cells. This interferes with the transmission and refraction of light. The ciliary muscle, which governs the convexity of the lens, decreases in length and replaces its muscle with collagen. The collagen causes stiffness of the ciliary muscle and, together with the lens changes, compromises the focusing or *accommodation* of the lens. This change results in the condition called presbyopia or farsightedness.

Presbyopia is the reason many older adults must wear glasses or bifocals for reading or close work. The lens becomes more opaque, resulting in a scattering of light and sensitivity to glares. Blue-green (the cool colors) discrimination becomes more difficult as the lens becomes more opaque and yellowed. The brighter colors of red, yellow, and orange are more easily seen. Using these bright colors contrasted with the cool ones helps to minimize difficulties with depth perception and discernment of fine details (Staab & Lyles, 1990). The increase in lens opacity decreases the ability to focus on fine details as the visual reflexes slow and results in the common frustration of being blinded when rapidly moving from dark to light. The pupils become smaller. This, along with changes in lens opacity, reduces the light reaching the retina, which results in changes in dark adaptation.

Older adults take longer than younger ones to reach the same level of dark adaptation. The danger inherent in their slower response is obvious. When entering a dark room from a brightly lithted one, or after passing an oncoming car with bright headlights, older adults require more time for the eye to recover to a level of sensitivity equal to that of a younger adult. Bathroom falls occur more frequently as one ages. The falls have to do with loss of night vision and sluggish pupillary response that is more typical in the elderly (Oberlink et al., 1997).

Peripheral vision and depth perception decline with age. The scope of visual field narrows markedly in older adults, who may lose as much as 15–30 degrees of lateral vision (Miller, 1990, Ebersole & Hess, 1998). Visual field is important in the performance of tasks like driving and walking in crowded places, which require a broad perception of the environment and moving objects. Depth perception is the visual skill that is responsible for localizing objects in three-dimensional space. Depth perception enables a person to use objects effectively and maneuver safely in the environment. Alterations may lead to falls and mobility problems because of miscalculations about the distance and height of objects.

Another aspect of declining visual function involves the loss of acuity. This is due in part to a decreased amount of light reaching the retina because of changes in the lens and decreased hydration of vitreous humor. This causes absorption and scattering of light, blurred retinal images, and reduced resolution. It may cause an increase in *vitreous floaters,* the benign tiny specks or webs often seen in the field of vision.

Age-related Conditions

Most older adults have impaired vision. There is a variety of widespread changes, the most common being presbyopia. The nurse must discuss the relationship between environmental factors and normal age-related deficits to determine if the change is pathological. Loss of accommodation and loss of elasticity in the lens capsule cause the common symptoms of not being able to see near objects clearly, headaches, and eyestrain after doing close work. Fortunately, presbyopia is easily corrected by wearing glasses or contact lenses.

Cataracts seem to be an almost inescapable consequence of old age. Risk factors other than age include: diabetes, poor nutrition, cigarette smoking, long term exposure to ultraviolet radiation, exposure to high doses of infrared radiation, and some drugs (Flowers & Baker, 1998). Any clouding or opacity occurring in the normally clear crystalline lens is a cataract. Although opacities may not disturb vision in the early stages, as opacification increases, visual acuity diminishes. The earliest change may be an increase in myopia, with progression to disturbed distance vision and yellowing of colors. There may be susceptibility to glare and a general darkening of the world. Cataracts usually develop bilaterally. The only treatment is surgical removal and replacement with an intraocular lens, contact lenses, or glasses. The decision to operate is influenced by the location of the cataract, the degree of visual impairment, and the effect on the individual's quality of life and his or her ability to carry out activities of daily living.

The prevalence of glaucoma increases with age. It is characterized by increasing intraocular pressure (presumably resulting from some impairment in the outflow of aqueous humor from the eye), degeneration and cupping of the optic disc, atrophy of the optic nerve head, and loss of peripheral visual fields. Left untreated, it can result in visual field abnormalities and irreversible blindness. Treatment may be with eye drops, surgery, laser coagulation, or a combination of these, depending on the disease.

Senile macular degeneration involves degeneration of the macula due to decreased blood supply and tissue atrophy, which results in diminished sharpness of "central" vision. Although those affected cannot see straight ahead, they can see peripherally and do not become totally blind. They see a gray shadow in the center of their field of view, making impossible any "fine" or close work such as reading, watching television, sewing, or painting. Eyeglasses are not effective for improving vision, but some "low-vision aids," which are essentially magnifiers, are available to help patients use their remaining vision more effectively. Treatment is aimed at arresting the process of retinal destruction by using laser photocoagulation.

Some elderly experience dry eye because of diminished tear production and alteration in the composition of the tears. Many prescription and over-the-counter drugs can contribute to or cause dry eyes. Symptomatic relief can be obtained from daily use of over-the-counter artificial tears, especially if used before reading and other activities that cause frequent eye movements. Application of cold compresses and increasing home humidity can decrease evaporation of eye moisture and add to eye comfort. Older adults who experience dry eye should avoid irritants, such as smoke, paints, and hair sprays, as well as hot rooms and high winds. Some relief can be obtained with protection of the eyes from wind and dust by wearing wraparound glasses when outdoors.

Nursing Assessment

Nursing assessment of visual deficits should provide information that will assist in planning care. The assessment should identify risk factors that can be eliminated, functional consequences of any vision changes, the psychosocial consequences of visual impairment, and negative attitudes towards treatment or adaptation to limitations. Assessment of vision should include a check of visual acuity, depth perception, color contrast, peripheral vision, and the ability to adapt to dark and light. If the person wears glasses, these should be clean and well-fitted. A standard Snellen chart can be used to test for vision measured against the normal value of 20/20. Older adults can be asked to read a newspaper with various sizes of print to test for near vision. Depth perception can be grossly determined by having the person reach for objects and noting whether the distance is accurately perceived. The confrontation test is a standard mechanism to provide an estimate of peripheral vision fields of the patient as measured against his or her peripheral vision. Peripheral vision is tested by bringing your fingers from the periphery to the patient's field of vision from several different directions while he or she keeps the eye fixed on a constant point straight ahead.

Adaptivity to light and dark is gauged by the level of vision achieved and the length of time needed to reach maximum ability to see in dim light. Older adults need more time to adapt to decreased illumination when moving from a brighter to a darker environment. The nurse should ask patients if they need extra time to focus when entering a darkened movie theater or facing the headlights of oncoming cars.

Nursing Caregiving Strategies

Nursing caregiving strategies should be based on helping visually impaired older adults correct vision problems, as well as cope with the difficulties created when this function cannot be fully restored. Visual acuity may be increased with the use of corrective lenses or bifocals. Sunglasses or tinted lenses reduce glare. When night-driving exposure to the newer "halogen" lights can cause an individual to lose two lines of acuity on a Snellen chart (from 30 to 50) for as long as 20 to 30 minutes (Oberlink et al., 1997). Some eye-care specialists recommend antireflective coating for night time lenses. It is important that all glasses be kept clean and free from scratches.

Reading materials should be on nonglare paper and printed large enough to be seen adequately. Large lettering on objects such as clocks, medicine bottles, and home appliances is helpful. Contrasting colors of red, yellow, and orange should be used to mark edges of steps, furniture, table napkins, and utensils. Blue and green should not be used next to each other.

The glare of shiny floors may cause a safety problem, making normal vision virtually impossible. Position dinnerware, medicines, and canes within the person's visual field. Leave objects in familiar places and do not move them unless it is more convenient for the patient. During social interactions and mealtimes, encourage older adults to face one another to permit optimal social interaction and communication.

Problems related to adjustment to light and dark should be discussed, particularly the hazards of night driving, going from a dark room into bright sunshine, and going into a darkened theater from daylight. Night-lights should be suggested for the home, particularly if nocturia is a problem. *Table 3-2* presents additional nursing coping and caregiving strategies.

Counseling regarding regular eye examination by an optometrist or ophthalmologist, surgery, drug therapy, or a combination of these treatments is critical. Even if restoration of completely normal vision is not possible, partial restoration may permit greater independence and a better quality of life.

LOSS OF TASTE

Physiological Changes of Aging

Older adults' frequent complaints of distortion and lack of taste have led investigators to speculate that this sense may diminish as a function of aging. After the age of 60, the taste buds seem to atrophy and lose some of their functioning. Studies to determine changes in the four senses of taste (sweet, sour, salt, and bitter) have yielded conflicting results.. Loss of taste buds begins in the sixth decade and proceeds slowly as neural degeneration occurs (Wilson, 1995). Changes in taste may be due to dental problems, medication use, protein deficiencies and smoking (Ebersole & Hess, 1998). Taste changes in the healthy aged are insignificant. The quality of taste may vary, but taste remains vigorous in the healthy elderly person.

There is a gradual and progressive age-related decline in gustatory ability, much of which occurs in the oral cavity. A decrease in salivary secretion with age results in *xerostomia,* or dry mouth. The tongue may atrophy slightly and become fissured. Beginning in middle age, the number of taste buds per papilla decrease. Taste cells have the ability to regenerate, but an age-related decline in the number of functioning taste buds does occur (Miller, 1988; Nelson & Franzi, 1992, Wilson, 1995). Increased amounts of salty, sweet, sour, and bitter substances are needed for the person to identify the particular substance offered. Possible reasons for diminished taste sensitivity in older adults include the presence of oral, dental, and systemic diseases; occlusion of the upper palate by dentures; an age-related slowing of taste cell regeneration; and the presence of age-related changes in the nervous system and neurotransmitter levels that influence the perception and processing of taste information. Increased stress may stimulate the autonomic nervous system to inhibit salivary and gastric juice

TABLE 3-2
Nursing Coping and Caregiving Interventions for Patients with a Visual Deficit

ISSUE	INTERVENTIONS
Patient and family education	1. Keep reading glasses properly fitted and clean. Some older adults cannot see well enough to notice spots or scratches. 2. Educate regarding cataracts, glaucoma, and senile macular degeneration development and treatment options. 3. Assist in locating community resources for large-print materials, talking books, and magnifying lenses. 4. Examine diabetic patients for defects in color vision before they are instructed in self-care blood sugar monitoring to avoid misinterpretation of glucose levels. 5. Acquire printed materials from local and national organizations that focus on people with blindness or partial losses in visual functioning.
Institutional adaptations	1. Paint door frames, baseboards, curbs, and steps in different colors to assist in depth perception. 2. For stimulation, use bright pictures placed at eye level on the walls. 3. Color-code hallways and stairwells by decorating with different colors assigned to each area. Be certain staff correctly use the color code when giving directions to older adults. 4. Leave some low-level light on at night in rooms and hallways to decrease accidents if patients awaken and get out of bed. 5. Use illuminated light switches. 6. Use felt-tipped pens rather than regular pens or pencils for written communications.
Aids for vision	1. Hand-held or standing magnifiers. 2. Large-print books, magazines, and newspapers. 3. Large numbers on telephone dials, rulers, playing cards, and thermometers. 4. Large-eye needles, high-intensity lamps. 5. Sunglasses, clip-on lenses, visors, sun hats, tinted lenses.

secretion and has a marked effect on digestion and appetite.

Most tooth loss in older adults is attributed to long-standing lack of preventive care. Tooth loss is combined with the loss of periodontium and atrophy of the bone and results in a shortening of the face and "tobacco juice" wrinkles that appear on either side of the chin. There is a loss of elasticity of the mouth and lips. Since food appeal is significantly influenced by flavor, texture, and the temperature of food, as the taste sense decreases, food tends to lose its appeal.

Age-related Conditions

Evidence suggests that decrements in taste sensitivity occur in older adults. In a malnourished or finicky patient, the diminution of taste can further inhibit eating. Diseases such as chronic rhinorrhea and sinusitis can affect this sensory loss, because clear, thin, or mucopurulent discharge may hinder the receptors of smell (Hoole, Greenberg, & Pickard, 1988). Periodontal disease, stomatitis, wearing dentures, and the condition of the mouth and dentition can alter the sense of taste. Loss of teeth and wearing of full upper dentures will diminish taste sensation, as they cover the taste buds located in the hard palate. The palate is the location of the neural response of the gustatory cells in the taste buds.

The quality and quantity of nutrient intake are determined by eating habits, which are influenced by food appeal; physical health; economic status; activity level; functional abilities; and psychosocial, cultural, and environmental factors. Changes in these factors may alter eating habits and affect the nutritional status of older adults.

Lifelong economic and cultural influences are important determinants of eating patterns and attitudes toward food and nutrition in older adults, much more so than in younger adults. An older adult who is experiencing adjustment problems to a new living situation may complain about or show a lack of interest in food. Age-related influences that affect eating patterns most directly are psychosocial factors; deficits in functioning of other areas of sensation, such as smell and vision; and changes in physical health and functional abilities because of illness. In older adults, depression and loneliness are common experiences and are sometimes accompanied by anorexia and loss of interest in food. Cultural patterns are reflected in the value and acceptability of food and influence food preparation and nutritional intake. Medical illnesses such as diabetes and hypertension, which require diet modification, may create barriers to nutritional therapy and balance.

Nursing Assessment

Nursing assessment should include determination of eating habits, usual eating patterns, and presence of risk factors that interfere with optimal nutrition or digestion. The interviewer should acquire information on age-related changes and environmental and social support factors that affect the procurement, preparation, and enjoyment of food. In addition to a complete nutritional history, nursing assessment should include physical examination of the mouth and oral cavity. The nurse should test the sensory portion of cranial nerves I and VII, because these function in taste sensation, mastication, and chewing. This can be achieved by having materials such as vinegar, peppermints, salt, and sugar for the patient to taste. Other "sip, spit, and rinse" tests can be useful and are easily stored. The nurse may want to include in the assessment height, weight, body build, and any laboratory data that may be available.

Nursing Caregiving Strategies

Sensory changes may intensify complaints of "tasteless foods." Nurses should encourage patients to eat with friends to decrease social isolation. Food should be visually appealing in addition to being tasty. The more aesthetically food is presented, the more likely it will be eaten. Each meal should contain foods of various textures and colors. Patients should be encouraged to use herbs or spices to enhance flavors of food rather than to compensate with increased salt or sugar. Sweeteners can be limited with a dash of cinnamon or allspice instead of sugar, and lemon or basil can help cut the desire for more salt. *Table 3-3* contains additional nursing interventions for older adults with taste deficits.

LOSS OF SMELL

Physiological Changes of Aging

Olfactory nerves are complex and are thought to be the only nerves capable of regeneration (Knapp, 1989). Accidents are the leading cause of diminished sense of smell. Normal aging, head trauma, influenza, brain tumors, and allergies can diminish this sense. The degeneration is not positively correlated with the age of the adult. There seems to be little change in olfactory sensation in healthy adults. With aging, there is a generalized atrophy of the olfactory bulb and the olfactory nerve fibers and a significant reduction in the number of olfactory neurons lining the nasal passages, which may reduce the awareness of odors. The ability to smell odors depends both on the perception of odorous vapors by the sensory cells in the olfactory epithelium and on central nervous system processing of that information (White & Ham, 1997; Miller, 1988). Damage to the olfactory system is more likely to be due to environmental factors such as smoking, airborne toxic agents, occupational odors, or the use of some drugs, rather than to degeneration of the central nervous system.

Age-related Conditions

Anosmia, decrement in the sense of smell, can affect such factors as appetite, social relationships, and detection of warning signals. As taste is highly dependent upon the ability to smell, olfactory sen-

sation plays a role in older adults' ability to recognize and appreciate the flavor of foods. Social isolation and rejection by others may be due to the inability of an older adult to detect offensive personal odors or offensive odors in environment. Another relevant problem involves the diminished ability to perceive "warning" signals, such as smoke, fumes from dangerous chemicals and gases, and the odor of spoiled food. Anosmia diminishes background smells that contribute immensely to the feeling of "being alive" and a part of "what's happening," such as perking coffee, the upholstery of a new car, newly cut grass, the fish market, and the bakery.

Senile rhinitis is a clear, continuous watery discharge from the nose that does not seem to be associated with underlying disease. The mucous membranes are thin and lacking in goblet cells and glandular structure. It may result from abuse of nasal sprays or nose drops, a tumor, or a polyp, but generally it occurs as a result of the aging process. This benign condition may be a social problem, as there is a constant nasal discharge that causes the person to sniff or blow his or her nose frequently.

Nursing Assessment

The assessment of smell must be a part of the history and physical of all older adults. The nurse should ask about past head and nose injury; head and nasal surgery; allergies; occupational toxin; or pollutants; and the ingestion of such drugs as streptomycin, nifedipine, and diltiazem HCl. Visually inspect the nose for symmetry and condition of the nasal mucosa. Check for engorged turbinates as a sign of vasomotor rhinitis. Palpate the nose for lesions and depressions, which suggest postnasal fractures. Palpate the sinuses for swelling or tenderness, which may indicate sinusitis or postnasal drip. Ask the patient to close his or her mouth, alternate occluding each nostril, and breathe to test the patency of the nares. Test olfactory nerve function by asking the patient to identify various smells

TABLE 3-3
Nursing Coping and Caregiving Interventions for Patients with a Taste Deficit

ISSUE	INTERVENTIONS
Coping with taste deficit	1. Make foods visually appealing. 2. Include a variety of textures in foods to assist with identification of food and dispel the monotony engendered by similarly textured foods. 3. Have "taste parties" or explore new restaurants to rekindle interest in food. 4. Add commercial food flavorings to increase palatability of foods. 5. Encourage patients to practice good oral hygiene, and have regular dental checkups. These can help prevent periodontal and gingival disease, which can distort the taste of food or make it offensive. 6. Recognize that some medications may influence taste-bud functioning and appetite control and that alcohol is an appetite suppressant.
Environmental influences on eating	1. Stress and anxiety can influence the physiology of digestion and the desire to eat. 2. Various psychosocial events, such as widowhood and change in living environment, can influence habits and food enjoyment negatively. 3. Cultural patterns and food customs may have harmful consequences on the diet of older adults. 4. Economic status influences food choices. 5. Inclement weather or lack of public transportation may prevent older adults from obtaining groceries. 6. Environmental conditions and food packaging in the grocery store such as cellophane wrappers, small labels, high-glare floors, and fluorescent lights maybe a problem for older adults.

with his eyes closed. Begin with mild scents such as vanilla extract and progress to stronger odors such as smoke, tobacco, and soap. "Scratch and sniff" tests can be purchased. Avoid testing with products that emit irritating fumes, such as bleach or ammonia.

Nursing Caregiving Strategies

Health teaching should focus on corrections of safety factors as well as on the psychosocial influences of smell. Install smoke detectors in the home and visually apparent gas-detection devices on heaters and stoves. Enlist family members or friends to check for spoiled food and pet wastes. An older woman might ask family members if her perfume is too "powerful" or to check for body odors.

Use "smell-enhancing" strategies to stimulate appetite, such as presenting food in a visually appealing manner. Ask the elderly to assist with food preparation to expose them to more smells while getting ready for meals. Discourage older adults from drinking alcohol before or with meals, as it is an appetite depressant, contains empty calories, and interferes with absorption of the B-complex vitamins. Discourage smoking, which impairs the sense of smell. *Table 3-4* includes nursing interventions helpful in dealing with patients with diminished olfaction. The nurse's awareness of diminished olfactory sensation in older adults will assist these patients and their families in preventing accidents and encourage nutritional and social well-being.

SUMMARY

There are a variety of factors that influence the aging process and produce a different course of aging in each person. For example, the genes we inherit, the food we ingest, the manner in which we handle stress, and all the environmental factors and insults to which we subject our bodies will play a role in our aging process. Aging is an individual process; however, there are some general changes in the senses that occur in many persons as they age, though they may not occur similarly in all persons.

Older patients differ greatly from younger patients. One of the ways nurses can prepare themselves for the unique factors that will confront them in providing care to older adults is to increase their understanding of the normal aging process and the resulting pathological conditions that are found in everyday nursing care situations.

Age-related sensory losses are a valid concern to nurses in their assessment and care of older adults. Nursing attention to sensory deficits can influence older adults' health-related behavior and ability to care for themselves in their home environment, be it a private residence or an institutional setting. Awareness of communication strategies can improve understanding and caregiving between the patient and the nurse.

TABLE 3-4

Nursing Coping and Caregiving Interventions for Patients with an Olfactory Deficit

ISSUE	INTERVENTIONS
Test for olfactory threshold	1. Commercially prepared flavored additives, such as cherry, grape, lemon, orange, tomato, bacon, cheddar cheese, and chocolate, can be used in testing for anosmia. 2. Use the traditional stimuli in the initial physical examination, such as coffee, peppermints, tobacco, and soap. 3. Be certain to test for nasal passage patency before proceeding to test for olfaction.
Helpful hints for coping	1. Encourage older adults to actively smell food items before placing the items in the mouth to help identify what they are eating. 2. Call attention to various "environmental" odors encountered during the day, such as smells from bakeries, restaurants, and industrial odors. 3. Add artificial flavorings to food to enhance appeal. 4. Enrich the environment with the more strongly scented fresh flowers or the aroma of baked goods to provide stimuli for diminished sensations. 5. Stop or decrease smoking to prevent further damage to olfactory sensation.

Coping with hazards	1. Accident-proof the home environment whenever possible:
	   a. Install smoke alarms with loud buzzers.
	   b. Put blocks over gas jet handles to prevent their being turned on accidentally.
	   c. Secure potentially toxic agents such as ammonia or cleaning fluids from accidental spillage.
	2. Rigorously maintain personal and environmental hygiene.
	3. Check frequently for food spoiling in the refrigerator; encourage patients not to keep leftovers more than 3 days or to label the leftovers with the date.

CHAPTER 3
Questions 21–30

21. A major cause of conductive hearing loss in older adults is

    a. accumulated cerumen.

    b. noise damage.

    c. presbycusis.

    d. tinnitus.

22. Tinnitus is an example of which type of hearing loss?

    a. Conductive loss

    b. Sensorineural loss

    c. Mixed loss

    d. Unexplained loss

23. Loss of subcutaneous fat around the orbit of the eye affects vision by

    a. limiting upward gaze.

    b. limiting downward gaze.

    c. decreasing peripheral vision.

    d. decreasing central vision.

24. Decreased pupil size results in

    a. presbyopia.

    b. less light reaching the retina.

    c. night blindness.

    d. less color in the iris.

25. Arcus senilis refers to

    a. yellowing of the conjunctiva.

    b. whitish-grey ring visible in the eye.

    c. loss of pigment in the iris.

    d. pallor of the limbus of the eye.

26. Some elderly persons experience dry mouth, otherwise known as

    a. presbyopia.

    b. xerostomia.

    c. anosmia.

    d. stomatitis.

27. Changes in the sense of taste as one ages is

    a. caused by increased salivary secretion.

    b. caused by an increased number of taste buds.

    c. significant in the healthy aged.

    d. caused by a decline in the number of functioning taste buds.

28. Mrs. T. has been assessed for visual acuity by asking her to read various sizes of print in a newspaper. She is able to read only the largest headlines. Which of the following is the most likely cause of her deficit?

    a.   Senile macular degeneration

    b.   Cataracts

    c.   Presbyopia

    d.   Xerophthalmia

29. Mr. S. seems to have difficulty hearing during conversation. The nurse has determined that he has sensorineural hearing loss. The best way to communicate with Mr. S. is to

    a.   speak loudly to Mr. S.

    b.   speak softly to Mr. S.

    c.   use "home helpers" such as chimes and lights.

    d.   speak while facing Mr. S.

30. Mr. S. may also have hearing impairment related to accumulated wax in the ear canal. The best way for the nurse to clear the canal of wax is to

    a.   soften the wax with drops, then lavage with warm water.

    b.   clean the canal with a water pick and warm water.

    c.   remove the wax with a curette.

    d.   wash the canal with a washcloth, soap, and water.

CHAPTER 4

PHYSIOLOGICAL CHANGES: COPING AND CAREGIVING STRATEGIES

by

John Lantz, RN, PhD

CHAPTER OBJECTIVE

After studying this chapter, the reader will be able to distinguish normal physiological changes that occur with aging and recognize risk factors that these normal physiological changes present for activities of daily living for an elderly person.

LEARNING OBJECTIVES

After studying this chapter, the reader will be able to:

1. List the general physiological effects of aging.

2. Discuss the components of risk and their relationship to physiological changes of aging.

3. List four risk factors that contribute to impaired functional status.

4. Relate anatomical alterations in the cardiovascular system to decreased activity level.

5. Explain why elderly persons are at risk for the development of respiratory failure during stressful situations.

6. Specify physiological changes of bones, muscles, and joints that affect functional capacity of elderly persons.

7. Specify physiological changes in the nervous system that alter sleep patterns.

8. Define the concept of self-integration and its relationship with appearance and sexuality.

INTRODUCTION

It is generally agreed that there is no single known factor that causes aging or prevents the process. Hampton (1991) agrees, stating, "A most conspicuous feature of an aged population is the range (i.e., variability) of function seen in any given age group... This variability is not trivial to the understanding of age changes." "The rate of aging among different body systems within one individual may vary, with one system showing marked declines, while another may demonstrate no significant changes" (Eliopoulos, 1995). A variety of degrees of physiological changes, capacities, and limitations can also be found within a given age group. These changes and losses demand multiple adjustments for the elderly and they are important for the healthcare provider to consider as a foundation for assessment and a framework for care.

Aging is said to begin at conception, and it is a complex, multidimensional, natural phenomenon. All factors, physiological, psychological, and socioenvironmental, are interrelated in the process (Featherman & Peterson, 1986; Hampton, 1991). Aging is an experience of life, and it is highly individualized. Chronological age alone is not a predictor of individual performance or appearance. Lifestyle variables like physical activity, eating, drinking, smoking, and personality characteristics apparently affect the aging process (Geokas, 1990).

It is important to note that being old is not the same as being ill, and aging is not a disease. Some factors that predispose a person to disease also influence that persons responses to aging. They include heredity, culture, race, nutritional status, and environmental factors. Experts sometimes have difficulty distinguishing changes that occur with normal aging and those that are caused by disease processes. An important difference generally agreed upon is that aging changes are irreversible, whereas those that occur as a result of a disease can generally be reversed (Yurick et al., 1989). Although aging is not disease, the physiological changes that occur may make a person more susceptible to illness and disease.

Overall the aging process does not follow a specific and predictable pattern. The changes are gradual; one does not wake up one day, look in a mirror and say, "I'm old." Aging should not be considered a decline, but should be considered a phase of normal development, and as a phase of development, it can be defined as patterns of change that are qualitative rather than quantitative. It becomes a time of transformation rather than a time of stagnation, total decline, and loss.

In this stage of life, the elderly have a unique set of developmental tasks that are commensurate with the capacities of aging. Butler and Lewis (1977) define the following four developmental tasks:

1. Clarification of the value and significance of a lifetime of experience.

2. Conservation of strength and physical and emotional resources.

3. Adjustment to changes and losses.

4. Enjoyment of the achievement of being "a completed human being."

It is important for health care providers to consider these tasks as they evaluate the health status of an elderly person. Two of these tasks, conservation of strength and physical resources and adjust-

ment to changes and losses, are directly related to the physiological changes that occur with aging.

PHYSIOLOGICAL CHANGES

In order to stay alive, your body must live on the wings of change. The skin replaces itself once a month, the stomach lining every five (5) days, and the skeleton every three (3) months. By the end of this year, 98% of the old atoms in your body will have been exchanged for new ones (Chopra, 1993).

Overall physiological changes as one ages can be traced to basic cellular changes. It is estimated that an older person possess 30% fewer cells than younger adults (Eliopoulos, 1995). This is partially due to generalized slowing of cell division. This loss of cells accounts for substantial weight reduction in a number of body organs. Cells also change in their ability to perform specialized integrated function and tend to combine in irregular patterns. These changes may be attributed to cellular changes including lipofuscin accumulation; decreased cytoplasmic RNA; and cell nucleus changes, with DNA not being replaced after final developmental mitosis.

An additional overall change is a decrease in both intracellular and extracellular fluids. This total body fluid decrease makes an elder more susceptible to dehydration and affects the dilution ability of the body when certain kinds of drugs are used.

These cellular changes contribute to the fact that physiological changes are universal, progressive, decremental, and intrinsic (Ebersole & Hess, 1998). These changes do not hinder an elder in the task of daily living under normal, nonstressful conditions. A person adapts to needs and functional ability, and special consideration may be necessary in times of stress, illness, and overexertion. Major physiological aging can be analyzed through parameters such as cardiac output, pulmonary function, and glomerular filtration. Other authors present or analyze these physiological changes by body systems. In both cases, it is important to consider the person as a whole and to always remember the whole is more than the sum of its parts.

RISK: A FRAMEWORK

A risk is a condition that may compromise a person's health or longevity (Hill & Smith, 1990). One may conclude that a major difference exists between morbidity and mortality between the young and old because of differences in risks. These risks have "to do with situations in which an individual is exposed to an increased possibility of emotional, social, or physical injury" (Wold, 1990). Risk factors may be actual, potential, or perceived and threaten a person's health or well-being. From a physiological perspective, risks may be due to structural and functional changes of aging. They may decrease a person's ability to maintain homeostasis.

The conceptual model for risk reduction proposed by Blum (1980) provides a good beginning to determine the needs of individuals and groups of older adults. Nurses have an important role in fostering a level of self-care, self-responsibility, and self-determination in decreasing risk, adapting to change, and promoting wellness. This role is important in all settings: hospitals, nursing homes, community settings, and other settings that provide healthcare to the elderly. Effective nursing care planning recognizes potential risks and strategic ways to intervene rationally to reduce these risks. It is important to note that risks are not an all-or-none situation, and nurses must consider and deal with degrees of risk (Wold, 1990).

Risk Factors Contributing to Impaired Functional Status

Many evaluate their health state in relation to their functional ability or activity status. Society tends to translate a person's value and worth into what the person does and contributes. For an elderly person, what is done and contributed might differ from what it was as a younger adult. As one ages, functional status is affected by capabilities and limitations, as well as external factors mandated by society. Successful aging is often evaluated in terms of the ability of the person to stay active, maintain activities, and continue to be involved in life. Maintaining independence is a major goal for elderly persons, and a major issue is the fear of becoming a burden or becoming dependent. For nurses, the inclusion of functional status as part of an assessment shifts the delivery of care from a curing-of-disease focus to improving function. Such an approach has an indirect and a direct impact on a person's daily quality of life.

As a group (a macro perspective), one in five of persons 65 years or older have mild degrees of functional impairment. These mild limitations affect basic needs, such as eating, dressing, toileting grooming, ambulating, and bathing. Some persons may also have difficulties in maintaining themselves in the community. This might be reflected as an inability to do things such as shop, clean house, do laundry, or use transportation. Of this group, 4% have major impairment defined as impairment in performing five to six of these defined activities, and 5% are homebound. As one advances in age, the probability of multiple or severe functional impairment develops. It is estimated that by the age of 85, these impairments increase fourfold (Aging America, 1985; Walker, 1991).

As a group, the elderly are a microcosm of society. Overall, many in our country live a sedentary life, which makes it increasingly difficult to remain or become active. The right amount of exercise in old age is "more exercise than yesterday" (Hall, 1997). It is estimated that only 8% of the elderly are regularly active. Regularly active is generally defined as engaging in activities lasting at least 20 min, three times per week. This kind of regular activity requires motivation, and the pace must be adjusted to watch for fatigue, muscle pain, and cramping. Less efficient management may cause shortness of breath, muscle weakness, severe fatigue, and decreased range of motion. It is important to note that regular, ongoing activity facilitates the functioning of the respiratory, circulatory, and musculoskeletal systems. Impaired functioning of these systems affect a person's ability to stay actively involved and may affect cognitive abilities.

Activity can be compromised because of physiological changes. Under normal circumstances, a person's activity level progressively slows, and he or she exhibits a methodical manner that allows him or her to engage in normal activity while conserving energy, preventing undue fatigue, and providing balance. Persons with insufficient physiological energy to ensure or complete required or desired daily activities may be experiencing "activity intolerance" (Bowles, 1991).

According to Bowles (1991), the following are common contributing factors to activity intolerance:

- Compromised oxygenation
- Neuromuscular limitations
- Progressive decreased activity
- Bed rest and immobility
- Generalized weakness or fatigue

From a systems perspective, the following may be **risks** to maintaining an active state and may cause potential activity intolerance:

- Decreased cardiac output
- Decreased breathing capacity and efficiency
- Decreased muscle mass, strength, and movement

- Demineralization of bone; deterioration of cartilage and surface of joints
- Altered neurological functioning inhibiting regulating activities, such as skeletal movement.

What physiological changes may contribute to each of these?

PHYSIOLOGICAL CHANGES OF THE CARDIOVASCULAR SYSTEM

As one ages, the heart and blood vessels change in several ways. From middle age, the prevalence of cardiovascular disease continues to be the major cause of death. Because normal changes occur independently of pathological processes and because of a high incidence of cardiac disease, it is often difficult to determine which changes are age related and which are associated with disease. As with other bodily changes, cardiovascular changes are slow and insidious (Stanley & Beare, 1995). Major influences on these changes in the cardiovascular system are arteriosclerotic changes, which increase with aging and are considered by many a normal aging process, because it develops in everyone to some extent. The cardiovascular system adapts to these processes, and most exhibit no health problems related to these processes. Arteriosclerotic changes begin soon after birth and are characterized by progressive thickening of the arterial lumen and collagen and calcium accumulation. The process of arteriosclerotic disease is used as an umbrella covering three separate processes: Mönckeberg's sclerosis, atherosclerosis, and arteriolosclerosis. Most persons have more than one of these changes occurring at one time, but it is believed that the changes can occur independently of each other. Mönckeberg's sclerosis is the accumulation of calcified salts in the mediae of arteries. Arteriolosclerosis is the thickening of the arterial lumen or thickening of the arteries. Atherosclerosis is the presence of plaque composed primarily of fat on the artery walls. This last process is the major cause of cardiovascular disease (Esberger & Hughes, 1989).

In general, the arteries, which are pliable and elastic when young, become less elastic, dilated, and elongated. These physiological changes make the heart work harder to push blood into the less elastic arteries. It is important to note that research studies conclude that persons from urban areas consume six times more sodium chloride than those in rural areas, and this increase accelerates age-related arterial stiffness (Avolio, Deng, & Li, 1985). Overall arterial changes appear to be widespread and result in diminished circulation to all organs and tissues. A major impact is the reduced circulation to the brain and kidneys, but adaptive responses contribute to age-related normal functioning. Factors like stress and exercise increase cardiovascular workload on this stabilized, maintained system. It is estimated that cardiovascular workload increases as much as four or five times during stress (Geokas, 1990).

The impact of aging on the heart influences the total cardiovascular system. The heart, as a muscular organ, changes as muscle fibers are replaced by fibrous tissue. Collagenous buildup can almost encase the heart in a collagen matrix. These anatomical changes lead to diminished contractibility and filling capacity (Bullock & Rosendahl, 1984; Hampton, 1991). Heart valves tend to increase in thickness, and calcium salt deposits may occur on certain valves. These changes may modify the normal closing of the valves, causing murmurs or abnormal heart sounds. An overall adaptive response may be myocardial hypertrophy. This response is made in an attempt to maintain normal heart volume and pump function. Considerations must be given to cardiac strength, efficiency, and the decreased stroke volume. Despite these adaptations, cardiac output does

decrease. Some experts estimate that a person's cardiac output decreases 1% each year, beginning at approximately age 25 (Eliopoulos, 1995; Hampton, 1991). It is estimated that the cardiac output decreases as much as 50% by the age of 80. The normal average output of 5 liters/min decreases below 3 liters/min (Forbes & Fitzsimmons, 1981). This diminished cardiac output again becomes significant when an elderly person is physically or mentally stressed by illness, disability, activity, worry, loss, or excitement.

A frequent cardiovascular measure is blood pressure. It is debatable as to how aging and these physiological changes affect this measure of cardiovascular status. Some believe normal blood pressure for older persons is in the range of 140mm Hg systolic and 90mm Hg diastolic. The Fifth Report of the Joint National Committee on Detection, Evaluation, and Treatment of High Blood Pressure (1993) states that both young and old have similar blood pressure. The definition of hypertension, according to this committee, is a systolic pressure at or above 140mm Hg and a diastolic pressure at or above 90mm Hg. 50% of over age 65 individuals are estimated to have blood pressure greater than 140/90mm Hg (Frohlich, 1995). Others think systolic increases are due to decreased aortic elasticity, and others believe that peripheral resistance in the vessels causes an increase in both systolic and diastolic pressure. Caird, Dall, and Williams (1985) indicate that the elderly may not manifest true hypertensive disorders, but may normally have a blood pressure range of 200–210mm Hg systolic and 100–115mm Hg diastolic. These different beliefs reinforce the importance of establishing a baseline normal for each elderly person. Hypertension can be a major health problem for the elderly, because it is the primary risk factor for strokes and is a contributing factor for myocardial infarctions (Menscer, 1997). The usefulness of treating hypertension in the elderly is still being studied. Most elderly people will want to be treated if it is relatively inexpensive and the side effects of the treatment not too bothersome. Lifestyle and dietary changes should continue along with drug therapy.

Another measure of cardiovascular evaluation is the electrocardiogram (ECG). The ECG reveals changes in heart functioning as affected by exercise. For example, during exercise, S-T segment shifts may point to inadequate oxygen metabolism possibly due to partial coronary occlusion. Extra beats of the ventricles may be precipitated by exercise. The frequency of an abnormal exercise ECG increases with age and is present in about 30% of persons 65 and older (Hampton, 1991). Conduction is also affected by a decrease in the total number of pacemaker cells in the sinoatrial node. Alterations may include blocks or irregular discharges. The baroreceptors in the aortic and carotid arteries also become less sensitive to pressure changes with aging. This results in low response to postural changes, and changes in position may cause dizziness or syncope (Menscer, 1997). Elderly persons who are taking vasodilators, diuretics, or beta blockers should be observed for this orthostatic response in the form of hypotension.

In summary, with advancing years, the physiological changes of the cardiovascular system affect and alter the function of the whole body. Under normal circumstances, the cardiovascular system adapts and allows the person to maintain a "normal" level of functioning, but the effect of these changes may alter activity level. *Table 4-1* is a summary of the contributing cardiovascular changes.

PHYSIOLOGICAL CHANGES OF THE RESPIRATORY SYSTEM

Respiratory health is vital to the elder's ability to maintain a physically, mentally, and socially active life style. It can make the difference between whether or not a person will maximize opportunities to live life to the fullest or be too fatigued and uncomfortable to leave the confines of his or her home (Eliopoulos, 1995).

Often the frightening and anxiety-producing feeling of breathlessness is accepted as a situation associated with growing old. To prevent this subjective feeling, a person may diminish activity (Stanley & Beare, 1995). Breathlessness is the most common physiologic response to exercise of a sedentary person. It is estimated that the maximum oxygen consumption rate during stress and moderate exercise can increase nine times for an elderly person. For an elderly person whose physiological changes of the respiratory system are both structural and functional, respirations tend to be shallower and more frequent, and control becomes less precise. Maximum breathing capacity is diminished 50% by age 60, and actual air flow is reduced 20–30%. Older men and women have a lower total lung capacity and vital capacity. A 20-year-old man has a vital capacity of 5.20 liters compared with 4.00 liters for those 60 years old. Women's values are 4.17 and 3.29, respectively. This change requires the elderly to move 50% more air than younger persons. By age 90, most lungs have enough alveolar destruction to meet the strict criteria for a diagnosis of emphysema. These changes are related to loss of elasticity in the chest wall, calcification of cartilage in rib joints and vertebrae, destruction of the alveoli, and general wasting of muscles, including those required for respiration (Hampton, 1991; Kenney, 1985).

Respiratory system changes, as in other body systems, are gradual. Problems develop more easily and are more difficult to manage. Immobility, due to fractures, depression, weakness, a fear of falling, and a multitude of other reasons, is a major threat to pulmonary health.

TABLE 4-1
Factors Contributing to Cardiovascular Change

The heart

Elasticity decreases.

Rate at rest and maximum achievable rate declines.

Decrease in rate is compensated for by an increase in stroke volume to maintain cardiac output.

The conduction system loses cells and fibers and becomes infiltrated with fat.

Intrinsic contractile functioning declines.

Diastolic murmurs increase (more than 50% of older adults have such a murmur).

Vascular

Compliance decreases due to changes in proliferation and fibrosis, mediae elastin fragmentation, and calcification.

Peripheral resistance increases.

Systolic blood pressure increases, with lower rate of increase in diastolic pressure.

Pulmonary health becomes even more compromised when a person becomes bedridden, even for a short period. This problem is due to the fact that although lung capacity is not significantly altered, a redistribution occurs with lung expansion and inflation at the lung base, which is dramatically decreased. A loss of cough strength reduces mucus transport, which also complicates the situation. In addition to monitoring the respiratory status of any patient who is bedridden, healthcare providers need to be concerned about medications that the patient may be taking. Many medications cause problems and affect the somewhat compromised respiratory system. Cough suppressants and analgesics may cause depression of respirations and sputum retention. Sedatives and tranquilizers may also depress respirations. These potential drug responses reinforce the fact that a drug inventory, including over-the-counter drugs, is essential.

Under normal circumstances, the elderly can engage in activities of daily living without evidence or concern for the changes in the respiratory system. It is important to note that these changes have been affected by an accumulation of environmental factors such as air pollution, tobacco smoking, and

infection. The prevalence of respiratory abnormalities tends to be much higher in the elderly population than in other segments. (Reddy & Thadepalli, 1998). Respiratory status can be assessed best from interview, observation, and auscultation. The following are some of the questions that should be asked during the initial assessment:

- Do you have wheezing, chest pain, coughing, phlegm, a heavy feeling in your chest, or shortness of breath after a walk?

- Do you frequently get a cold or flu? How often during the season?

- How many pillows do you use?

- Do you smoke or have you ever smoked?

- Have you ever worked in a job that may have caused you to be short of breath or caused you to cough? What kind of job was this?

Always remember that respiratory system limitations may not be apparent when the patient is at rest.

Esberger and Hughes (1989) categorized respiratory system changes into four aspects: airway clearance, immunity or defense mechanism alteration, physical properties, and respiratory control. Analysis of important changes includes structural and functional changes as well as defense mechanism changes. These changes include alterations to those organs directly related to the respiratory system as well as supportive and facilitating associated organs. Cardiac output is also directly related to pulmonary function, endorsing and supporting the interrelationship of body systems.

Structural changes reduce maximum breathing capacity. Some of these changes include changes in the thoracic cage, reduced lung elasticity, and pulmonary artery changes as in the cardiovascular system. Lung expansion is altered by configuration changes of the thorax, calcification of the costal cartilages, and changes in posture and abdominal girth. The chest diameter from anterior to posterior may increase, and a transverse measure decrease. This alteration is called *kyphosis.* Reduced lung elasticity is another major structural change associated with a cross-linkage in collagen and elastin fibers around the alveolar sacs. The primary fibrous connective tissue proteins of the lungs are collagen, elastin, and reticulum. With aging, the ratio of elastin to collagen is increased (Hampton, 1991). This causes a reduction in elasticity, altering the alveolar ducts and stretching the alveoli, which decreases the amount of surface available for oxygen diffusion.

The main functional respiratory problems in the elderly who do not have pulmonary disease are reduced ventilation of all alveoli, especially at the bases of the lungs, and reduced oxygen postural pressure in the arterial blood. From a physiological perspective, these changes are seen as alterations in supportive or ancillary function as well as altered lung mechanics and ventilatory function. The major functional changes are alterations in respiratory muscle functioning, associated loss or decreased elastic recoil, and alterations in lung volumes and breathing patterns (Stanley & Beare, 1995). Although total lung capacity does not dra-

matically change, residual volume increases, and a decrease in vital capacity also occurs. The older person's response may be noticed as incomplete exhalation, inhibiting lung inflation and promoting secretion collection (Farrell, 1990). *Table 4-2* summarizes the physiological changes of the respiratory system.

These alterations place the elderly at risk for impaired functional status. It is also important to note that the maintenance of respiratory functioning is enhanced by the maintenance of functional status at the highest level possible.

PHYSIOLOGICAL CHANGES OF THE MUSCULOSKELETAL SYSTEM

The general integrity of the musculoskeletal system is related to its physiological functions of protection of internal organs, body shape, **mobility,** stability, coordination, and balance. Maintenance of the machinery requires an appropriate level of activity, adequate rest of its parts, and adequate nourishment (Esberger & Hughes, 1989).

The decrease of muscle mass, strength, skeletal inflexibility, loss of equilibrium, and limited ability to provide movement are most often seen as the major contributors to impaired functional status. The physiological changes of the musculoskeletal system are among the earliest and most obvious to the person affected. Posture and structural changes occur primarily because of calcium loss from bone and atrophy of cartilage and muscles (Ebersole & Hess, 1998). Alterations are affected by circulatory and respiratory function. The changes affect mobility and may force an elderly person to become more dependent on others and may diminish his or her life span.

TABLE 4-2
Factors Contributing to Respiratory Change

Decreased pulmonary elasticity and recoil as a result of collagen and elastin changes

Accessory muscle atrophy of pharynx and larynx

Respiratory muscle strength decrease

Chest wall compliance decrease, due to stiffness of chest wall and costal cartilage calcification

Increased anteroposterior diameter of chest

Alveolar duct and sac enlargement and less total alveolar surface for gas exchange

Fewer alveoli in lungs and thickening of the alveolar membranes

Decreased diffusion

Decreased mucociliary escalator

Increased trapping of air

Decreased blood flow in pulmonary circulation

Increase in residual volume and functional residual capacity

Decrease in vital capacity and expiratory flow rates

Decrease in arterial PO2

An analysis of the physiological changes that occur in the musculoskeletal system must consider each component that contributes to a healthy system. These three components are muscle, bone structure, and joints. These three form an integrated system, adapting to meet the needs of a person.

Muscle

Muscle change during aging is an individualized process with a high degree of variability. The muscles undergo a great amount of atrophy with age, and there is a gradual decrease in both the number of muscle fibers and their individual bulk. This muscle mass reduction may make it more difficult to control movement. A diminished storage of muscular glycogen may cause a loss of energy reserve, which contributes to a rapid onset of fatigue. Patterns of adaptation to this physiological change include taking frequent rest periods and taking and allowing more time to go somewhere or to do something.

As noted, muscle fibers decrease and atrophy as age progresses. This process begins by age 40, and fibrous tissue gradually replaces muscle tissue, because muscle cells do not regenerate (Hampton, 1991). This process is influenced by diet, especially potassium, and ineffective oxygenation. Cellular changes occur in the muscles. Muscles are composed of postmitotic cells, and these cells are dependent on the inclusion of neural components (Ebersole & Hess, 1998). These cells become depositories for **lipofuscin,** the refuse of cellular function. Muscle mass is altered by extracellular increases in fat, collagen, and interstitial fluid. Extracellular water, chloride, and sodium are increased in the muscles of the elderly. Regular exercise, even if started in later life, improves muscle strength, tone, and stamina, but generally it is speculated a man of 70 has 50% the strength of a man of 30. By 80 years of age, strength and stamina decrease to 65–85% of the maximum strength that a person had at his or her peak of 25 years of age.

Bone Structure

Around the age of 40, bone mass and density shift and begin to decline. In addition to affecting mobility, these changes also predispose the elderly to accidents. Bone mass changes are associated with age, sex, and race. Other influencing factors include nutrition; sedentary life style; alcohol abuse; immobilization; and diseases such as diabetes, chronic renal disease, hyperthyroidism and adrenal hyperactivity (Ebersole & Hess, 1998). Women are more vulnerable to bone loss; men have approximately 50% of the age-related bone loss than women do. This bone loss in women occurs especially in the decade following menopause. Ethnic differences have also been seen. Blacks have a higher peak bone density than whites, and hispanic women have lower bone density than black women, but higher than white women (Bauer, 1993).

The changes of bones are gradual and are due to reabsorption of the interior matrix of the long and flat bones. The external surface of the bones also begins to thicken. These changes are not observable but are evident by alterations in posture and stature. A human being loses 1.2 cm of height every 20 years. The decrease in height occurs in both men and women but is greater in women. It presents itself in the characteristic short trunk and long extremities seen in elders. This change is caused by osteoporotic vertebral narrowing. Two additional factors contributing to this shortening of stature are kyphosis and osteoporosis. It is important to note that this change alters a person's center of gravity. Reaching and climbing may become more difficult. Stooped posture may also cause a decrease in the visual field.

Joints

Joints are the articulating surfaces of a adjoining bones. Deterioration of these surfaces begins at age 30 and is exaggerated by injury, obesity, and excessive use. By age 70, an evaluation of the joints reflects a lifetime of wear and tear. Overall, the joints become less mobile, because the cartilage tends to lose water, and the joints fuse at the cartilage surfaces.

In summary, the musculoskeletal changes can be analyzed by looking at changes in muscles, bone structure, and joints. A summary of these changes is outlined in *Table 4-3.*

Five characteristics may be seen in various degrees. These are muscle wasting, lack of strength, lack of endurance, lack of agility, and complaints of fatigue. Assessment of these characteristics should include consideration of the following:

* Posture, stance, gait (length of stride), and pace
* Speed when walking
* Difficulty sitting and standing
* Ability to climb and descend stairs

These elements may give clues to musculoskeletal integrity and its relationship to a person's level of physical activity.

PHYSIOLOGICAL CHANGES OF THE NERVOUS SYSTEM

It is difficult to identify with accuracy and exactness the impact of aging itself on the nervous system, due to the dependence of this system's function on other body systems (Eliopoulos, 1995).

This relationship and the complexity of function of the nervous system make it difficult to differentiate changes that are caused by aging or disease. The changes that do occur in the nervous system may be unnoticed and nonspecific and progress slowly. They may be vague, abstract complaints, and alterations in thinking, feeling, reasoning, and remembering. Alterations of the nervous system can affect activities of daily living, contribute to impaired functional status, and modify the quality of life.

The cells of the nervous system do not regenerate, and they are never replaced (Hampton, 1991). This loss of cells begins at birth, is not uniform

---

TABLE 4-3

Factors Contributing to Musculoskeletal Change

Decrease in muscle weight and lean muscle mass, and muscle cell atrophy

Decrease in muscular strength, endurance, and strength associated with a decrease in the number of muscle fibers

Shortening of trunk due to intervertebral space narrowing

Bone loss (universal and highly variable, more rapid in women after menopause)

Decrease in water content of hyaline cartilage lining joint surfaces

Hardening of ligaments, tendons, and joints, leading to an increase in rigidity and a decrease in flexibility

Decrease in muscular glycogen storage, causing loss of energy reserve

---

throughout the system, and has little impact on the functioning of that system. The changes in the nervous system are primarily the result of two things: diminished blood flow to the brain and loss of nerve cells (neurons). It is estimated that a person loses several thousand neurons a day. Dendrite spines decrease, and the rate of nerve impulse conduction decreases about 10% (Hampton, 1991). It has also been found that with aging, glucose and protein synthesis decreases in the neurons. The total system of brain, nerves, and spinal cord exhibits decreased vascularity and fibrotic changes.

Accompanying aging is a slow, progressive loss in brain size. Over a normal life span, a 10% or greater loss of brain weight can be anticipated. Losses occur in both gray and white matter, more so in gray matter. Cerebral cortical cell loss is notable after age 50, and by age 90, the loss in some cortical zones (frontal and superior temporal regions) is about 50% (Hampton, 1991). The coverings of the brain, dura mater, arachnoid, and pia mater gradually thicken and become more fibrous. These changes are summarized in *Figure 4-1*.

A person interacts with the environment through his or her nervous system. It is an organizing and communication interaction, composed of receiving, processing, and responding. These functions occur through a complex system of connections and interconnections of neurons. Two major concerns regarding neurological changes and

abnormalities are related to cognitive impairment and the slowing of certain behaviors. Cognitive impairment is addressed in a following chapter with the exploration of dementia and the syndrome of Alzheimer's disease.

Nervous system changes basically affect all voluntary or automatic reflexes, making the reflexes slower. The slowing of certain behaviors is viewed as one of the most significant age-related functional changes of the nervous system (Katzman & Terry, 1984; Hampton, 1991). It is composed of both slower reflexes and delayed responses to multiple stimuli (Eliopoulos, 1995; Hampton, 1991). Examples of these changes were explored by Katzman and Terry (1984). They identified a number of simple motor skill alterations attributable to age related changes in the nervous system. Between ages 25 and 75, up to a 40% decline occurs in the following areas:

- Rising from a chair without support
- Putting on a shirt
- Buttoning a button
- Zipping a garment
- Cutting with a knife
- Writing quickly
- Standing on one leg with eyes closed

These changes can be frustrating to a hurried healthcare provider who may find it easier to do for

FIGURE 4-1
Aging Changes in the Brain

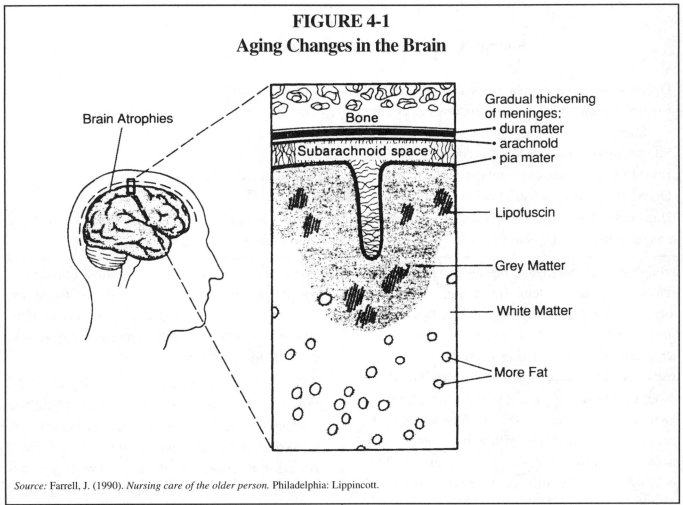

Brain Atrophies

Bone

Subarachnoid space

Gradual thickening
of meninges:
• dura mater
• arachnoid
• pia mater

Lipofuscin

Grey Matter

White Matter

More Fat

Source: Farrell, J. (1990). *Nursing care of the older person.* Philadelphia: Lippincott.

patients rather than to have them do it for themselves. It is important to note that these changes may be exhibited in a well, active, alert elderly person. An example given by Katzman and Terry (1984) was of a man 80 years of age who could walk, run, and do calisthenics but could not safely stand on one leg with his eyes closed. An analysis of delayed reaction time or psychomotor speed should consider the following three interrelated causes (Eliopoulos, 1995):

1. Vision impairment

2. Decreased number of axons in the nerves (especially the fast conducting axons)

3. Changes at the synapses, which lowers conduction

As previously stated, one in five persons 65 years of age or older has mild degrees of functional impairment; many of these are related to functional changes of the nervous system. It is also important to stress that the relationship of the cardiovascular, respiratory, and musculoskeletal systems to the nervous system is essential. In fact, the interrelationship of these systems provides the motivation, the ability, the resources, and the response for an activity to occur. It is the basis for a person to live an active life. As providers of healthcare, we need to recognize that body systems slow down and change in structure. Tissues become thicker, or thinner, and often inelastic. Despite these changes, a person continues to be a functional whole, with **risks** that require recognition and adaptation. *Table 4-4* lists factors that contribute to changes in the nervous system. The following nursing strategies can assist the elderly in coping with factors that may impair functional status (Rogers-Seidl, 1991):

TABLE 4-4
Factors Contributing to Nervous System Change

- Slowing of voluntary or automatic reflexes with a decreased ability to respond to multiple stimuli
- Moderate cortical atrophy
- Lower nerve conduction velocity
- Loss of neurons in neocortex, substantia nigra, and limbic system
- Decrease in number and size, of peripheral nerve fibers with a decrease in motor and sensory nerve conduction
- Less kinesthetic sense
- Accumulation of lipofuscin
- Decrease in binding sites for dopamine and serotonin
- Decreased blood flow to the brain

- Assess activity tolerance (evaluate heart and respiration rate).

- Encourage the person to increase muscle strength and endurance.

- Report fatigue and weakness.

- Encourage self-care activities.

- Encourage good posture and alignment when ambulating or in bed.

- Teach energy conservation.

- Evaluate environment for safety (i.e., throw rugs on slippery floor).

- Encourage a balance in rest and activity.

RISK FACTORS CONTRIBUTING TO IMPAIRED REST OR SLEEP

It is often said that an elderly person may stay in bed longer but tends to get less sleep. This statement is probably both accurate and reflective of the changes that occur with age. Rest and sleep are activities of daily living that provide a person with the opportunity to regenerate. To maintain a reasonable level of activity, one requires time for sleep and rest (Ebersole & Hess, 1998). Alterations in sleep patterns can be a response to aging or a symptom of more serious problems. Inadequate exercise or activity during the waking hours may result in an imbalance in the sleep-wake cycle (Rogers-Seidl, 1991). It is important to note that women have more resistance to age related sleep changes (Yura, 1978).

Three areas of sleep change can occur with aging. They are length of sleep, distribution of sleep throughout the day, and changes in sleep-stage patterns (Yurick et al., 1989). The following are specific examples that reflect these changes. An elderly person:

- Is more easily awakened.

- Takes longer to fall asleep.

- Awakens more often during the night.

- Spends more time lying in bed awake.

- Has more frequent sleep-stage changes.

- Is more susceptible to stress-related sleep disturbances.

- Does not have a decreased need for sleep.

Sleep patterns change with aging. At age 50, stage 4 sleep is reduced by 50% of what it was at age 20. It is replaced by stage 2 and 3 sleep. This alteration increases spontaneous awakening (Hampton, 1991). Frequent awakenings cause a minimal amount of lost sleep. This fragmentation occurs even for healthy elderly. These alterations reflect a decline in delta-wave sleep from 1.5 hr to a few minutes. REM sleep decreases from 2 hr to 1 hr. A response to this and other alterations may be that the elderly person may take short naps. Napping is a normal pattern that seems to increase with age (Ebersole & Hess, 1998). Hayter (1985) reported that there is an increase in time spent both taking naps and being awake during the night. He also found that these two are independent of each other, and although naps are needed, they generally do not cause wakeful nights.

Often older persons need to be taught to cope with age-related changes in sleep cycles. Medications are often advertised as the solution, and they are frequently used by elderly persons. Medications should be the last resort. Some medications frequently used, such as barbiturate, pentobarbital, and pheonobaribital, should be avoided. These drugs may cause adverse reactions of delirium or restlessness. Overall, medications tend to interfere with sleep by depressing REM sleep. An elderly person may feel tired and unrested from a drug-induced sleep. As a health care provider, one needs to help the elderly person to become an efficient sleeper. The following are some helpful suggestions to induce sleep:

- Avoid stimulants after 4 P.M. (coffee, chocolate, things that contain caffeine).

- Avoid alcohol.

- Eat a light snack before bedtime (bread or fruit an hour or two before bedtime).

- Learn to quiet your thoughts and practice relaxation techniques.

- Take a warm bath.

Elderly persons frequently complain that they did not sleep well. In fact, insomnia is a fairly common complaint. To assess if a person has slept well and long enough, the key question to ask is, "When you woke up this morning, did you feel rested?" This is the key to adequate rest.

RISK FACTORS CONTRIBUTING TO ALTERED SELF-INTEGRATION

The final area that is briefly covered in this chapter is risk factors that affect a person's ability to maintain self-integration. These are factors that tend to tear down the integrated self, the feelings of value, self-worth, and one's place in society. The basis for self-integration is one's personal philosophy and response to the perceptions of others. A number of factors tend to tear down the integrated self: diminished physical beauty, loss of status, and altered sexual identity are just a few.

Appearance

Most people take great satisfaction in their physical appearance and attractiveness to others. They may be disconcerted at the sight of wrinkles. Such physiological change may require readjustment of a person's feelings of self-worth to some other personal characteristics, activities, or relationships. For women, it may be perceived as a loss of beauty, and for a man, it is analogous with loss of physique and physical prowess. This may be the most demanding part of aging especially in a society where youth translates into beauty.

The skin presents the most readily observable signs of aging. These changes are both universal and progressive. It is especially true of exposed skin such as the face and hands. Skin resilience, turgor, and elasticity are influenced by diet, health status, heredity, and exposure. Sun is known to accelerate these changes and cause pigment change. As one ages, the skin dries, sebaceous glands secrete less material for lubrication, and the outer layers of the skin become more fragile. Along with changes in the epithelial layer, the elastic collagen fibers shrink and become more rigid. This loss of elasticity affects blood vessel integrity (Ebersole & Hess, 1998). Loss of subcutaneous fat

---

TABLE 4-5

Factors Contributing to Skin and Connective Tissue Change

Skin elastic collagen fibers shrink and become rigid.

Subcutaneous fat becomes altered.

Skin losses dermal thickness, making the skin appear more transparent and thin.

Melanocytes in epidermis decrease in number and activity, making the skin more sensitive to ultraviolet in the sunlight.

Epidermis turnover decreases, which contributes to slower wound healing.

Sebaceous and sudoriferous (sweat) glands decrease in number, size, and function.

The vascular beds decrease in their ability to respond (and sweating), which predispose an elder to hypothermia and hyperthermia.

---

results in lines, wrinkles, and sagging. Other visible signs of change are hair loss and graying. *Table 4-5* summarizes these physiological changes. It is important to note that the appearance of the skin reflects a client's well-being and may be the first indicator of less than optimum health.

Sexuality

Sexuality encompasses more than the physical sex act and is the way an older person feels about his or her identity. Body image and self-concept may discourage sexual activity, (Eliopoulos, 1995), and persons may be controlled by misconceptions and prejudices as to how aging and sex should be interrelated. It is an integral part of self and reflects the worthiness of affection by others. "Am I attractive and desirable?" It is through these feelings, beliefs, and attitudes that an expression of intimacy occurs. This intimacy is love, warmth, caring, and sharing between people.

In women, menopause begins between the ages of 45 and 50. This beginning denotes the end of menstruation and the child-bearing period. Estrogen production wanes, but androgen production continues, which maintains the libidinous aspects of sexuality. For a man, alterations of sexual functioning occur at a more gradual pace, varying from person to person. The changes that take place in the average aging male often look like impotence. It

appears that all phases of the sexual response can be affected (Ham, 1997). The excessive use of alcohol and other drugs can significantly affect functioning. *Table 4-6* summarizes the physical changes that may affect sexual functioning.

Age-related physical changes experienced by both sexes do not prevent sexual function, and it does not alter the pleasure of sex or inhibit desire. Sexual dysfunction is not an end result of aging, but it occurs more often as a person ages. It is often associated with chronic illnesses and disabilities. Common causes of sexual dysfunction in older adults have been defined by Barash (1991). These are identified in *Table 4-7*. It is through understanding that problems with sexual function can be diagnosed and treated.

It is important to note that medication regimens are common causes of sexual dysfunction. Decreased libido or potency may be caused by diuretics, tranquilizers, sedatives, tricyclic antidepressants, and some hypertensive medications.

Sexuality for the elderly is a way to share and become intimate with others. It is important and requires patience and, sometimes for the elderly person, perseverance. It is an essential component of the integrated whole person.

In this chapter, we have explored a multitude of physiological changes that occur in association

---

TABLE 4-6
Factors Contributing to Sexual Function Change

Women

The vaginal opening narrows, and vaginal tissue loses its elasticity.

With menopause a rapid decline of estrogen and progesterone occurs.

Hormonal changes cause atrophic changes of the uterus, vagina, external genitalia, and breasts.

Vaginal secretions become more alkaline as glycogen content increases and acidity declines.

Vaginal epithelial lining atrophies, causing narrowing and shorting.

A diminishing of breast tissue occurs.

Sexual activity decreases, but the exact relationship to biological changes and sociocultural factors are unknown.

Men

Obtaining and maintaining an erection becomes more difficult.

Prostate increases in size because of hyperplasia.

Testosterone levels decrease.

Erectile and ejaculatory function declines.

Phases of intercourse become slower.

Testes decrease in size.

Sperm decreases.

Viscosity of seminal fluid diminishes.

---

with aging by using an approach to make the changes client focused and to stress the importance of the interrelationship of the body systems to one another. One must always recognize that the whole is more than the sum of its parts and the physiolog-ical changes contribute to a person's uniqueness. Not all body systems are included in this chapter because a number of systems are analyzed in other chapters. However, *Figure 4-2* summarizes a number of these changes. For health providers, it is

---

TABLE 4-7
Common Causes of Sexual Dysfunction in Older Adults

Diabetes mellitus	Colostomy
Decreased hormone production	Fear
Chronic renal failure	Fatigue
Arthritis	Absence of sexual teaching
Myocardial infarction	Anxiety
Congestive heart failure	Pain
Peripheral vascular disorders	Cancer
Lack of partner availability	Altered body image
Liver disease	Alcohol
Cerebrovascular accident	Radiation therapy
Ileostomy	Medications

Source: Barash, R. A. (1991). How aging affects sexual functioning. *California Nursing.* May-June, pp. 25–28.

important that these changes be a basis for assessment and be considered in planning and delivery of care.

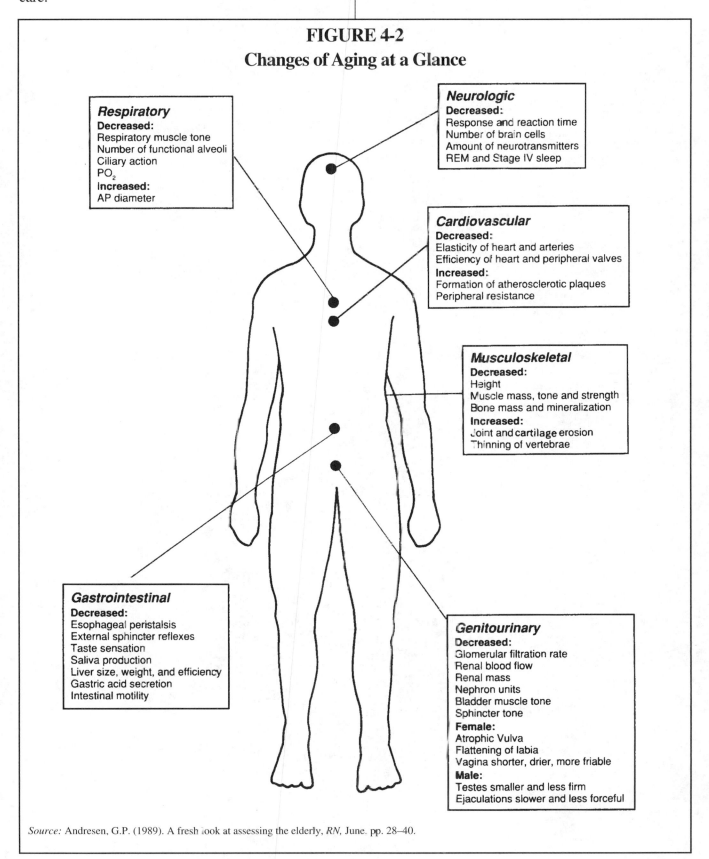

FIGURE 4-2
Changes of Aging at a Glance

Respiratory
Decreased:
Respiratory muscle tone
Number of functional alveoli
Ciliary action
PO_2
Increased:
AP diameter

Neurologic
Decreased:
Response and reaction time
Number of brain cells
Amount of neurotransmitters
REM and Stage IV sleep

Cardiovascular
Decreased:
Elasticity of heart and arteries
Efficiency of heart and peripheral valves
Increased:
Formation of atherosclerotic plaques
Peripheral resistance

Musculoskeletal
Decreased:
Height
Muscle mass, tone and strength
Bone mass and mineralization
Increased:
Joint and cartilage erosion
Thinning of vertebrae

Gastrointestinal
Decreased:
Esophageal peristalsis
External sphincter reflexes
Taste sensation
Saliva production
Liver size, weight, and efficiency
Gastric acid secretion
Intestinal motility

Genitourinary
Decreased:
Glomerular filtration rate
Renal blood flow
Renal mass
Nephron units
Bladder muscle tone
Sphincter tone
Female:
Atrophic Vulva
Flattening of labia
Vagina shorter, drier, more friable
Male:
Testes smaller and less firm
Ejaculations slower and less forceful

Source: Andresen, G.P. (1989). A fresh look at assessing the elderly, *RN*, June. pp. 28–40.

CHAPTER 4
Questions 31–40

31. Which statement best describes the relationship of aging and disease?

    a. It is easy to distinguish changes that occur with normal aging and those that are caused by disease processes.

    b. Aging denotes disease.

    c. Disease automatically occurs with aging.

    d. Some factors that predispose a person to disease also influences the person's response to aging.

32. Overall physiological changes of aging can be traced to

    a. basic cellular changes.

    b. heredity.

    c. body system changes.

    d. alterations in the integrated whole.

33. A risk can best be defined as

    a. a stressful event.

    b. a condition that may compromise a person's health or longevity.

    c. an actual threat to a person's health or well-being.

    d. Alterations in functional ability or activity status.

34. Regularly active is generally defined as

    a. jogging daily.

    b. engaging in strenuous activity at least 30 min/day.

    c. engaging in activities lasting at least 20 min, three times per week.

    d. walking a mile three times a week.

35. Which of the following specific conditions is the major cause of cardiovascular disease?

    a. Arteriolosclerosis

    b. Arteriosclerotic disease

    c. Atherosclerosis

    d. Mönckeberg's sclerosis

36. It is estimated that by age 80 cardiac output has decreased as much as

    a. 5%.

    b. 10%.

    c. 25%.

    d. 50%.

37. By age 90, most lungs have enough alveolar destruction to meet the criteria for a diagnosis of

    a. black lung disease.

    b. cancer.

    c. emphysema.

    d. pneumonia.

38. Which of the following is a major component to analyze in evaluating musculoskeletal function of an elderly person?

    a. Cartilage

    b. Bone structure

    c. Tendons

    d. Posture

39. The functional description that best summarizes the physiological changes of the nervous system is

    a. frustration.

    b. loss.

    c. slowing down.

    d. impairment.

40. Which of the following is true regarding sleep and elderly persons?

    a. It's hard to awaken them once they have fallen asleep.

    b. They have fewer sleep-stage changes.

    c. They need less sleep.

    d. They awaken more often during the night.

CHAPTER 5

DISEASE PROCESSES: COPING AND CAREGIVING STRATEGIES

by

Angela Simon Staab, RN, MN, CGNP

CHAPTER OBJECTIVE

After studying this chapter, the reader will be able to recognize the manifestations of coronary artery disease/myocardial infarction, congestive heart failure, hypertension, cerebrovascular accident (stroke), osteoarthritis, osteoporosis, gout and HIV/AIDS in older adults. The reader will also be able to specify appropriate coping and nursing caregiving interventions for these conditions.

LEARNING OBJECTIVES

After studying this chapter, the reader will be able to:

1. Describe the manifestations of coronary artery disease, congestive heart failure, hypertension, cerebrovascular accident, osteoarthritis, osteoporosis, gout and HIV/AIDS as they differ in older adults.

2. Select nursing interventions for caregiving in older adults with these specific problems.

3. Specify nursing strategies for establishing coping mechanisms of patients and their families in the care of older adults with these problems.

INTRODUCTION

Older adults experience an increased prevalence of chronic illness as their normal abilities and resources begin to decline. Approximately 85% of the aged population have at least one illness, and a larger percentage have multiple chronic conditions (Eliopoulos, 1995). Acute illnesses are less common in older adults and are usually a flare-up of a chronic illness. Today's older adults are a reflection of lifelong health practices, family traditions, and relationships. The hope is that nursing interventions today will modify health practices of the future. Family and friends must be involved to provide motivation to change.

This chapter examines some common health problems of older adults and offers specific nursing strategies and interventions for coping and caregiving. (The student is referred to a medical-surgical textbook for general information on nursing care of adults for each specific health problem.) Pathological conditions may be modified or intensified by age because of a decrease in "functional reserve," decreased efficiency of body systems, and a decreased ability to respond to environmental demands, which result in an inability to adapt to stressors, a compromised homeostasis, and difficulty in returning to a previous level of functioning.

Nurses must attend to some of the psychosocial problems as well as physical problems specific to the elderly that interfere with compliance. Some of these problems include resistance to change or the use of medication, inadequate transportation, solitary lifestyle, sensory impairment, mental confusion or depression, low fixed income, and difficulty opening safety caps on medication bottles and interpreting medication regimens. Stress and anxiety are sometimes the greatest obstacles to change. During periods of physical stress and anxiety, we tend to regress to old habits and patterns of behavior, many of which are dysfunctional. In working with older adults, it is essential to differentiate normal changes requiring assistance with adjustment and adaptation from pathological changes requiring special medical and nursing interventions (Brummel-Smith, 1998; Sloane, 1997).

CARDIOVASCULAR CONDITIONS

Cardiovascular disease is the most common health problem in the older adult population, and the most important risk factor for cardiovascular disease is arteriosclerosis. This is defined as a thickening and rigidity of the cardiac valves and blood vessels throughout the body that occurs with aging. It is a contributing factor in the total number of deaths occurring each year in persons over the age of 65, 40% of whom have cardiovascular disease and 15% of whom die of cerebrovascular disease (stroke). Age-associated alterations in the cardiovascular system are manifested by a progressive decline, particularly in the body's adaptation to stress and increased physical demand. The heart works harder but is less efficient. Cardiovascular disease may be manifested by a decrease in stroke volume and resting cardiac output, with subsequent decrease in blood supply to the organs, along with a decrease in cardiac reserve, decreased heart rate response to stress, and an increase in vascular resistance. Aging of the neuromuscular conducting system of the heart may

cause increased irritability manifested by multiple extrasystole and arrhythmias.

Coronary Artery Disease/Myocardial Infarction

Coronary artery disease (CAD), also known as ischemic heart disease, increases in prevalence, complications, intensity, and mortality as persons become older, and may lead to myocardial ischemia or myocardial infarction (Staab & Lyles, 1990). The same factors that cause stress and strain on the younger heart cause stress in the aged and are considered to represent risk for cardiac ischemia or infarction. These factors include continuation of a diet high in animal fat (elevated serum lipid levels), salt, and calories; excessive weight or obesity; a high pack-a-day smoking history; physical inactivity; internalization of emotions; exposure to high-density air pollutants; and various existing medical conditions such as infection, anemia, pneumonia, cardiac dysrhythmia, poorly controlled hypertension, surgery, fever, diarrhea, hypoglycemia, malnutrition, avitaminosis, circulatory overload, renal disease, and prostatic obstruction. Tachycardia produced by fever, emotion, exercise, or other conditions may cause cardiac decompensation and heart failure in older adults who have underlying CAD.

Myocardial oxygen supply is affected when arteriosclerosis or occlusion causes narrowing of coronary arteries. Atheromatous material in the coronary arteries causes decreased oxygenation to the myocardium and decreased coronary blood flow. Ischemia can result when myocardial oxygen supply through coronary arteries fails to meet oxygen demand and myocardial tissue is forced to change from aerobic metabolism to anaerobic metabolism, which is less effective. Tissue anoxia and necrosis can result from a myocardial infarction (MI).

Signs and Symptoms

Over the lengthy process of coronary artery disease, the elderly frequently experience less pain (or no pain) from myocardial ischemia than younger persons, leading to "silent" coronary artery disease. Older adults generally have better myocardial collateral circulation related to gradual progressive coronary artery narrowing. Because of limited activity, older adults may not experience typical exertional chest pain. This phenomenon may also be the result of reduced pain perception and memory deficits experienced by older adults. Elderly patients with acute MI may present with confusion or anxiety and unexplained behavior due to changes associated with cerebral insufficiency. Older adults are more likely to complain of shortness of breath, dyspnea, nausea or gastrointestinal discomfort, and mental or neurological symptoms such as nightmares, compared with younger adults, who will experience severe to excruciating chest pain and shortness of breath (a more catastrophic feeling). Frequently, older adults may have "silent myocardial infarctions" that go undiagnosed, or some may have signs and symptoms as ischemia progresses. As coronary occlusion or myocardial infarction occurs, chest pressure may become severe. Retrosternal pain radiating to the neck, jaw, arms, or back may be precipitated by exertion, excitement, cold weather, or heavy meals and may be described as "discomfort" rather than acute pain. The occurrence of substernal "indigestion-like" discomfort in an older adult after a large meal should not be discounted, because hypoperfusion of the myocardium with the shunting of blood to the gastrointestinal area during the digestive process might be a factor in the precipitation of myocardial ischemia or infarction.

Assessment

Nursing assessment of severe coronary ischemia or myocardial infarction may reveal tachycardia (sinus bradycardia or heart block may be present); hypotension or hypertension; cool, clammy, and pale skin; possible ECG changes (ST segment depression and arrhythmia); and S3 or S4 gallop. Chest radiographs may be used to screen for cardiac enlargement, valvular abnormalities, and pulmonary congestion. Radionuclide imaging can be used to assess the amount of myocardial ischemia present during rest and activity. Isotope studies are useful in patients who may not tolerate full treadmill testing. Exercise treadmill testing (ETT) is most useful if the person can complete the study; however, even limited studies are useful if the results confirm ischemia. Cardiac catheterization can be used to visualize the coronary arteries to quantify arterial insufficiency and assist in selection of further treatment, such as percutaneous transluminal coronary angioplasty, coronary artery bypass surgery (the goal of any treatment is symptomatic relief and improvement in the quality of life), and optimization of medical management.

Treatment

Treatment strategies are aimed at reducing the workload on the heart and decreasing myocardial oxygen demand. Older adults often have aggravating and contributing diseases such as hypertension, congestive heart failure, arrhythmias, anemia, infections, and thyroid disease that need to be evaluated. The primary treatment for myocardial ischemia with angina in older adults is coronary relaxation and vasodilatation with nitrates, beta-blocking agents, and calcium channel blockers. Anticoagulant therapy may be necessary.

Intervention

Complete bed rest treatment has been modified by having patients sit up beside the bed and gradually increase activity. This is believed not only to prevent many problems from immobility but also to decrease the work of the heart by preventing blood from pooling in the pulmonary vessels. Use of minimal patient energy during transfer and arm support while out of bed are essential. Control of anxiety and stress can be approached by helping patients identify areas of stress and secure assistance in reduction techniques. Encourage rigorous risk factor interventions *(Table 5-2),* and, if there are no significant cardiovascular contraindications to exercise, encourage regular, moderate, physical activities such as walking, dancing, bowling, swimming, yoga, and golfing.

Congestive Heart Failure

Congestive heart failure (CHF) indicates a decompensation in the pumping ability of the heart, and is sometimes called *presbycardia.* It is not an uncommon finding in older adults with arteriosclerosis; the prevalence of this condition increases with age, occurring in 75% of ambulatory patients over 60 years of age (Staab & Lyles, 1990). CHF is usually due to underlying conditions, particularly CAD, MI, mitral stenosis, long-standing or poorly treated hypertension, subacute bacterial endocarditis, bronchitis, pneumonia, and hypothyroidism. Decreased cardiac output and stroke volume compound this condition, as does the tendency toward hypernatremia, which can occur as a result of reduction in total body water. These reductions are seen with normal aging. The term congestive generally relates to the development of edema in the lungs or in the extremities, with the end result of an increased workload on the myocardium. CHF may develop in the older adult when they are confronted with lesser stresses than those producing failure in the younger person.

Signs and Symptoms

Older adults may not have the classic signs and symptoms of shortness of breath or fatigue if they engage in only limited activity; they may assume the edema is from noncardiac reasons, and the chronic, nonproductive cough may be interpreted as a viral infection. The nurse should observe the patient for anorexia, nausea, bilateral ankle edema, progressive dyspnea on exertion, dry hacking cough, interference with routine activities of daily living, oliguria, confusion (may be the result of cerebral edema), chronic fatigue, insomnia, and generalized weakness.

Pulmonary edema is a significant complication of CHF. Respiratory involvement can be determined by the presence of persistent, moist, basilar rales, crepitations, or wheezing. Other significant complications in older adults include the lack of response to treatment (recurrent CHF and dysrhythmia) and consequences of drug treatment, such as hypokalemia and toxic effects of medications.

Assessment

Diagnosis is based on history, physical examination, ECG, chest x-ray, and laboratory examination, including thyroid function tests. The history may have to be carefully elicited by the nurse, as most older adults, until questioned, do not realize they have been gradually slowing down their activities. Progressive weight gain over a short period may be the only sign the older adult associates with the illness. Edema is gravity dependent. In an ambulatory patient, it usually forms in the feet and ankles and the basilar areas of the lung. In a bedridden patient, it is more likely to occur in the sacral area. An S_3 gallop may be present, indicative of left ventricular volume overload and dysfunction.

Treatment

Treatment strategies are aimed at searching for and ameliorating precipitating factors, reducing the workload of the heart, increasing myocardial performance, and decreasing sodium and water retention. Diet should aim to reduce obesity and cholesterol levels and restrict foods high in sodium (about 2g daily). Cardiac workload can further be reduced with an altered lifestyle that includes bed rest interspersed with periods of therapeutic, planned mobilization.

All medications should be adjusted to the lowest level needed to control failure and be evaluated for causing myocardial depression. The patients

TABLE 5-2 *(1 of 3)*
Nursing Interventions for Elders With CAD or MI

ISSUE	INTERVENTIONS

Risk factor reduction	1. Counsel patient and patient's family regarding lifestyle modifications such as:
	  a. Weight control
	  b. Mild salt restriction
	  c. Moderate daily activity
	  d. Cessation of smoking to decrease vascular constriction
	  e. Diet low in cholesterol and fats
	2. Encourage vigorous treatment of concomitant conditions such as diabetes, hypertension, thyroid disease, and renal disease.
	3. Counsel to reduce stress by emphasizing relaxation techniques and the need to externalize emotions.

Use of transdermal patches	1. Teach patient how to:
	  a. Open the container
	  b. Apply the patch
	2. Review prescribed regimen of where to apply patch and time span for removal and replacement.
	3. Be certain patient understands that the old patch must be removed before a new one is applied.
	4. Teach rotation of site and application of mild lanolin lotion should skin irritation occur.

Use of sublingual nitroglycerin	1. Have the patient sit or lie down after taking a tablet to avoid falls from hypertension. 2. Be certain the drug stings when placed under the tongue to ensure activity. 3. Encourage proper storage in a dark container. 4. Advise patients to keep a small bottle of the drug in a pocket or handbag at all times. 5. If more than three tablets are needed in an hour, the patient should call a physician or go to the emergency department. 6. Caution the patient that nitroglycerin tablets disintegrate quickly and must be replaced every 6 months if the bottle has not been opened. They must be replaced every 3 months if the bottle has been opened.

TABLE 5-2 *(2 of 3)*
Nursing Interventions for Elders With CAD or MI

ISSUE	INTERVENTION
Family education	1. Evaluate the patient's home situation to determine if someone in the home can administer CPR if needed. 2. If family members have physical or emotional handicaps, select a close neighbor to assist with caregiving. 3. Teach family members pulse and blood pressure monitoring. 4. Caution older adults to make turns slowly and avoid sudden turns of the head or position changes. Instruct them to rise from bed or to a sitting position slowly. 5. Caution patients with carotid sinus hypersensitivity to avoid falls by not reaching for objects from high shelves, washing windows and walls, and hanging clothes on a line. These may cause dizziness or faintness.

Specific nursing care	1. Avoid inadvertent carotid massage with bathing, pulse taking, and physical examination of the neck and lymph nodes.
	2. Acquire accurate blood pressure readings by measuring pressure in both arms and in at least two positions.
	3. Advise patients to protect feet by:
	   a. Using adequate foot covering in cold weather to prevent frostbite
	   b. Avoiding garters or stockings with tight bands at the top
	   c. Elevating legs on long trips or after extended periods of standing or sitting to prevent venous pooling

Tips to decrease sodium	1. Advise patients to do the following:
	   a. Use fresh or frozen fruits and diet vegetables (Staab and Lyles, 1990).
	   b. Read labels on products for identification of sodium or salt content. Often families or friends do the grocery shopping for their disabled family members. The nurse should involve them in the planning and teaching.
	   c. Acquire lists of foods high in sodium.
	   d. Use low-salt products or seasonings in powder, dried, or flake form, not "salts," which are high in sodium. Place a variety of spices in an attractive basket for the table to encourage use.
	   e. Avoid drinking or cooking with water from a home water softener, as these appliances add sodium to the water.

TABLE 5-2 *(3 of 3)*
Nursing Interventions for Elders With CAD or MI

ISSUE	INTERVENTION
Tips to decrease sodium	f. Refrain from adding salt to food at the table.
	g. Be aware that most canned and dried soups are very high in sodium.
	h. Avoid pickles and olives.
	i. Use condiments like ketchup, soy sauce, and mustard sparingly, if at all.
	j. Avoid cured meats such as packaged luncheon meats, ham, sausage, and hot dogs.
	k. Avoid snack foods.
	l. Limit fast food meals.
	2. Stress care in use of sodium-potassium combination products, because the tendency will be to add extra, thereby increasing salt load.

---

should be aggressively monitored for hypokalemia, especially if they are taking digoxin.

Intervention

Nursing interventions should be aimed at modifications of lifelong health practices, family traditions, and relationship practices of the elders. Family and friends must be involved to provide the motivation to change. Even though the impact may be less than on younger patients, risk factors such as smoking cessation, decreased sodium and cholesterol in diet, and an exercise program fitted to age and abilities are important to control (*Table 5-2*).

Hypertension

Historically, hypertension (HBP) in the elderly is the persistent elevation of the arterial blood pressure to levels greater than or equal to 95mm Hg diastolic and 160mm Hg systolic. However, in 1993 the publication of the Fifth Joint National Commission report redefined hypertension as: diastolic blood pressure readings of at least 90 and systolic readings of greater than 140 for all ages.

Decreased aortic elasticity and increased peripheral resistance contribute to compromised left ventricular function and diminished autonomic baroreceptor response. Isolated systolic hypertension (pressures greater than 160mm Hg) is common in the elderly. Systolic blood pressure values between 140 and 160 are, at the very least, borderline and warrant treatment in persons under age 85 (Menscer, 1998). In older adults, wide, temporary fluctuations of blood pressure can result from anxiety, stress, or activity, and rapid lowering of blood pressure may produce complications. Consequently, treatment of hypertension in the elderly requires more attention to detail.

Signs and Symptoms

Risk factors for HBP are similar to those for other cardiovascular diseases but also include heredity and stress. Hypertension can adversely affect all systems of the body, resulting in heart and kidney failure, blindness, and cerebrovascular accidents. Early pathological changes of the body that can be associated with HBP include dull, occipital headaches that are more severe in the morning

TABLE 5-2 *(1 of 2)*
Nursing Interventions for Elders with CHF

ISSUE	INTERVENTIONS
Administration of diuretics	1. Renal failure and renal changes related to the aging process may cause dosages to vary greatly. 2. Monitor carefully if patient has history of gout. 3. Use early morning dosage schedule to avoid insomnia or falls that occur when a patient gets out of bed at night to go to the bathroom. 4. Stress the need to maintain oral fluid intake. 5. Stress the importance of taking diuretics regularly, as noncompliance may result in recurrent illness. 6. If the patient is taking potassium-depleting diuretics, observe for malaise, muscle weakness, leg cramps, faint heart sound, and "gassy" abdominal distension.
Administration of digoxin	1. Lower maintenance dosages are generally needed for older adults. 2. Teach family and patient to monitor heart rate and rhythm closely. Older adults have decreased cardiac output and stroke volume, and digoxin increases oxygen demand of the heart. 3. Determining serum levels may be useful to detect noncompliance and narrow therapeutic or toxic levels that may occur due to decreased renal function. 4. Teach patients the signs and symptoms of the toxic effects of digoxin. 5. Monitor patients for interaction with other medications (particularly quinidine and verapamil) and for hypokalemia if the patients are also taking diuretics.
Administration of vasodilators	1. Calcium channel blockers may be especially useful for patients with coexisting angina or hypertension. 2. Observe patients more closely for potential hypotension by taking blood pressures when the patients are lying and standing.
Fluid overload	1. Teach the patient's family the signs of bilateral, nontender, pitting, and dependent edema. 2. If fluid restriction is ordered, observe for signs of dehydration such as poor skin turgor, dry mucous membranes, body temperature elevation, and mental status changes.

TABLE 5-2 *(2 of 2)*
Nursing Interventions for Elders with CHF

ISSUE	INTERVENTIONS
Fluid overload	3. Weigh the patient daily. Weight should not vary greatly except if fluid is in imbalance. 4. Teach the patient about commonly used over-the-counter drugs that contain sodium or influence salt and water reabsorption, such as antacids and ibuprofen.
Need for potassium supplementation	1. Encourage compliance in taking potassium if the patient is taking a potassium-depleting diuretic, as tablets are usually large and difficult to swallow and most liquids are impalatable. 2. Advise the patient that eating bananas or drinking orange juice *will not* supplement loss. Use of salt substitutes that contain potassium chloride *will* help replace loss. 3. If a potassium-sparing diuretic such as spironolactone or triamterene is used, observe patient for hyperkalemia.
Need for emotional and physical rest	1. Emotional rest is as important as physical rest for the CHF patient, so comfort and stress reduction measures should be initiated by the patient's family, such as coordinating rest periods and visitors. 2. Advise the patient to plan and space activities with rest periods to avoid fatigue and to conserve energy. 3. Counsel overweight patients about weight reduction to decrease cardiac workload.

upon rising, nosebleeds, light-headedness, and impaired memory or confusion.

Assessment

Diagnostic studies are done to obtain a baseline for treatment and to detect secondary causes of HBP. The best assessment technique for the nurse and the patient's family is to take blood pressure measurements in *both arms* when the patient is supine or sitting (at least two positions). Lower the mercury column *slowly* when measuring blood pressure to detect irregularities in heart rate, and use a larger cuff on a larger arm, otherwise readings may be artificially elevated. In older adults,

pump the blood pressure cuff high enough to detect systolic hypertension.

Treatment

Treatment for HBP in the elderly is aimed at a gradual reduction in blood pressure to 140/90mm Hg or less, to achieve comfort and function, while avoiding overtreatment or hypotensive reactions such as dizziness, syncope, lightheadedness, or mental confusion. Reduction must be *gradual* to permit cerebral autoregulation to reset. This enables blood flow to the brain to be maintained at lower levels of pressure, thereby avoiding hypotensive reactions, which can lead to falls and even death. Patients and their families must be counseled on nonpharmacological approaches, including rest combined with mild activity; stress reduction; weight reduction, if indicated; no smoking; and, most important, dietary salt restriction.

Interventions

Because many times HBP is asymptomatic, the nursing interventions must stress these caregiving techniques to both patients and patient's families in order to ensure compliance with the treatment regimen *(Table 5-3)*.

Cerebrovascular Accident

Cerebrovascular disease is most commonly manifested as a cerebrovascular accident (CVA), more commonly known as stroke. After age 60, stroke frequency increases, with women affected twice as often as men. Over age 75, the prevalence is 95 per 1000 population (Baum and Manton, 1987). Seventy-five percent of strokes occur in patients over age 65, with an annual incidence of 2% (Ferri, 1997). According to Baum and Manton, between 20% and 40% of CVAs result in death. Of those who survive a stroke, 55% are disabled but able to perform activities of daily living with assistance, and 15% are fully dependent on others for care.

Stroke occurs as a result of cerebral ischemia, hemorrhage, or infarction. Eighteen percent of strokes are caused by intracranial hemorrhage, and 82% are caused by cerebral infarction (Ferri, 1997). Stroke is the term used to describe neurological deficits resulting from an interruption of the blood supply to the brain. Cerebral thrombosis (most common) is the formation of a blood clot in a vessel supplying cerebral tissue. The term *hemorrhagic stroke* refers to neurological deficits that occur as a result of bleeding within the cranial cavity. The brain, which requires more than one-fifth of all cardiac output, suffers inadequate oxygenation and tissue death occurs. The severity of neurological deficits depends on the extent of brain damage. The specific signs and symptoms are determined by the precise location of the cerebrovascular involvement and the extent of brain damage.

Signs and Symptoms

A transient ischemic attack (TIA) is referred to as a "little stroke" that results from a temporary lack of blood to the brain. It may be a warning of an impending stroke. Risk factors of CVA include TIAs, arteriosclerosis, HBP, heart disease, obesity, tobacco smoking, and elevated levels of serum lipids. Stroke can also occur as a result of a fat embolism after a long-bone fracture. The TIA may completely resolve in 15 min, may persist for up to 24 hr, may be ignored or go unnoticed by the patient, or may be symptomatic. Older adults may complain briefly of slurred speech, blurred or double vision, dizziness, numbness of the hands and fingers, or mental confusion. Brief periods of speech loss, limb weakness, and unconsciousness are warning signs of CVA. Permanent one-sided (hemiplegia) or two-sided (paraplegia) paralysis, speech loss (aphasia), visual and sensory loss, disturbances in perception of self and environment, emotional problems, and incontinence are the most common outcomes of CVA. The location of a CVA determines its manifestations and consequences (see *Table 5-4* for specific clinical features).

Assessment

Diagnosis of stroke involves a complete history and physical examination and various diagnostic procedures, which might include computed tomography (CT), cerebral angiography, lumbar puncture, skull x-ray, electroencephalography, and positron emission tomography (PET). These tests are selected to determine antecedent conditions, risk factors, prognosis, and need for rehabilitation.

Treatment

Treatment is centered on basic supportive measures and control of the atherosclerotic disease, to prevent recurrence and treatment of concomitant

TABLE 5-3 *(1 of 2)*
Nursing Interventions for Elders with HBP

ISSUE	INTERVENTIONS

Avoid sudden drop in blood pressure	1. Teach patients to do the following:
	   a. Rise slowly from bed and sit on the edge for a few minutes before ambulating.
	   b. Rise slowly from chairs.
	   c. Sit or lie down if light-headedness occurs.
	2. Help patients and their families plan individual modifications to reduce stress and provide restful environment.

Compliance with diet	1. Explain reason for dietary measures. 2. Evaluate motivation to follow prescribed diet, and offer methods for compliance with diet. 3. Pursue patients' sociocultural background and lifelong habits, and explain dietary measures and foods consistent with a low-sodium diet. 4. Discuss uses of food spices and seasonings that can be used freely. 5. Caution patients about drinking water that has been softened or conditioned (generally not sodium-free).

Compliance with medication	1. Educate patients to avoid potential reactions to antihypertensive drugs by:
	   a. Moving slowly when changing positions, turning slowly to allow time for vascular system to adjust to changes.
	   b. Avoiding immobility after exercise, standing motionless, hot baths, and excessive alcohol consumption, as all cause vasodilatation and possible fainting.
	   c. Using caution driving equipment or doing work activities that require hyperextension of the neck.
	2. Be alert to noncompliance suggested by missed appointments, vague recollection of regimen, erratic prescription refills, no weight reduction, or continued smoking.
	3. Keep patients' memory deficits and isolation in mind when designing reminders for a drug regimen, especially if there are multiple drugs or dosage times.

TABLE 5-3 *(2 of 2)*
Nursing Interventions for Elders with HBP

ISSUE	INTERVENTION
Need for long-term therapy for an asymptomatic disease	1. Increase patients' compliance by providing an unhurried exchange of information and establishing a long-term relationship between nurses, patients, and patients' families. 2. Help patients and their caregivers understand that high blood pressure is a chronic condition that can be controlled but not cured by lifelong therapy, whether asymptomatic or requiring adaptation to physiological changes. 3. Teach patients and their caregivers about home blood pressure monitoring and the need to record blood pressure at least weekly, but not daily. Have them note day, time, and the patient's position to show to nurse or physician. 4. Teach patients and their caregivers to monitor for dizziness and fatigue, which might indicate hypotension or the need to review drug regimen. 5. Be certain patients understand that they play the crucial role in maintaining health, and that their families and caregivers play a crucial role in assisting with compliance.

conditions such as HBP, blood disorders, and arrhythmias. Bed rest is used only in the initial stage of the stroke. Rehabilitation begins in the hospital but is generally performed in the home or in a specialized hospital unit or facility. Since there may be motor and sensory losses, the course of rehabilitation generally includes the establishment of a definitive diagnosis, prevention of secondary disability, and development of the patient's function to include maximal use of remaining abilities and compensatory mechanisms. Stroke rehabilitation programs optionally incorporate encouragement of self-help, control of incontinence, prevention of contractures (including muscle training and locomotion therapy), assessment of parallel bar use and supportive devices, gait training, and wheelchair independence.

Nursing assessment of the extensiveness of cerebral damage by monitoring all body systems and mental status is the most important intervention. Other nursing interventions include neurological assessment, social assessment, and active involvement in all phases of the treatment and rehabilitation processes, as well as in-home care and the support and instruction of the patient's family and caregivers in the various procedures that need to be performed in the transition from institutional discharge to home care.

Interventions

Interventions begin early in the care of patients evaluated with extensive cerebral damage. These include monitoring of all body systems; assessment of mobility; management of nutritional, bowel, and bladder status; assessment of communication and cognition; assessment of self-care; and management of sensory and perceptual alterations *(Table 5-5)*. Older adults should *not* be disqualified from rehabilitation programs because of age.

TABLE 5-4 *(1 of 2)*
Clinical Features of Stroke

PROBLEMS	MANIFESTATIONS
Sensory and perceptual disturbance	• Decreased response to pain, temperature, and touch • Disturbance in proprioception, or awareness of body movements or position in space • Agnosia, or impaired ability to recognize common articles • Inability to recognize sounds in the environment
Visual deficits	• Diplopia, or double vision • Homonymous hemianopia (e.g., the left visual field is absent in both the right and left eye) • Decreased acuity of vision • Inability to identify common objects through visual input
Disturbances in perception of self and environment	• Lack of awareness of paralysis • Lack of awareness of a body part or a side of the body, neglect of that side • Apraxia or agnosia • Temporal or spatial disorientation
Bowel and bladder disorders	• Incontinence • Constipation as a complication of paralysis and immobility
Emotional problems	• Emotional instability or lability • Depression, withdrawal, anger • Confusion • Maladaptive behavior such as exposing oneself, using profanity
Communication disorders	• Expressive aphasia • Receptive aphasia • Global aphasia
Cognitive problems	• Short-term or intermediate memory loss • Tendency to be easily distracted, attention deficits • Difficulty in planning components of problems or tasks, difficulty in sequencing information • Little recall of learning

TABLE 5-4 *(2 of 2)*
Clinical Features of Stroke

PROBLEMS	MANIFESTATIONS
Cognitive problems	• Inability to think abstractly, inability to perform mathematical computations • Impaired judgment • Disorientation to time, place, person
Motor deficits	• Hemiparesis or hemiplegia • Dysphagia, or difficulty swallowing • Dysarthria, or difficulty speaking • Apraxia, or inability to carry out skilled movements on command when no paralysis is present (such as the inability to dress oneself), or locomotor apraxia (inability to carry out a task when asked to demonstrate a specific act)

MUSCULOSKELETAL CONDITIONS

Musculoskeletal conditions are commonly seen in older adults. More than 100 different entities can produce joint and muscle signs and symptoms. These conditions are of great importance, for they affect a person's lifestyle as well as general feelings of health and wellness. They are generally associated with pain, stiffness, and disturbances of gait, all of which can alter the functional status of older adults. Emotional factors can exacerbate the disease and contribute to increased morbidity. The gradual bone loss that occurs with aging, beginning in late midlife, causes bones to become weakened, making them more susceptible to fracture. Changes in the cervical and thoracic curves of the spine may impair balance and walking. Aging causes an atrophy of all muscles, with a consequent decline in muscle strength, tone, mass, endurance, agility, and efficiency. A decrease in elasticity of tendons and ligaments results in a generalized stiffening of the joints, particularly the knees, hips, and spine. Even with these changes, most older adults remain mobile and independent unless an underlying disease process develops.

Osteoarthritis

Osteoarthritis is a noninflammatory, progressive, degenerative disorder of the movable, weight-bearing joints. This disease is extremely common among older adults (Hampton, 1991; Studenski & Laird, 1998) and is a universal phenomenon of aging. It affects 50% of persons in their sixties and 85% of those over age 75. It is a low-grade inflammatory condition that can have a dramatic impact on a person's lifestyle, with effects that vary from simple irritating aches to excruciating pain and total immobility (Dalton, 1995). Severe osteoarthritis can be present without pain and tends to develop in joints that have undergone previous injury (Sloane, 1997).

Signs and Symptoms

Osteoarthritis has been associated with various factors, including aging, mechanical trauma to joints, obesity, genetic predisposition, congenital abnormalities, joint infection or inflammation, immobility, normal daily wear and tear, and neuro-

TABLE 5-5 *(1 of 6)*
Nursing Interventions for Elders with Stroke

ISSUE	INTERVENTIONS

Care of patient on anticoagulant therapy	1. Familiarize the patient's family about possible interactions among frequently prescribed anticoagulants, salicylate, cimetidine, sulfonamides, and allopurinol.
	2. Suggest that the patient minimize alcohol intake.
	3. Encourage compliance with drug taking and frequent prothrombin time testing.
	4. Improve compliance by suggesting use of a calendar to make alternate drug dosage differences, prothrombin times, and dosage alterations.
	5. Teach patients to prevent bleeding by:
	   a. Using a soft toothbrush to prevent gum injury.
	   b. Using a soft tissue, not fingers, to clean the nose.
	   c. Using an electric razor for shaving.
	   d. Avoiding situations likely to cause an injury or cut.
	   e. Informing the doctor, dentist, or healthcare worker that they are taking anticoagulants before they undergo surgery, dental work, or treatments (Staab & Lyles, 1990).
	6. Teach the patient's family to report any evidence of bleeding, such as nosebleeds or increased prevalence of bruising.

Need for safe performance of diagnostic procedures to acquire definitive diagnosis of stroke	1. Although older adults have decreased immunological responses compared with younger persons, ascertain hypersensitivity to injected contrast medium before CT or PET scanning is done. 2. After PET or CT scanning with contrast medium, encourage patients to drink extra fluids to assist urinary excretion of isotope or contrast medium. (Older adults have a reduction in total body water and therefore a greater potential for fluid volume deficit.) 3. With PET scan, since renal excretion is slower in older adults, ensure that the patient has not had alcohol, tobacco, or caffeine for at least 20 hr before the procedure is done. 4. Because a blindfold and earplugs will be used during PET scanning, offer psychological support and frequent orientation to the procedure, because of sensory alterations common with aging.
Need to effectively communicate with patients with deficits	1. Approach and treat the patient as an adult; determine type of aphasia if present.

TABLE 5-5 *(2 of 6)*
Nursing Interventions for Elders with Stroke

ISSUE	INTERVENTIONS
Need to effectively communicate with patients with deficits	2. Discuss with patients and their families the nature of the impairment and the treatment available. 3. Control the environment to minimize distractions and maintain quiet and calm. 4. Be aware of nonverbal communications and avoid raising your voice if the patient's hearing is not impaired; maintain eye contact. 5. Use direct contact and other visual aids (pictures, photos) when talking with the patient; face the patient and gain attention. 6. If the patient's reading comprehension is intact, use written materials. 7. Ascertain that vision and hearing are intact to prestroke levels through provision of patient's previously worn eyeglasses and/or hearing aid. 8. Be aware that poorly fitting dentures may inhibit speaking ability. 9. Use simple, direct sentences addressed to the unaffected side to enhance understanding. 10. Teach the patient's family as many communication techniques as possible before hospital discharge. 11. Be calm and unhurried with the patient. Allow adequate time for the patient's responses; some patients may take up to 30 seconds to process information and respond (Bronstein, Pupovich, and Amider, 1991). 12. Encourage the patient's family to engage the patient in conversation; educate the family in methods to cope. 13. Encourage patients to use rhythmic chanting or singing to increase their ability to speak. 14. Communicate with rehabilitation team members to determine progress and promote reinforcement. 15. Refer any psychological problems such as depression, withdrawal, rejection of therapy, or social isolation to appropriate persons.

Home caregiving	1. Assist the patient's family or seek counseling to help them deal with the emotional stress of a long-term or terminal illness. Consider the following:
	  a. Alterations in lifestyle
	  b. Changing family roles
	  c. Financial problems
	  d. Access to systems of home care and healthcare

TABLE 5-5 *(3 of 6)*
Nursing Interventions for Elders with Stroke

ISSUE	INTERVENTIONS
Home caregiving	2. Acquire family, church, and community support for the patient. 3. Counsel patient's on the continued pursuit of previously pleasurable activities that remain in their physical limitations. 4. Encourage attendance at group activities such as physical fitness, educational programs, and church. 5. Teach family members how to obtain emergency assistance in the community.

High risk for pulmonary complications	1. Follow up on any direct complaints of respiratory difficulty, but be aware of physical findings such as cyanosis, nasal flaring, and restlessness.
	2 Auscultate the lungs and report and note for clarity of sounds, any rales or rhonchi.
	3. Note the patient's ability to handle secretions, and determine whether the gag reflex is present.
	4. Focus on prevention of respiratory complications and provision of respiratory support:
	  a. Position the patient upright, but monitor for hypotension, which will contribute to additional ischemia and neurological deficit.
	  b. Encourage early mobilization to minimize the risk of pneumonia and other hazards of immobility.

Effect of stroke on mobility	1. To facilitate care, explain to patients and their caregivers that strokes produce various levels of immobility, from mild weakness to severe paralysis, and can cause ataxia, tremor, spasticity, and flaccidity (Bronstein et al., 1991). 2. Assess muscle strength, deep tendon reflex, and cerebellar function. 3. While the patient is at rest, assess muscle tone (move joints through normal range of motion), and inspect major muscle groups for abnormal movements such as tics, fasciculations, jerking, and tremors. 4. As a part of general nursing and caregiver care, prevent complications of immobility including skin breakdown and loss of functional mobility.

TABLE 5-5 *(4 of 6)*
Nursing Interventions for Elders with Stroke

ISSUE	INTERVENTIONS
Effect of stroke on mobility	5. Begin formal or informal rehabilitation programs, focusing on improvement of the patient's functional ability and promotion of independence. 6. Teach the patient's family how to participate in the recovery process and the reasons behind carrying out the necessary exercises. 7. As a step to rehabilitation, increase the patient's awareness and use of the affected side. Place some of the patient's necessary items on that side, and deliver nursing care and activities from the affected side. 8. Teach patients and their families transferring techniques.
Techniques to assess and prevent complications of immobility (Staab & Lyles, 1990)	1. Change the patient's position frequently to facilitate breathing and prevent skin breakdown. 2. Position the patient on the affected side frequently to begin weight-bearing on that side, to stretch out contracted muscles of the trunk, and to encourage use of both sides of the body. 3. To avoid having the patient's head tilt toward the affected side, bring the patient's shoulders forward and extend the arm on that side, with the palm facing upward. When the patient is positioned on the unaffected side, flex the affected hip and knee. 4. To help prevent contractures on the affected side, place a small pillow or towel under the patient's trunk at the waist. 5. Use pillows and rolls to support all the patient's body parts and joints. 6. Use strict skin hygiene, foam mattresses, special beds, and padding techniques to promote comfort and prevent skin breakdown. 7. Monitor elimination and skin cleanliness. 8. Encourage fluid intake, if not contraindicated. 9. Institute a program of active and passive range of motion, to maintain joint mobility and body alignment and to prevent foot drop and contractures. Encourage the participation of patients and their caregivers. 10. Have the patient strengthen muscle groups by working on sitting balance, standing balance, transfers, and gait training.

TABLE 5-5 *(5 of 6)*
Nursing Interventions for Elders with Stroke

ISSUE	INTERVENTIONS
Techniques to assess and prevent complications of immobility (Staab & Lyles, 1990)	11. Provide for patients safety. Advise them to avoid the use of heating pads, requesting assistance getting out of bed, and use side rails and overhead bars. 12. Involve the patient and the patient s family and caregivers in the patient's care whenever possible to teach them how to manage the problems of immobility created by a stroke.
Feeding and nutritional management	1. Assess the patient's ability to swallow and chew foods and monitor for dysarthria (slurring, slowness of speech, rhythm), which would indicate impaired neuronal control of the oral musculature. 2. If the patient can safely be fed orally, but has swallowing difficulty, feed only thick or pureed foods with thick liquids (add a thickening agent to liquids to increase consistency). 3. Encourage the patient to sip from a cup rather than use a straw. 4. Sit the patient upright for feeding; maintain him or her in the same position for a short time after feeding. 5. Clear the patient's oral cavity after each feeding, food tends to accumulate in a pocket on the affected side. 6. Provide good mouth care before and after feedings.
Management of bowel and bladder problems	1. Assess the patient for adequacy of voiding, need for bladder training, and the development of neurogenic bladder. 2. Offer a bedpan, or place it on bedside commode at regular intervals to establish a schedule. 3. Whether bowel problem is temporary or permanent, institute a constipation and fecal impaction prevention program (increased liquid and fiber, suppositories, and digital stimulation).
Management of psychological and emotional responses to stroke	1. Assess the patient's extent of impairment to orientation, memory, attention span, self-esteem, body image, and role changes. 2. Encourage the patient's family to provide familiar objects (photos, calendars, clocks, newspapers, and information about family activities and current events) to assist with the patient's orientation and decrease social isolation. 3. Provide resocialization through group attendance. 4. Encourage verbalization of fears, concerns and feelings about deficits; accept feelings of fear, rejection, and hostility.

TABLE 5-5 *(6 of 6)*
Nursing Interventions for Elders with Stroke

ISSUE	INTERVENTIONS
Management of psychological and emotional responses to stroke	5. If the patient has severe brain injury causing behavioral changes (weeping, swearing, exposing self, sexual advances), reassure the patients family and caregivers that it is not under the patient's control and will eventually resolve. 6. Support patients and their families in identifying realistic outcome expectations; suggest support group attendance.
Management of sensory and perceptual alterations	1. Assess the patient's awareness of stimuli such as hot, cold, sharp, and dull. 2. Provide stimulation with familiar sounds, smells, tactile surfaces such as rough and smooth, and changes in light intensity and color. 3. Be certain care includes touch and that the patient's family provide touch and affection. 4. Continually orient patient to location of affected body parts.
Plan for long-term rehabilitation	1. Teach performance of activities of daily living to maximize strengths and minimize defects. 2. Help the patient do tasks by breaking them down into simple components. 3. Avoid doing too much for the patient in order to increase independence. 4. Assess the patient's home setting by interviewing caregivers or with home visit; suggest adaptations to provide maximum rehabilitative care. 5. Assess appropriateness of the individual rehabilitation programs to permit the patient to regain maximum functioning and independence. 6. Reinforce strategies presented by the rehabilitation team. 7. Encourage patients to dress in street clothes rather than pajamas or hospital gown to encourage participation in rehabilitation and decrease image of sickness.

pathic and endocrine and metabolic disorders such as diabetes mellitus. The disease process includes destruction of the articular cartilage and changes in ligaments, tendons, and synovial fluid, with pain resulting from synovitis, inflammation, and spasm. Loss of bone density and erosion usually lead to increased calcium production and the formation of osteophytes, or bony spurs, in the joint. The pain resulting from these osteophytes is caused by formation of a mechanical block, synovitis, inflammation in the articular capsule, contracture, and spasm. Osteophyte formation and cartilage deterioration are mechanical deformities that frequently lead to pain and enlarged, stiff, and immobile joints. The most common signs and symptoms include stiffness after a long period of immobility; morning stiffness, which usually subsides in less than 30 min; joint pain that occurs with activity; bony enlargement or deformity, particularly Heberden's nodes, bony enlargement's found on the distal interphalangeal joints (DIP), and Bouchard's nodes, found on the proximal interphalangeal joints (PIP); limitation of movement and crepitus; aching or nagging discomfort, usually experienced with motion, weight-bearing, or activity; and "flare-ups" of the disease that are associated with the use or abuse of the joint or trauma and are often relieved with rest.

Assessment

Assessment is based on signs, symptoms, and radiological changes. Examination may show crepitus during range-of-motion tests, with bony enlargements seen more frequently than soft-tissue swelling. Pain is a mechanical type in the lower extremities and weight-bearing joints, particularly hip pain in the groin radiating to the thigh and knee pain that is generally worse with walking, stooping, or stair climbing. Laboratory assessment generally consists of x-rays of the affected joints. These may show joint-space narrowing secondary to cartilage loss and spur formation.

Treatment

The major goals of treatment include preservation of function, reduction of pain, and minimization of further damage to involved joints. Because of the irreversibility of the condition, treatment is medical, with aspirin and nonsteroidal anti-inflammatory drugs (NSAIDs) as the main pharmacological agents prescribed. In addition, range-of-motion and physical therapy exercises to correct muscle atrophy; cold and heat therapy; weight reduction (if needed); and support with a cane, crutches, or splints may be used along with rest and elimination of trauma to involved joints. If the conservative approach is unsuccessful, surgical intervention may be necessary in the form of joint fusion, prostheses, or total joint replacement. The joint replacements are reserved for severe joint destruction and pain or a disability that has been refractory to conservative treatment; these are usually total hip or knee replacements.

Interventions

Nursing coping and interventions specific to older adults with osteoarthritis *(Table 5-6)* should include ways to protect affected joints, encouragement of mobility as much as possible, and providing a balance between rest and supervised exercise to maintain and improve joint function and to strengthen muscles and ligaments.

Osteoporosis

Osteoporosis is one of the most common metabolic bone disorders of aging (Staab & Lyles, 1990). Osteoporosis has reached epidemic proportions in this country with 25 million people affected by the disease and over 1.5 million related fractures annually (Lyles, 1998). The universal loss of bone that occurs with aging is the result of the uncoupling of the relationship between osteoclastic bone resorption and osteoblastic (new bone) formation. Other compounding factors of aging include decreased physical activity, and changes in phosphorus and vitamin D metabolism that accompany

TABLE 5-6 *(1 of 2)*
Nursing Interventions for Elders with Osteoarthritis

ISSUE	INTERVENTIONS
Potential for falls and fractures	1. Prevents falls by evaluating the patient's strength, joint stability, and gait for muscle atrophy or decline in strength due to aging factors. 2. Teach patients environmental alterations, such as removal of throw rugs, installation of hallway and bathroom grip bars, and use of nonglare lighting. 3. Teach use of assistive load-shifting devices such as canes, crutches, a brace, or walker. 4. Use caution when transferring, moving, or ambulating frail older adults. 5. Protect institutionalized patients by providing close observation, side rails, and frequent orientation and teaching. 6. Include in the therapeutic plan an evaluation of how the disease affects the patient's life and a weight reduction program to attain ideal body weight. 7. Teach the patient that a proper balance between rest and exercise helps maintain and improve joint function and strengthen muscles and ligaments. 8. Acquire and distribute free patient education literature from the Arthritis Foundation.
Aching and pain in affected joints	1. Teach patients that mild exercise is appropriate but not to stress degenerating joints. 2. Develop and teach a low-intensity exercise program that begins with muscle strengthening and simple flexibility exercises, done without weights, that the patient can perform daily or on alternate days. 3. Combine the exercise programs with other options such as water aerobics, stationary biking, walking, and low-impact sports such as golfing and swimming. 4. Explore changes that can be made in the patient's home to conserve his or her energy. 5. Teach lifestyle adjustments, proper body alignment, and good body mechanics to decrease wear and tear on affected joints. 6. Advise rest, heat and/or cold applications, and gentle massage to affected joints.

TABLE 5-6 *(2 of 2)*
Nursing Interventions for Elders with Osteoarthritis

ISSUE	INTERVENTIONS
Aching and pain in affected joints	7. Apply heat to the patient's joints by means of hot packs, paraffin baths, heating pads, blankets, whirlpool, or ultrasound to alleviate muscle spasms, decrease pain and stiffness, and make exercise easier.
Use of aspirin or NSAIDS	1. If aspirin is ordered, advise patients to use it cautiously for pain relief to avoid side effects.
	2. Teach the patient to take drugs with food to decrease gastric irritation.
	3. Observe patients closely for tinnitus and gastrointestinal discomfort or bleeding, and be aware that the potential for toxic effects is high in older adults, because of lower levels of serum proteins to bind the salicylate and decreased renal function, which slows excretion.
	4. Be aware that older adults may not experience tinnitus at toxic levels of drugs or may not be able to recognize tinnitus as different from the noise made by their otosclerosis.
	5. Observe patients for unique toxic reactions such as confusion, memory loss, and an inability to think clearly.

changes in renal function. Some older adults increase dietary protein intake, causing an increase in urinary calcium excretion and a nutritional calcium deficiency. There is ongoing investigation into the relationship between male and female gonadal function, vitamin D metabolism, and calcium balance. Other factors that may be associated with reduced bone mass include ethnicity (whites, Asians), alcohol consumption, and cigarette smoking (Lyles, 1998). Bone loss ultimately leads to structural failure of the skeleton, resulting in fractures and much pain. Osteoporosis is a type of osteopenia that often results in hip fracture, causing death, or disability or costly treatment. The disorder may be preventable, but once established, it is almost impossible to correct (Kirkpatrick et al., 1991).

Signs and Symptoms

Bone mass is affected by nutrition, exercise, race, and sex. Postmenopausal osteoporosis is a decrease in bone mass mostly in trabecular bone that occurs more rapidly in women up to about 70 years of age. Age-related osteoporosis affects both trabecular and cortical bone loss in people greater than 75 years of age. The disease is a silent crippler that does not become apparent until midlife when a fracture occurs, often a vertebral compression fracture or a Colles' fracture of the wrist. Fractures occur during normal activities such as lifting, bending, stepping off a curb, or coughing or with minimal trauma such as an aggressive hug or bumping a bedside table.

The risk profile of factors that predispose a woman to the development of osteoporosis includes alterations in nutrition, exercise or fitness, menopause, ancestry, and some disease processes *(Table 5-7)*. Mechanisms involved include calcium loss, calcium deficiency from insufficient intake, lactose deficiency or impaired absorption, deficiencies adrenals sexual hormones or parathyroid hormones, and decreased physical activity.

Many dietary factors are linked to osteoporosis. Lifelong inadequate calcium intake is a major contributor, with milk being critical to the formation of adequate bone density. Ninety-nine percent of body calcium is in the bones. The average daily intake of elemental calcium in the United States is 450–550mg, although the Registered Dietary Association (RDA) recommends 1,000mg (Windhem, 1983). Recent research confirmed that a calcium supplement of 1,000mg daily had a positive effect on bone density in postmenopausal women (Reid et al., 1993). Ettinger's study (1987) concluded that average menopausal women need 1,500mg of elemental calcium to maintain calcium balance. Separate research by Baran, Sorensen, and Grimes (1990) and Reid et al. (1993) supports that normal premenopausal women who received at least 1,500mg of calcium per day did not lose bone. Even high calcium levels are not sufficient treatment. Vitamin D is essential for calcium absorption and metabolism (Heaney, 1993; Wood, 1992).

Assessment

Diagnosis is usually made clinically; as there are no absolute diagnostic studies, it may not be established until the disease is radiologically evident. Detection of osteoporosis is frequently made only after a fracture has occurred, although loss of height and back pain may signal the onset of this condition long before then. The disease is far advanced when loss of bone tissue becomes apparent on plain radiographs, since by then about one third of bone mineral loss has occurred. More sophisticated methods of measuring the degree of

bone loss include single and dual photo absorptiometry, quantitative CT, and ultrasound of the patella. Patients relate a history of pain that may include weakness in the arms and legs, stiffness in the hips and shoulders, and unsteadiness in walking. The pain is more severe during activities including sitting or standing and is relieved with rest; it may subside for a month or two or may be persistent. Pain and the fear of fracture may lead to reduced activities, affecting the patient's personal and social functioning. Recurrent fractures and thoracic kyphosis or dowager's hump will lead to a progressive loss of body height, which is the late hallmark of osteoporosis.

Treatment

Treatment consists of regulating calcium intake, vitamin D, estrogen, and exercise, with the goal of retarding the progression of the disease and preventing complications. In addition to estrogen, two drugs are approved by the FDA (Food and Drug Administration) for treatment of osteoporosis: calcitonin and alendronate. These drugs act by decreasing bone resorption, and their use can assist in maintaining bone mass or decrease the rate of bone loss (Lyles, 1998). This disease is one in which comprehensive nursing assessment and caregiving interventions can be the trademark for treatment and prevention *(Table 5-8)*. Older adults who stay indoors, have a sedentary lifestyle, do not eat dairy products, or drink well water are at high risk for osteoporosis. Treatment assessment should include data on the type of water consumed and the hormonal replacement. Studies have found that persons who drink water high in fluoride and who have moderate physical fitness show enhanced bone density. Both exercise and fluoride seem to enhance bone density. Do not recommend calcium supplements simultaneously with fluoride because the two elements form an insoluble complex that is not absorbed. In female patients, estrogen replacement therapy after menopause can reduce bone

TABLE 5-7 *(1 of 2)*
Risk Factors for Osteoporosis

RISK FACTOR	RATIONALE
Female sex	Men have greater skeletal mass, and women lose bone earlier and at an accelerated rate after menopause.
Aging (over 65 in men)	Midlife changes continue with age. Older adults have a reduced ability to absorb calcium.
Leanness/thin habitus	Small women have low original bone mass. Other physical characteristics include fair complexion, blond hair, and freckles (Lindsay, 1989).
Caucasian and Northern or European extraction	Black people have greater initial skeletal mass.
Inactive lifestyle	Bone formation is stimulated by stress, such as weight bearing on long bones. Bone resorption increases with limited activity.
Family history of the disorder	A genetic predisposition to osteoporosis exists.
Calcium deficiency	Calcium stored in bone is reabsorbed in deficiency states; increased calcium loss in urine; inadequate calcium intake, malabsorption; lactose intolerance.
High stress	The body's response to stress may be to decrease calcium absorption and increase calcium urinary excretion.
Excessive caffeine intake	More than 4 to 6 cups of coffee or soda per day interfere with calcium absorption and increase urinary calcium excretion.
Changes related to menopause	Decreasing or low levels of sex hormone accelerate bone loss.
Smoking	Occurrence of osteoporosis is great in women who smoke.
Excessive fiber intake	Very high levels of fiber increase the rate at which food passes through the intestines, causing a decrease in intestinal calcium absorption.

TABLE 5-7 *(2 of 2)*
Risk Factors for Osteoporosis

RISK FACTOR	RATIONALE
Excessive protein intake	Excess dietary protein may increase urinary loss of calcium.
Long-term steroid use	All glucocorticoids increase calcium excretion and decrease bone density. Other drugs included are heparin, thyroxine, and alcohol (Kirkpatrick et al., 1991).
Hyperthyroidism	Excess of thyrocalcitonin has the effect of lowering plasma calcium and phosphate, in a manner that opposes that of parathormone.
Hypoparathyroidism	Excess destruction of hypoparathyroid glands leads to reduction of parathormone and a resultant calcium loss.
Cushings's syndrome	This disease causes an excess of catabolic hormones.
Changes related to gastrectomy	Malabsorption after gastrectomy can lead to inadequate calcium levels.

resorption and slow or halt menopausal bone loss (Ettinger, 1987; Riggs & Melton, 1992).

Interventions

Nursing caregiving interventions should attempt to secure a comprehensive assessment uncovering the specific factors that place individuals at risk for the silent changes of osteoporosis *(Table 5-7)*. They should also teach the patient and the patient's family about lifestyle behaviors, menopausal factors, medical and nutritional histories, densitometry analysis, and self-protective behaviors *(Table 5-8)*. Yearly physical examinations must be encouraged, as well as a safe living environment that minimizes the risk of falls. Nurses must seek out older adult women early in menopause and counsel the women to take steps to protect the women's health. Waiting until the first fracture occurs to seek medical help may be too late.

Gout

Gout is a crystal-induced arthritis that is the most dramatic and painful form of nonseptic arthritis. Gout is the most common inflammatory disease in men over age 40 and may occur in postmenopausal women, especially in the small joints in hands previously affected by degenerative arthritis (Yeomans, 1991). Gout is a disease of purine metabolism characterized by hyperuricemia (a serum uric acid level greater than 7.0mg/dl). In recurrent attacks of acute arthritis, the hyperuricemia is due either to a metabolic overproduction of uric acid or to a renal undersecretion. Gout is common in patients with a family history of the disease, obesity, hypertension, or alcoholism.

Signs and Symptoms

Classical signs and symptoms include extremely severe constant pain with redness, swelling, and warmth over the gouty joint. Inflammation can occur in almost any single or combination of synovial joints, but it most often

TABLE 5-8 *(1 of 2)*
Nursing Interventions for Elders with Osteoporosis

ISSUE	INTERVENTIONS

Need for calcium supplementation	1. Encourage the patient to maintain a diet with an adequate intake of elemental calcium by eating or using the following:
	  a. Tablets of 1500mg/day of calcium carbonate that can be acquired at food, drug, and health food stores
	  b. 200mg of calcium in one serving of broccoli, green leafy vegetables, kidney beans, sardines, or almonds
	  c. 100mg of calcium in one serving of kale or mustard or turnip greens or two eggs
	  d. About 400mg of calcium in 8 oz. of plain yogurt.
	  e. About 150mg of calcium in 1 oz. low-fat cottage cheese or mozzarella.
	  f. 200mg of calcium in 1 cup of soft-serve ice cream.
	2. Remind patients that milk is a major source of calcium and vitamin D.
	  a. One 8 oz. glass of milk contains 300 mg of calcium.
	  b. Advise patients and their families to avoid whole milk. Skim, 1/2%, and 1% have increased calcium and the same vitamins and minerals as whole milk but fewer calories and less butterfat.
	  c. Persons with a lactose intolerance may need to avoid milk and supplement calcium and vitamin D in another manner.
	3. Advise patients that calcium can be acquired by taking TUMS antacid (6 tablets gives 1200mg of calcium).

Need for vitamin D	1. Advise patients that supplementation of approximately 400 units of vitamin D orally per day is necessary. 2. Teach patients that the daily dosage of vitamin D can be acquired along with other necessary vitamins and minerals in one daily multivitamin. 3. Since the ultraviolet rays of the sun produce vitamin D, the adult requirement for the vitamin can be achieved with 15–30 min/day exposure sure to sunlight. Encourage older adults to go outdoors, even in a wheelchair, or to spend time in a sun room.
Need for exercise	1. Encourage older adults to maintain a daily or alternate daily schedule of mild weight-bearing exercises such as walking, stationary biking, swimming, water aerobics, golf, low-impact aerobics, or exercise on machines.

TABLE 5-8 *(2 of 2)*
Nursing Interventions for Elders with Osteoporosis

ISSUE	INTERVENTIONS
Need for exercise	2. Teach patients and their families that physical exercise enhances bone formation.
	3. Teach patients lifestyle adjustment, proper body alignment, and good body mechanics to decrease wear and tear on the affected joints.
	4. Protect patients from sudden movements or falls. With bone loss and joint instability, falls can be major accidents.

---

involves the feet, ankles, and heels. Classically, the great toe is involved; this is called *podagra.* Onset of an attack is over a few hours, peaking in intensity in 24–36 hours and subsiding spontaneously in 3–10 days. A low-grade fever may also be present. Gouty attacks usually recur at variable intervals, especially if provoked by trauma, medication noncompliance, severe dietary indiscretion, or alcohol ingestion.

Chronic gout occurs after the patient has experienced sustained inflammation, joint damage, secondary osteoarthritis, and the development of tissue deposits of monosodium urate (tophi). The patient is almost never pain-free (Chenitz, Stone, & Salisbury, 1991). (Tophi are nodules that contain deposits of monosodium urate crystals; they appear most commonly on the helix of the ear, the olecranon bursa, the feet, and the eyelids. Their rate of formation is directly related to the level and duration of the periods of hyperuricemia.) Gout in older adults is frequently related to hyperuricemia secondary to the use of diuretics (thiazides, furosemide), which partially block the excretion of urates by the kidneys.

Assessment

Diagnosis is based on the results of synovial fluid assay for urate crystals and increased white blood cells. X-ray films are not diagnostic except in untreated gout, in which tophaceous deposits with bony erosion of the joints may be evident. In the early, acute stage, x-rays may show soft-tissue swelling. Gout is often confused with other forms of arthritis and cellulitis.

Treatment

The goals of treatment for gout include termination of the acute attacks as quickly as possible; prevention of recurrent attacks; prevention of complications such as kidney stones; and reversal of hypertension, obesity, and alcoholism, which may contribute to the disease. Treatment for the acute attack is administration of colchicine, nonsteroidal anti-inflammatory agents (particularly indomethacin), or intraarticular steroids. Nonsteroidal anti-inflammatory drugs are preferred for treatment in the elderly. These drugs have fewer gastrointestinal toxic effects, but they may cause renal impairment if used over a long period of time. Intraarticular or systemic steroids may be used for patients unable to take colchicine or NSAIDs. In chronic gout, the goal of therapy may be to lower the serum uric acid levels by increasing renal excretion of urate or by decreasing uric acid synthesis. The most commonly used uricosuric drugs are probenecid and sulfinpyrazone. Allopurinol may be given to regulate the production of uric acid. The nurse must counsel the patient to follow medication dosage correctly, because if the drugs

TABLE 5-9 *(1 of 2)*
Nursing Interventions for Coping with Gout

ISSUE	INTERVENTIONS
Need for monitoring medication compliance	1. Advise patients that use of colchicine is associated with serious side effects, particularly nausea and diarrhea, which can be problems for older adults. 2. Advise patients to take indomethacin with food to prevent gastric irritation. 3. Prevent systemic toxic effects of drugs by lowering the dose given to elderly patients and avoiding use of drugs in patients known to have renal and/or hepatic insufficiency. 4. Advise patients that the most common side effects of uricosuric drugs include gastrointestinal intolerance, rash, and fever. 5. Teach patients that the drugs used to treat gout have serious adverse interactions with other drugs, both synergistic and toxic effects, so the patients should check with the nurse or pharmacist before taking any other drugs. 6. Be certain the patient does not take thiazide diuretics that may trigger a gout attack

Patient education	1. Provide information about medication dosage side effects and the toxic effects of drugs.
	2. Advise dietary modification only if diet is extremely high in dietary purine, more than 150mg/day.
	  a. Recommend that patients limit food rich in proteins to two or three servings per week.
	  b. Advise patients to avoid foods containing large amounts of purine, such as anchovies, herring, liver, sardines, kidney, and wine sauces.
	  c. Emphasize that a purine-free diet is not necessary.
	3. Encourage patients to drink 2 quarts of fluid a day to promote good renal function.
	4. Advise patients to reduce or avoid activity, particularly sustained activity, during an attack.
	5. Encourage patients to eliminate alcohol intake or limit it to one drink per day.
	6. Instruct patients to report attacks immediately, so that treatment will not be delayed.

TABLE 5-9 *(1 of 2)*
Nursing Interventions for Coping with Gout

ISSUE	INTERVENTIONS
Patient education	7. Be sure patients are aware that some physicians prescribe that anti-inflammatory agents be kept on hand to begin therapy at the first sign of an acute attack and abort serious recurrences. 8. Provide patients with educational materials on medication, diet, and complications. 9. Teach patients to prevent attacks by avoiding dehydration, fasting, binge drinking, low-dose aspirin, and thiazide diuretics. 10. Inform family members of the toxic effects of drugs. Instruct them to stop medication and seek medical consultation if they note any changes in mental status or behavior of the patient.

are started during an acute attack, they can magnify the intensity of the gout.

Nursing interventions should center on patients education as the key to the treatment of gout. Patients should be informed of the chronic nature of the disease and the importance of adhering to the prescribed therapy to prevent serious complications. The nurse should monitor the patient for complications such as renal failure and toxic drug effects and teach self-care measures, for gout can be controlled by proper care.

HIV/AIDS: The Great Imitator

About 60,000 Americans over age 50 have AIDS (Acquired Immune Deficiency Syndrome), and about 10% of all new AIDS cases occur in this age group according to the Centers for Disease Control (Johnson, Haight & Benedict, 1998). These figures have remained the same for years and, yet, older persons and their health care providers do not recognize the threat.

Signs and Symptoms

AIDS in the elderly has been called the "great imitator" because it can appear as a dementia such as Alzheimer's disease or some other chronic ill-

ness. Careful assessment is critical. HIV/AIDS in the elderly is often not recognized or diagnosed until in a later stage of the disease than it is in a younger person. The reasons for this are more social than physiological or biological. Sexual stereotypes of older adults are that they are sexually inactive. These same stereotypes prevent older gay men from seeking treatment when they may have spent their whole lives hiding their sexual orientation. Defining HIV/AIDS as a condition of certain social groups has led to a stigmatization of any one associated with the disease. This stigmatization has been particularly harmful to older adults.

Assessment

Nurses involved with gerontological clients need to be aware of the factors that may keep them from recognizing AIDS (Mueller, 1997). HIV/AIDS dementia should be considered for any cognitively impaired adult when seen by a primary care provider. One of the major differences, clinically, between Alzheimer's dementia and HIV/AIDS dementia is the rapid onset of the dementia with HIV/AIDS as opposed to the slow onset of Alzheimer's dementia (Whipple & Scura, 1996). It may cause extrapyramidal symptoms resembling parkinsonism without the resting tremors. Confusion and difficulty concentrating may be intermittent. In HIV/AIDS dementia the aphasia is usually not present. The difference in clinical signs between HIV/AIDS dementia and Alzheimer's dementia is based on the variation in the pathology. HIV/AIDS typically involves the subcortical structures while Alzheimer's affects the cerebral cortex. Of course, other medical conditions and even the use of some medications can mimic or mask the symptoms. Comprehensive laboratory tests to rule out other causes of dementia should be completed as well as a history to determine the possibility of exposure to HIV.

Treatment

Once a positive diagnosis for HIV has been established using the ELISA (enzyme-linked immunosorbent assay) and subsequent Western Blot testing, a trial of medication such as zidovudine is attempted. Since elderly individuals are generally more prone to adverse effects of drugs, close monitoring is essential. Granulocytopenia or anemia are two potential toxic reactions (Whipple & Scura, 1996). Other drugs may be used in combination to manage or prevent opportunistic infections. However, polypharmacy in the older person produces major adverse effects due to drug interactions. Underlying pre-existing conditions, such as kidney and heart conditions, potentiate these effects. Safety and quality of life are two of the overall considerations when closely observing the elderly individual with HIV/AIDS. Nursing interventions have the goals of preventing further infections and maintaining the individual's quality of life. Diarrhea and other gastrointestinal problems may result from HIV-related conditions or from adverse drug effects or interactions. Symptom-management is paramount to the individual. Good nutrition practices emphasize a high-protein, high-carbohydrate diet with rest and exercise to promote physical and emotional fitness and wellness. Offering support through either a support group for

HIV older adults or by enlisting family support is important. Most elderly persons with HIV/AIDS feel isolated and need nursing support and assistance to access other support systems. As nurses we have the chance to recognize the "great imitator," HIV/AIDS dementia.

SUMMARY

This chapter discusses several common healthcare problems in older adults, including cardiovascular diseases and musculoskeletal disorders as well as HIV/AIDS. How patients and families perceive the situation and mobilize their resources may affect how they cope with the stress of an illness. Coping is the way in which humans react and respond to the environment. It is a process involving cognitive, emotional, and behavioral components, and it includes the efforts a person makes to master conditions of harm or threat.

One of the goals of the nurse is to facilitate the patient's coping and help the patient's family understand changes they may see in the patient and to provide patients every possible chance to understand and live with the illness. Nurses have a major responsibility for careful assessment and evaluation of findings so that appropriate care, support, and teaching can be initiated. They must help elderly patients adapt to and cope with age-related changes and provide direction for the management of pathological conditions.

Problems that chronically ill persons face include preventing and managing medical crises, controlling signs and symptoms, managing health regimens, dealing with social isolation, and changing available resources. The goal of nursing intervention is to facilitate coping by maximizing patients' and families' resources to enable them to maximize the situation. To accomplish this goal, the nurse must accurately assess what the patient and the patient's family need and then implement the appropriate interventions. Nursing interventions generally include developing a professional relationship with the patient's significant others, engaging them and the patient in the patient's care, addressing their concerns, and identifying sources of hope. The information presented in this chapter relates implications for care of older adults and stresses consideration of changes that occur because of the normal aging process.

EXAM QUESTIONS

CHAPTER 5
Questions 41–50

41. Which of the following statements is true concerning transient ischemic attacks (TIAs)?

    a. TIAs are caused by rapid lowering of serum lipids.

    b. TIAs always result in permanent brain damage.

    c. TIAs are high risk factors for CVA.

    d. TIAs are irreversible.

42. To establish communication with Mrs. Smith, 78, who is recovering from a right-sided CVA, the nurse should do which of the following?

    a. Limit verbal communication.

    b. Use only visual aids.

    c. Speak in a very loud voice.

    d. Speak in simple direct sentences to Mrs. Smith's unaffected side.

43. Mrs. Green, 81, who has osteoarthritis in both knees, is taught by the nurse to do which of the following?

    a. Swim or ride a stationary bike for exercise.

    b. Walk vigorously for at least 1 mile per day.

    c. When discharged, begin an exercise program that uses weights.

    d. Incorporate isotonic exercises into her lifestyle.

44. The preferred treatment for osteoporosis includes:

    a. Skeletal traction for 3–4 weeks.

    b. Calcium, vitamin D, and estrogen replacement.

    c. Bed rest for a week at a time before ambulating again.

    d. Calcium, vitamin A, and vitamin E supplementation.

45. Patients with CHF who are taking digitalis are closely monitored for which of the following conditions?

    a. Hypermagnesemia

    b. Hyperuricemia

    c. Hyponatremia

    d. Hypokalemia

46. Which of the following is correct about elderly patients with hypertension?

    a. They are always placed on drug therapy.

    b. They are allowed to follow a normal diet with mild salt restriction.

    c. They might receive tranquilizers.

    d. They are placed on a severe weight reduction diet.

47. Two toxic reactions to HIV/AIDS drugs in the elderly are

    a. weight loss and hair loss.

    b. dementia and decreased urine output.

    c. granulocytopenia and anemia.

    d. bleeding and hypokalemia.

48. The dementia that may occur with HIV/AIDS is likely to

    a. affect the individual in the early phases of the disease.

    b. have a fairly rapid onset.

    c. come on slowly over months.

    d. affect the cerebral cortex.

49. Mr. Smith's ECG shows evidence of an acute myocardial infarction. When telling him what to expect over the next few days, the nurse will base explanations on the knowledge that

    a. rest is important to decrease the heart's workload.

    b. Mr. Smith will soon feel much better.

    c. Mr. Smith will have frequent x-ray studies.

    d. Mr. Smith will be unable to see his family.

50. Mrs. Long has CHF. To most accurately determine whether she is retaining or losing fluid, the nurse should do which of the following?

    a. Check degree of ankle edema.

    b. Listen for rales in the lungs.

    c. Record Mrs. Long's urinary output.

    d. Check Mrs. Long's weight daily.

CHAPTER 6

GENERAL PRINCIPLES OF DRUG THERAPY IN THE ELDERLY

by

Marcie Lepkowsky, PharmD

CHAPTER OBJECTIVE

After studying this chapter, the reader will be able to discuss physiological changes that affect drug disposition and how different drugs are used for geriatric patients.

LEARNING OBJECTIVES

After studying this chapter, the reader will be able to:

1. Specify the physiological changes that occur with aging and affect the disposition of drugs.

2. State common reasons why patients are non-compliant with prescribed medication use.

3. Discuss the reasons why elderly patients are at risk for adverse drug reactions.

4. Select the appropriate indications for antipsychotic drug use as described by the Omnibus Budget Reconciliation Act of 1987.

INTRODUCTION

The challenge of healthcare professionals in regard to care of geriatric patients is to balance the professionals' own concept of quality of life with what is important to the elderly. In the area of geriatric pharmacology, this is particularly difficult, because the clinician has the ever-present desire to cure and treat with the useful yet potentially dangerous drugs. The elderly, however, must incorporate the use of these medications into a lifestyle that maximizes independence and balances other aspects of life, including financial security, symptomatic cognitive and psychological well-being.

Recent reviews have shown that whereas those over 65 years of age constitute only 11–12% of the total population in the United States, more than 30% of all drugs are prescribed for this age group. This population is expected to increase to more than 20% of the total U.S. population and consume 40% of all drugs by the year 2030. This disproportionate use of medications has not, unfortunately, been accompanied by adequately prioritized mandatory education at the undergraduate, graduate, and postgraduate levels of training in medical, nursing, pharmacy, or related healthcare fields. Only recently, the awareness of the physiological changes that occur with the natural aging process has influenced the approach to clinical drug trials and utilization reviews. The Food and Drug Administration is becoming more aware that new drug trials at Phase II and III should include a reasonable sample of patients over the age of 65, especially when the drugs are intended for use in disease states seen primarily in this age group. This should include performing clinical trials in the elderly who have the disease that the drug is intended to treat as well as in the healthy elderly (Jaffe, 1987). Results should be analyzed for the possible effects of age on end-organ response and the need for dose adjustments in this age group. More information concerning drug response is needed in all patients over 65 years old, but with the recognition of the increasing heterogeneity of populations with age, the frail elderly and very old patients over 85 years of age, in particular, must be included in investigational drug trials.

PROBLEMS THAT COMPLICATE DRUG THERAPY IN THE ELDERLY

Care of geriatric patients is often complicated by the atypical presentation of disease that may occur in elderly persons. Signs and symptoms of disease may be insidious in onset, nonspecific, or masked by the patient's or the clinician's assumption that they are part of the normal aging process. Often diagnosis is difficult because disease in one organ system can cause signs and symptoms in another, especially the central nervous system (CNS). In other situations, the patient may be asymptomatic because of impairment of homeostatic control mechanisms.

Although there is a high prevalence of chronic diseases in older patients, especially with continued advances in modern medicine, there is some controversy as to the extent to which diseases are inevitable with aging. Several diseases show an increased prevalence with increasing age but are not part of the normal aging process. An elderly person, therefore, may be at increased risk for the development one of these diseases but is not destined to have the disease. These include malignant neoplasms, hypertension, and diabetes. Other diseases, not aging processes themselves and which may not show an increased prevalence with age, may result in greater morbidity as a person ages. Respiratory infections and the sequelae of falls or accidents, for example, may be more likely to cause death if they occur in the elderly. A third group of diseases are those previously thought part of the aging process and inevitable in that they develop if a person lives long enough. More recently, however, the inevitability of diseases such as atherosclerosis, degenerative joint disease, and osteoporosis, has been the subject of much research. Perhaps factors such as diet and lifestyle contribute to disease onset and progression. Elderly patients may have multiple diseases including cardiovascular disease, renal, malignant tumors, arthritis, diabetes, osteoporosis, glaucoma, and dementia. The onslaught of disease often results in a patient's requiring multiple medications. Polypharmacy, including prescription as well as over-the-counter medications, contributes to the potential for noncompliance and adverse drug reactions in these patients.

AGE-RELATED PHYSIOLOGICAL CHANGES: PHARMACOKINETICS

Several basic principles highlight the physiological changes with aging that affect how a drug is utilized in the body and the response to the drug.

Absorption

The path of a drug may be traced from absorption to elimination. Whereas a drug may enter the circulation by many routes *(Table 6-1)*, the oral route of absorption is best studied in the elderly.

Drug absorption may be influenced (delayed or hastened) by many factors, including coadministration of food or other drugs, gastric pH, lipid or water solubility of the drug itself, stomach emptying time, enteric coating, and vomiting for oral products; local conditions such as edema, abrasions, and presence of hair for topical administration; and retention time for enemas. The total amount of orally administered drug that enters the system, or the bioavailability of the medication, is

TABLE 6-1
Routes of Absorption

- Inhalation
- Otic
- Intramuscular
- Rectal
- Intranasal
- Subcutaneous
- Intravenous
- Sublingual
- (peripheral or central)
- Topical
- Ophthalmic
- Vaginal
- Oral

usually unaltered with aging. This is true for most drugs that passively diffuse into the circulation. The rate of absorption, therefore, may be affected by age *(Table 6-2)*, but the extent of absorption is usually not changed for drugs taken by mouth. Some drugs, however, such as propranolol (Inderal), are extensively metabolized by the liver before they reach the systemic circulation. This process of absorption from the gastrointestinal tract directly into the portal system and subsequent metabolism, called the first-pass effect, appears to be decreased in the elderly, making more of the drug available for systemic circulation.

Distribution

Once a drug has been absorbed into the systemic circulation, it is distributed throughout body tissues. This distribution is highly dependent on how lipid soluble or water soluble a drug is, as well as the extent to which the drug is bound to plasma proteins. Changes in body composition from aging are accompanied by significant changes in drug distribution. Unfortunately, an increase in fat-to-muscle ratio occurs gradually with age so that fat content accounts for approximately 15% of the younger person's body, and increases to more than 30% in the elderly. In addition to this increase in total body fat, a decrease occurs in total body water as well as a decline in lean body mass. These changes are reflected in corresponding variations in drug distribution. As expected, water-soluble drugs, having less water to distribute into, become highly

concentrated in an elderly patient who receives the same dose per kilogram as a younger patient. High plasma concentrations are reflected in higher drug blood levels when monitored, but more importantly, reflected in increased prevalence of drug side effects and toxic reactions. Lipophilic drugs distribute into the fatty tissues of the body and may accumulate over time. Even after a medication is discontinued, patients may experience prolonged evidence of the presence of the drug or toxic effects as the stores are slowly eliminated. This is seen dramatically with the drug diazepam (Valium), which has a half-life of approximately 20 hours (it takes 20 hours for the plasma drug concentration to decrease by one-half) in a patient who is 20 years old but 48–96 hours in a patient who is elderly, with the half-life extending with age (Ferri & Fretwell, 1997).

Many drugs, such as phenytoin (Dilantin), are highly bound to plasma proteins. The distribution of these drugs is influenced by the concentration of plasma proteins, the affinity of the proteins for the drug, and the presence of other substances that compete for binding. It does appear that the concentration of albumin, one of the primary binding proteins, decreases with age. Drugs that are highly bound to albumin show a corresponding increase in free fractionation of the drug. This increase in the unbound, active portion of the drug may result in a greater prevalence of adverse side effects or toxic effects if drug doses are not lowered accordingly.

Metabolism

The primary organ for metabolic biotransformation is the liver. Through enzymatic activity, the liver attempts to convert foreign substances such as drugs and alcohol to products that are more easily eliminated. Metabolism may be influenced by several factors, including smoking, other drugs, altered blood flow to the liver, disease states such as congestive heart failure, and age. Although liver function test results do not appear to change as patients

TABLE 6-2
Changes That May Alter Oral Drug Absorption

CHANGE	CONSEQUENCE
Increase in pH secondary to decrease in acid production	Altered solubility of certain drugs, altered absorption of drugs requiring an acid or basic environment for absorption
Decrease in intestinal perfusion of 40–50%	Delay or reduction in absorption
Decrease in gastric emptying (increase in gastric emptying absorption or increased time)	Delay or increase in degradation secondary to acid
Increased prevalence of duodenal diverticula	Possible malabsorption

become older, interpretation of the results in the elderly should include consideration of age-related alterations in metabolism (biotransformation). In the elderly, reduced liver blood flow may account for a decrease in first-pass metabolism, which allows more drug to reach the systemic circulation. Age-related changes in the liver are variable and should be considered when prescribing drugs eliminated primarily by the liver. Because of this variability, it is difficult to predict the need to alter a drug dose for patients without overt liver disease. Monitoring serum drug levels can be useful for several drugs with toxic potential, such as phenytoin, that are used by older persons (Ives, 1992). Although further studies are needed in the area of metabolism, it seems that drugs that are metabolized via oxidation pathways, such as many psychotropic drugs, anticonvulsants, oral anticoagulants, and oral antidiabetic agents, require lower doses in elderly patients, whereas drugs such as isoniazid, procainamide, and hydralazine, which are biotransformed in the liver, may not require dose adjustment. One can see that generalizations concerning complex metabolic activity in older persons are difficult to predict, and currently there are no exact specifications for the dosing of these medications in geriatric patients. These changes

suggest, however, that initial doses of drugs that are highly metabolized should be decreased for the elderly. Increasing doses slowly while titrating to clinical response is the safest method of dosing for these patients.

Elimination

Although there are many routes by which drugs can leave the body, including the skin, lungs, and via the bile to feces, the ultimate elimination of a drug or its metabolites from the body is predominantly though the kidney. Age-related changes in the renal pathway of elimination are well understood. Renal elimination may be affected by disease, altered blood flow to the kidneys, urinary pH, and the presence of other drugs. In addition, it is well known that a physiological decline in renal function occurs with aging. An age-related decline of approximately 1–2% per year of age is seen after maturity. Even in the absence of active intrinsic kidney disease, renal clearance is decreased in the elderly to about half that of a younger person. This decline is reflected in a corresponding decrease in creatine clearance. Fortunately, clinicians have a method of assessing renal function based on easily accessible information. One method, formulated by Cockcroft and Gault

(1976), uses serum creatinine (SCr) levels to determine the clearance (CrCl):

$$\frac{(140 - age)\ (body\ weight\ in\ kg)}{72(SCr)} \quad (\times\ 0.85\ for\ females)$$

Results from one study that compared young and elderly ambulatory patients showed good correlation between the estimated, calculated CrCl and CrCl determined by using 24-hr urine collections. Values for younger women best correlated with the proposed equation, when the results were multiplied by 0.85, which accounts for a decreased muscle mass in women, whereas renal function in elderly women was underestimated when this factor was used. The CrCl for elderly women correlated best when the equation was not adjusted by the factor of 0.85 (Rho & Wong, 1998). Perhaps this is a reflection of postmenopausal changes affecting fat to lean body mass ratios. It is suggested, therefore, that clinicians use the same equation for both elderly men and elderly women. In addition, the study showed that the majority of elderly patients had SCr within normal limits but calculated and actual CrCl of less than 60 ml/min. This suggests that CrCl and not SCr should be used as a guideline for determining doses of renally cleared drugs such as digoxin (Lanoxin) and aminoglycoside antibiotics such as gentamicin (Rho & Wong 1998). When used in the elderly patient, these medications have a longer half-life and require lower doses, longer time between doses (increase in dosing interval), or both to attain the appropriate serum levels and clinical response.

AGE-RELATED PHYSIO-LOGICAL CHANGES: PHARMACODYNAMICS

An individual's response to drug therapy does not rely simply on the concentration of the substance in the blood. Study of the pharmacodynamic response of a drug reviews the actual receptor response at the target tissue. Little information is available on the changes that occur at the receptor and postreceptor levels with aging. The data that are available are variable: Age-associated increases in sensitivity to several drugs have been noted, particularly, CNS-acting drugs, warfarin (Coumadin), heparin, and narcotic analgesics. For these drugs, target serum concentrations, dose, or dosing intervals may have to be adjusted. In contrast, although higher serum levels may be achieved with the same dose/per kilogram, elderly patients may actually require higher doses than younger patients for some medications such as captopril (Capoten). One can see that generalizing in this age group is difficult. It is still best to initiate new medications at lower doses for an elderly patient, and with small increments, increase the dose by slow titration to achieve clinical response. One must not be surprised, however, if normal or high-normal doses are required to treat the patient effectively. These doses must be achieved, however, only if tolerated well by the patient and not at the cost of toxic effects.

AGING AND ALCOHOL

Alcohol is a potent drug. Toxic effects due to its abuse can affect almost any organ system in the body. Older persons may have a greater potential for the toxic effects of alcohol because of decreasing metabolic function and the concurrent use of other drugs that may have similar CNS side effects or that may compete for metabolic elimination. Given the availability and social acceptability of alcohol, it is not surprising that the estimates of alcohol use in the elderly are quite high. Although reports are difficult to compare because of different definitions of how many drinks or ounces are required to label someone as an alcoholic, percentages of elderly alcoholics range from 1% of women and 12% of men over age 60 who have serious problems with alcohol abuse and up to 20% of persons in nursing homes who are alcoholics (Kaplan & Saddock, 1994).

It is possible that an entirely different set of criteria should be established for the diagnosis of alcoholism in the elderly compared with younger persons. Often an older person may drink less in terms of quantity and frequency. The amount of alcohol consumed may decrease yet result in a higher blood level (because of decreased total body water with increasing age) than in a younger person, bringing on increasingly stronger effects with age. Diagnosis may be further complicated in that the elderly may have atypical signs and symptoms. Rather than complaints of gastritis or findings of hepatic dysfunction, the older patient may have a history of falls, incontinence, psychotic behavior, malnutrition, social isolation, dementia, self-neglect, myopathy, diarrhea, or accidental hypothermia. Alcoholism is distinctly related to dementia and estimates are that 10% of the dementia in older persons are alcohol-related (Campbell, 1997). Studies have shown that physicians miss the diagnosis of alcoholism in older patients almost twice as often as in younger patients, especially if the patient is white, female, and has completed high school (Ebersole & Hess, 1998). To complicate matters further, underreporting among older persons may occur, because the elderly are more likely to be isolated from situations that make abuse visible. Younger persons may experience difficulties resulting in poor job performance, automobile accidents, marital and legal problems, while the elderly may be retired from work, less mobile, and less likely to be out in public. In addition, loving, well-meaning family members may try to protect their elderly relatives from the possible ridicule or embarrassment that may accompany a diagnosis of alcoholism. Unfortunately, delayed diagnosis may account for the high percentage of elderly patients with alcoholic liver disease who have cirrhosis and the poor prognosis of these patients. Although only 7% of cirrhotic patients under the

age of 60 die in the first year after diagnosis, as many as 50% of the elderly patients with cirrhosis die in 1 year (Scott, 1989).

Although most self-reports indicate that persons tend to continue with the same drinking patterns they had before 60 years of age, about one third of elderly alcoholics are considered late-onset drinkers (*started* drinking after the age of 50). For these late-onset alcoholics, it is possible that susceptibility to social and psychological pressures of aging contributed to the beginning of a drinking problem. Losses that may be associated with old age include loss of health, loved ones, social supports and job and distance from family members (Campbell, 1997).

The interactions between alcohol and medications are complicated. At the metabolic level, short-term binges of alcohol may cause a competitive inhibition between alcohol and drugs that require metabolic clearance. This will result in a decreased clearance of drug, a potentiation of clinical effect, and an increased potential for toxic effects. For example, the use of acetaminophen is generally considered to be safe. In combination with alcohol, there is an increased risk of adverse drug reactions and side effects, especially drug-induced hepatotoxic effects. In contrast, long-term alcohol use causes an induction of the enzymes that normally metabolize drugs, increasing metabolic clearance and decreasing clinical efficacy.

Another type of alcohol-drug interaction is the potentiation of drug-induced side effects. The sedative effect of alcohol, when used in combination with medications that also may cause drowsiness, may increase the risk of accidents and falls. These drugs include phenytoin, barbiturates, benzodiazepines, antidepressants, antipsychotics, opiates, and even nonsteroidal anti-inflammatory agents. In addition, the use of alcohol with agents that have local or systemic effects on clotting mechanisms, such as aspirin, may significantly increase the risk of bleeding.

Although treatment for elderly alcoholics is less likely to be recommended by physicians, it is fortunate that the elderly are particularly inclined to benefit from treatment of alcoholism when treatment is initiated early. Studies have shown that older patients are more likely to remain in treatment and maintain sobriety for longer periods than younger patients (Blazer, 1995). In addition, it has been found that elderly patients benefit most when treated in therapy groups that consist of others of similar age, rather than participating in treatment with mixed age groups.

Because of the alarming rates of misdiagnosis of alcoholism in the elderly, training for healthcare professionals needs to be improved. Screening tests designed to identify elderly problem drinkers should be developed and administered routinely. When a geriatric alcoholic is identified, and the diagnosis is confirmed by the clinician, the patient should be informed of and encouraged to participate in all treatment possibilities.

DRUG USE IN EXTENDED CARE FACILITIES

The financial constraints imposed on most government-subsidized extended care facilities have a definite influence on the appropriate use of medications. Physician visits occur as rarely as once per month per patient, and the tendency for the clinician to prescribe medications on an as-needed (prn) basis is great. There is an inclination toward polypharmacy, however, in regard to scheduled medications as well.

The amount of drugs consumed is directly related to the prevalence of drug-related problems. It is estimated that 75% of community dwelling elderly take at least 1 prescription medication and consume 12–15 medications daily if over-the-counter medications are included. Hospitalized elderly take an average of 9.1 medications, and between 3 and 6 drugs are taken by persons in long-term care facilities. Approximately one third of long-term care residents take as many as 8-16 drugs daily (Nolan & O'Malley, 1988; Stolley et al., 1991). The most commonly prescribed medications in long-term care facilities are phenothiazines and psychotropic drugs; cardiotonics, especially digitalis; diuretics; analgesics; and gastrointestinal medications (Stolley et al., 1991). One study in Massachusetts elicited startling information about drug prescribing in long-term care facilities: (1) 55% of the residents were taking at least one psychoactive drug; (2) 39% of these were taking antipsychotics, 18% taking two or more; and (3) physician participation in drug decisions (i.e., thorough investigation and assessment) occurred in less than half of the population (Avorn et al., 1989; Ray et al., 1993).

Generally, more drugs are prescribed for those over 65 years old than for younger patients. When the number of drugs per *institutionalized* patient is compared, the disparity becomes even greater. In a review of several surveys, the average number of drugs per elderly patient in household and family practice settings was 2.0–4.5, whereas the average for long-term care institutions was 3.7–7.2. In addition, prescribing patterns do not appear to be universal. The United States, for example, has higher averages of drugs per long-term care patient than does Great Britain or Australia (Ray et al., 1993).

Previously, extended care facilities were primarily regulated by Title 22, in the chapter Health Facilities and Referral Agencies. Among the guidelines for medication use set by Title 22 is the mandate that drugs can be used to restrain a patient only if the patient's behavior or manifestation of disordered thought process that was to be treated with the drug is indicated in the patient's chart. In addition, the patient's care plan must specify what data should be collected to determine the effectiveness of the drugs used. Title 22 also specifies that prn orders must include the indication for use of the drug, that medications shall not be used as punishment or for the convenience of staff, and that patients have the right to be free from chemical restraints unless the patient is a danger to himself or to others.

More recently, the Omnibus Budget Reconciliation Act of 1987 (OBRA '87) has expanded (but not negated) these requirements. OBRA '87 specifies that residents shall be free from unnecessary drugs. The word "unnecessary" is given a fairly broad meaning and includes drugs that are given in excessive doses, for excessive periods of time, or in the absence of a diagnosis or reason for the drug. Unnecessary drugs also include medications for which monitoring data or the presence of adverse side effects indicates that the dose be reduced or the drug eliminated entirely. More specifically, OBRA '87 also outlines the appropriate indications for the use of antipsychotic agents. Residents who have not previously used psychotropic drugs must not be given these agents unless therapy is necessary to treat a specific condition. Residents who are currently receiving antipsychotic drugs should receive gradual dose reductions or drug holidays in an effort to discontinue the medications, unless it is documented that this is clinically contraindicated.

The appropriate conditions, or diagnoses, that warrant antipsychotic drug use are specified by OBRA '87 *(Table 6-3)*.

In addition to indications for appropriate antipsychotic drug use, OBRA '87 also outlines unacceptable uses for these drugs *(Table 6-4)*.

More recent revisions in OBRA also target sedatives, hypnotics, and anxiolytics. The rules state that residents should not be prescribed long-acting benzodiazepines unless a shorter acting benzodiazepine has been tried and has failed. The rules go on to say that short-acting benzodiazepines

should not be used until a thorough assessment has elicited possible causes of agitation or disturbing behavior have been eliminated through environmental manipulation, interdisciplinary teamwork, care planning, and so on. These rules apply to sedatives as well. Interestingly, OBRA has made some exceptions to the rules. For example, if diazepam is prescribed for muscle pain rather than anxiety, the rules do not apply. Further, if diphenhydramine HCl is prescribed for sleep, the thorough assessment must be done and other non-chemical factors must be implemented first. However, if diphenhydramine HCl is prescribed as an antihistamine, the rules do not apply (Health Care Financing Administration, 1992).

In addition, OBRA requires that all behaviors be quantified and objectified before a psychoactive drug can be prescribed. The behavior must be identified specifically, such as kicking, biting, having auditory hallucinations, rather than a blanket statement stating that the resident is "confused." Each time the behavior is exhibited, it is documented. In this way, a thorough assessment can be made so that use of a psychoactive drug can be avoided. For example, agitated behavior may occur only at a certain time of day or when a certain caregiver is present. By avoiding overmedication, the patient is safer and more comfortable. OBRA also mandates continued documentation of behaviors to determine effectiveness and monitoring for side effects of all psychoactive drugs (Health Care Financing Administration, 1992).

Programs have been developed and implemented for systematic dosage reductions for antipsychotic drugs and antianxiety drugs (Ray, et al., 1993; DeMaggd, 1995). A 50% weekly progressive reduction is recommended in conjunction with education in new behavior management skills, a written behavior plan, and better communication between residents of nursing homes, their families and staff. The results have proven to be very successful. In fact, reducing the use of chemical

---

TABLE 6-3
Acceptable Indications For Antipsychotic Drug Use

Management of documented psychotic disorders
- Schizophrenia
- Schizoaffective disorder
- Delusional disorder
- Psychotic mood disorder, including mania and depression with psychotic features
- Acute psychotic episodes
- Brief reactive psychosis
- Schizophreniform disorder
- Atypical psychosis
- Continuous crying or screaming

Tourette's syndrome

Huntington's chorea

Organic mental syndromes with associated psychotic and/or agitated features, in which documented behaviors include the following
- The patient is a danger to him or herself.
- The patient is a danger to others.
- The patient's behaviors interfere with staff's ability to provide care.

---

restraints has often resulted in reduced use of physical restraints as well.

Another therapeutic approach to reducing drug use and potential toxicity by the elderly is the use of a "drug holiday" (Ebersole & Hess, 1998). This involves omitting a drug for one to two days during a week. The nurse needs to assess the benefits versus the risks with the resident and their family. The benefits may include increased energy, mental alertness, reduction in medication cost and increased ability to participate in certain activities, i.e.; walking. One risk that might be identified is that due to accumulations of some drugs in fat, a one or two day holiday would not have any noticeable effect. For many elders this is an option that, at least, should be presented by the nurse acting as an advocate for the elderly individual.

Mental status tests should be included as part of the initial assessment of patients and be periodically done throughout a stay at a facility. But the concern for drug misuse in the elderly should not

stop at the antipsychotics. In light of the considerable cost of drugs in terms of morbidity and money to the taxpayer, the patient, or a third party, the use of all medications should be monitored extensively. In addition to the use of psychotropics, use of cardiovascular agents, sedatives, analgesics, laxatives and vitamins increases with age (DeMaggd, 1995; Miller, 1996).

A rational approach to use of therapeutics in the elderly that is based on pharmacological, pharmacokinetic, and pharmacodynamic models is needed in extended care facilities. This includes the need for specific guidelines and policies for infection control, nutrition, medication use, nondrug treatments, and dentistry.

The prevalence of infection for elders is much higher than for younger persons, with significantly more nosocomial infections after the seventh day of hospitalization, pointing to the hazards of immobility (Stolley & Buckwalter, 1991). Epidemics occur frequently in long-term care facilities, most

---

TABLE 6-4
Unacceptable Indications for
Antipsychotic Drug Use

- Simple pacing
- Wandering
- Poor self-care
- Restlessness
- Crying out, yelling, or screaming
- Impaired memory
- Anxiety, nervousness, fidgeting
- Depression
- Insomnia
- Unsociability, uncooperativeness
- Indifference to surroundings
- Any indication for which the order is on an as-needed (prn) basis

---

commonly upper respiratory infections, diarrhea, conjunctivitis, and antibiotic-resistant bacteriuria (Stolley & Buckwalter, 1991). Many of the patients and residents of extended care facilities are already at risk of serious infections developing because of underlying disease. Predisposing factors to infections also include the sedative side effects of many drugs. The drowsiness caused by these medications may make it difficult for a patient to maintain maximum mobility. A diminished febrile response to infection in the elderly has been described in which either there is little or no fever response to infection or there is a delayed response of 24 to 48 hours (Fraser, 1997). Pneumonia and pressure ulcers are more likely to develop in a patient who is sedated than in one who is active, independent, and ambulating. In addition, infection is a major cause of hospital admissions from these facilities. The most common types of infections seen include pneumonia, urinary tract infections, infected decubitus ulcers, and conjunctivitis.

Infection control practices should include active prevention with immunization, staff education of prevention techniques (e.g., handwashing),

restricted contact between patients and ill employees or visitors, and appropriate isolation techniques when needed. Although controversial, influenza vaccine (administered annually) and pneumococcal vaccine are recommended for nursing facility patients. When outbreaks of type A influenza do occur, prophylactic treatment with low doses of amantadine HCl, 100mg daily, should be instituted unless contraindicated. It is important to remember, however, that detection of infection may be masked by the presence of atypical signs and symptoms in the elderly. For example, lack of fever, lack of sputum production, or previous treatment with antibiotics for another infection may make the diagnosis of pneumonia difficult. Pneumococcal vaccine should be given to all adults over age 65 and those with chronic diseases (Fraser, 1997). It can be repeated in 7 or 8 years. The vaccine is considered necessary because of the increased incidence of pneumococcal pneumonia in this age group.

Good nutritional care of elderly nursing home patients is vital, because weight loss in the elderly is a significant problem with grave medical and quality of life consequences for the older individual. Early recognition and intervention avoids the morbidities associated with malnutrition (Morley, 1998). When a nutritional or dietary problem is suspected, consultation should focus on evaluation, diagnosis, and treatment plans. Complete evaluation of the patient may include a psychological evaluation if depression is suspected, a medical examination to rule out underlying illness, and a review of medications to rule out drug-induced anorexia. Calorie counting; evaluation of swallowing mechanism; and consultation with a dentist, speech pathologist, and occupational therapist may be warranted. It may be necessary to supplement feeding orally, or in some cases, tube feeding may be required. In addition, one should not overlook the possibility that dehydration may contribute to weight loss. The elderly are particularly vulnerable to dehydration secondary to a decreased sense of thirst, inadequate water intake, and the frequent use of diuretics. Unfortunately, dehydration and weight loss may also be an indication of inadequate care.

The application of the interdisciplinary team approach to health evaluation and treatment of the elderly in extended care facilities would be ideal. Comprehensive assessment may contribute to improved diagnostic accuracy, enhanced functional status, reduced use of medications, decreased acute hospital admissions, and decreased costs in general. Although the physician's role in the nursing home remains crucial and should include care of patients as well as quality control within the institution, the nurse-patient dyad continues to be central to the outcome of good clinical care. Other members of the healthcare team and those available for consultation should include nursing aides; social workers; pharmacists; psychiatrists; dentists; and communication, speech, physical, occupational, and rehabilitation therapists as well as facility administrators.

It is also possible that a new approach to primary care in nursing homes should be considered. The use of nurse practitioners and physician's assistants as primary care providers may allow more frequent visits to patients in a cost-effective manner. Advanced practice nurse practitioner have demonstrated their value and expertise in working with the elderly (Ebersole & Hess, 1998). In one study of a large population of patients (Kane, Garrard, & Buchanan, 1991), comparisons of quality of care suggested that using nurse practitioners and physician's assistants provided equal or better care than physicians alone. In addition, the inclusion of nursing homes as part of the academic setting for geriatric medicine training will also enhance the quality of care with little additional cost.

ADVERSE DRUG REACTIONS

A review of the factors associated with the prevalence of adverse drug reactions (ADRs) indicates that, it is not surprising that the elderly are at particular risk. In addition to advanced age (over 75 years), small physical stature, excessive number of medications, change in medical condition, development of renal or hepatic dysfunction, and the presence of a high-risk medication all contribute to the increased possibilities of an ADR. In a review, more than 300 acute care hospital admissions, 16.8% were due to an ADR. This accounted for total hospital costs of more than $200,000 due to ADRs alone. Adverse drug reactions are also costly in terms of human illness and suffering. In this study (Col, Fanale, & Kronholm, 1990), admissions due to ADRs were related not only to increased number of medications used but also to higher medication costs and patients who lacked home services.

Estimates of the number of geriatric admissions to hospitals because of ADRs are approximately 10%. It is possible that although the elderly do take large numbers of drugs, the association with hospital admissions is due to the severity of illness, which may predispose this population to the adverse effects of drugs. Of all hospital admissions, 10% to 33% are caused by adverse drug reactions (DeMaggd, 1995).

There are many potent drugs with the potential to cause a variety of ADRs, ranging from minor, clinically insignificant reactions to severe, debilitating reactions that require immediate medical attention. The most common drugs producing adverse reactions leading to hospitalization include warfarin, digoxin, prednisone, diuretics, antihypertensives, insulin, and even aspirin. A review of the list of drugs implicated in ADRs shows that these medications are more often prescribed for the elderly. These drugs, along with their desirable clinical effects, have narrow therapeutic windows such that toxic levels are not too far from levels required for clinical efficacy. In addition, in geriatric patients signs or symptoms of ADRs and toxic effects may go unnoticed, or may be attributed to concomitant illness or the aging process itself.

Side effects from benzodiazepines (e.g., diazepam, triazolam), antidepressants, and diuretics are more frequent in the elderly than younger patients. Although benzodiazepines have been thought to have a higher therapeutic margin, the elderly are more susceptible to unwanted effects. Despite similar plasma concentrations, the extent and duration of the effects of benzodiazepine were more marked in older subjects. When the same drug doses were used, the half-life and duration of action of several benzodiazepines were increased such that daytime sedation was difficult (Nolan & O'Malley, 1989). When the use of a benzodiazepine is absolutely necessary, short-acting agents such as triazolam should be recommended. Still, caution must be taken with the use of these drugs. In a case report by Sullivan (1989), in an 83-year-old woman who inadvertently received 0.5mg of triazolam, severe respiratory depression developed that required 36 hr of ventilatory support. This dose, although four times the recommended initial starting dose of triazolam for the elderly, is within the adult dosing range suggested by the manufacturer. In an effort to guard against this type of error, the manufacturer no longer produces a 0.5mg tablet.

Undesirable side effects from antidepressants are seen more frequently in the elderly. In particular, anticholinergic effects such as urinary retention, dry mouth, constipation, and mental confusion are common. Some of these side effects may be difficult to differentiate as drug induced or may contribute to a preexisting condition. The higher sensitivity of older persons to antidepressant side effects may be due to decreased cholinergic function or to higher plasma levels. In addition, concomitant administration of other drugs with anticholinergic side effects may potentiate these unwanted effects. Such drugs include phenothiazines, antihistamines, and antiparkinsonian medications.

In addition to causing obvious inconvenience to the geriatric patient who may have decreased mobility, the use of diuretics may lead to serious electrolyte imbalances. Of particular concern is the loss of potassium. As diuretics are often prescribed along with digoxin for the treatment of congestive heart failure, drug-induced hypokalemia may contribute to the risk of digoxin-induced arrhythmias. Adequate monitoring of electrolyte and digoxin levels is crucial to effective and safe treatment with these agents.

Because elderly patients are so vulnerable to the ill effects of medications, considerable care must be taken to prevent the occurrence of ADRs. When the use of a medication is necessary, the nurse should undertake a complete review of the patient's medical history, including allergy history. Current prescriptions and over-the-counter drugs should be screened for potential duplication, and drug-drug, or drug-disease interactions. Once the most effective medication is determined, the clinician must determine the appropriate initial dose on the basis of the patient's age, weight, and renal and hepatic function. In the choice of the new medication, the clinician must determine that the drug regimen will not be so complicated that the patient cannot incorporate it into daily life.

Educating patients is a good safeguard against the development of adverse effects from medications. The patient must be provided with enough information to take the drug correctly, but not be so overloaded that taking the medication is impossible. The most effective means of communication for most patients is verbal information reinforced by written directions for review at home *(Table 6-5)*.

TABLE 6-5

Methods of Preventing Adverse Drug Reactions: Educating the Patient

- Name (generic and brand) and strength of the drug
- Intended purpose and benefits of drug use
- Dose, route, and frequency of administration
- Duration of treatment
- Clinically significant potential side effects
- Special storage instructions, if any

Periodic review of the patient's progress and response to the new medication is fundamental. The clinician must determine if the drug is effective, and if so, how long it should be continued. Patients should be asked in a nonjudgmental fashion how and when they are taking their medication. Avoid simple yes or no questions. This will help determine if a lack of response is due to inappropriate use or to the drug's being clinically ineffective in the patient.

NONCOMPLIANCE/ NONADHERENCE

Nonadherence to or noncompliance with prescribed drug regimens is an issue that plagues all patients, young and old. Historically, noncompliance has been the term used for deliberate misuse of medication. The nurse may become angry or frustrated with the person because of the noncompliance with the medical program or treatment plan. A less harsh and accusatory term to use when explaining why elderly individuals do not follow the expected treatment plan or take prescribed medications is nonadherence (Ebersole & Hess, 1998). This term implies that elders cannot and will not comply with a prescription or treatment plan when it interferes with their day-to-day life, when it causes as much or more distress, or when

misinformation or lack of information or disability hampers compliance. Nonadherence implies a responsibility for the health care provider, the elderly individual for whom the prescription is written, and the social support network of the person. Confusion results when directions are given too rapidly to be processed, not in the person's primary language or the directions are not heard or seen because of auditory or visual deficits. Systems to monitor and ensure compliance have been developed, but the primary responsibility lies with the health care provider to recognize that this is complex and affects the elderly persons quality of life as they see it.

Types of Noncompliance or Nonadherence

A patient may intentionally or unintentionally deviate from the drug regimen prescribed by the physician. Intentional departures are often related to the patient's perception of the medication, its benefit and side-effect profile, or its cost. These deviations may be trivial, or they may be clinically significant, compromising ideal therapy outcome.

There are several different types of noncompliance. Errors in frequency, correct intervals of dosing, or total dosage usually result in a patient's making an error of omission: They simply do not take a dose when they are supposed to, or they take too few tablets at the appropriate time. This leads to underdosing of medication. In contrast, a patient may take too many doses either at once or throughout the day, resulting in overmedication.

Another type of noncompliance involves taking a medication for the wrong reason. This may include medications prescribed for a specific reason (e.g., digoxin: take 1 tablet every morning for your heart) or, more frequently, medications that are prescribed "as directed" or on an as-needed basis, often without accompanying indications (e.g., triazolam: take 1 tablet as needed). In this case, the patient must remember several pieces of information (assuming the information was given to the patient in the first place), compounding the innate difficulties of prescription taking. Some of this assumed information includes what the medication is usually used for, how often it may be taken throughout the day, how many tablets are too many to take, and when to discontinue use.

Incorrect administration of medications includes several possible errors. A patient may fail to take a drug at specified times, by an indicated route, or under specific conditions. For example, a medication may be prescribed to be taken only at bedtime, placed under the tongue for sublingual absorption, not to be swallowed or chewed, or not be taken with milk products.

Premature discontinuation of a medication occurs most often with antibiotics but may occur with any prescription. This interruption of treatment may be intentional; the patient may no longer see a need for the medication or may find that undesirable side effects outweigh the potential benefits from continued use. This type of noncompliance may have dangerous consequences. Abrupt discontinuation of several antihypertensives, for example, may result in rebound hypertensive crisis.

Other types of nonadherence include the addition of other drugs (prescribed or over-the-counter), which may interact with the prescribed medication; the use of drugs prescribed for others; the use of outdated medications; or the complete failure to purchase or obtain the medication when it is prescribed.

Reasons for Noncompliance or Nonadherence

There are many reasons why a patient may unknowingly or consciously be noncompliant. Many times drug regimens are complicated or difficult to follow. The suggested scheduling of the medication or unpleasant side effects that develop may interfere with the patient's lifestyle or with daily living. There may be a lack of understanding

or a misinterpretation of instructions, with poor communication between the healthcare professional and the patient as a contributing factor. The patient may perceive the medication as unnecessary or harmful. In the elderly, multiple chronic illnesses, diminished vision, hearing loss, physical limitations; social isolation, and limited, fixed income may contribute to noncompliance. In some situations, memory loss or poor cognitive function may make it difficult for the patient to recall all the information given by the physician or pharmacist. Inadequate drug labels or hard-to-open drug containers may also contribute to decreased compliance. In addition, multiple providers and receiving medications at more than one pharmacy are associated with increased nonadherance. For all age groups, the greater the number of prescriptions taken, the more times medication must be taken in a given day; the greater the number of as-needed medications, the more likely the development of some kind of noncompliance.

Consequences of Noncompliance or Nonadherence

Serious medical problems may result from the incorrect use of medications. It is estimated that 5–35% of nonadherent elders endanger their health by taking medications other than as prescribed (Morrow, Leirer, & Sheikh, 1988). Potential repercussions of noncompliance include recurrence of illness, transmission of communicable disease (e.g., with premature discontinuation of antibiotics), unnecessary hospitalization, increased number of lost workdays, increased morbidity and mortality, and increased healthcare costs to the individual and society. In one review, 11.45% of hospital admissions for patients 65 years and older were directly due to noncompliance, with estimated costs of more than $75,000.

Strategies to Overcome Noncompliance or Nonadherence

Estimates of noncompliance in the elderly range from 25% to 60% or more (Col et al., 1990). In one study, elderly patients taking only one or two medications were noncompliant 27% of the time, and those receiving five or more drugs had a 63% rate of noncompliance. The elderly are at particular risk to experience some type of noncompliance, in part because of the presence of multiple chronic illnesses and the use of multiple medications. As this population is prone to the adverse consequences of nonadherence, it would seem that prevention of this occurrence should be a main focus of the healthcare professional.

Effective communication skills and devotion of sufficient time and effort is essential to the healthcare provider-patient relationship. An integral part of this communication is our anticipation of the patient's need for information. In particular, medication instructions should be complete, both verbal and written, and should include the following:

- Patient's name
- Physician's name and telephone number
- Medication name
- Purpose for medication use
- Warnings about food and drugs to avoid when taking this drug
- The form in which the medication is taken
- Medication dose
- How often to take the dose and at what times of day
- How long to take the medication and whether a refill is required or optional
- Date of issue and expiration date
- Most likely side effects
- Emergency telephone number (911)

This information is best remembered when presented in a numbered, line fashion rather than in paragraph form (Morrow et al., 1988). Information must be delivered clearly, loudly, and slowly for those with hearing impairment. Information should be explicit (not vague), therefore "p.r.n." and "use as directed" are inappropriate instructions. Written information should be provided in large, boldface type, in terminology appropriate for the patient. Package inserts for patients should accompany prescriptions to reinforce the instructions of the physician, pharmacist, and nurse.

Prescription label design used in current practice should be evaluated with the geriatric patient in mind. Labels should be redesigned to be larger so they may present the necessary information in large, high-contrast print. Prescription containers used for elderly patients should be large, with non-childproof caps unless contraindicated.

Strategies to prevent and treat noncompliance should include the use of a visual-graphic format and compliance aids. These products are currently available and include medication calendars, medication containers for daily and weekly use (Medisets), and medication diaries. Encouraging the patient's family members and friends to be involved with medication use builds a social support system for the patient that may alleviate some of the confusion and difficulties in remembering how to take multiple, complicated prescriptions. Whenever clinically possible, substitution with generic drugs, less costly drugs, or drugs available over-the-counter or the use of nondrug alternatives should be considered to counter the high costs of medications, which may contribute to noncompliance.

To encourage continued compliance, especially with medications requiring long-term treatment, follow-up visits with the physician and pharmacist should reinforce instructions. It is best to initially ask patients how they are taking each of their medications, if they have been started on any other new medications (prescribed or over-the-counter) by themselves or other providers, and whether they have missed doses of the drug. Again, these questions must be asked with a nonjudgmental approach or patients are most likely to respond with answers they think the clinician wants to hear! For example, one may ask, "Did you miss any doses of your digoxin this month?" Or this question may be rephrased as, "It is quite common to forget to take your medication once in a while. How many times this month would you say you forgot to take your digoxin?" This second question requires more than a yes or no answer and implies both humaneness and acceptance of noncompliance.

Home visits to the patient by a healthcare professional often disclose interesting and previously unknown drugs and drug-use behavior. During these visits, if prescriptions no longer required by the patient or outdated medications are found, it is best to ask the patient if they may be disposed of. With permission, this should be done at the home, in front of the patient, while explaining the goal of improved safety.

EXAM QUESTIONS

CHAPTER 6
Questions 51–60

51. What physiological change in the elderly is most likely to affect drug absorption?

    a. Increase in intestinal perfusion.

    b. Increase in gastric pH.

    c. Increase in fat to lean body ratio.

    d. Decrease in total body water.

52. Enzymatic biotransformation of drugs is an example of which type of pharmacokinetic activity?

    a. Elimination

    b. Distribution

    c. Metabolism

    d. Absorption

53. Which of the following statements about most elderly alcoholics is correct?

    a. Their alcoholism is of late-onset.

    b. Their alcoholism is easily diagnosed.

    c. They have started drinking before the age of 50.

    d. They drink more than their younger counterparts.

54. Long-term alcohol use results in

    a. an increase in drug clearance.

    b. a decrease in drug clearance.

    c. an increase in clinical effect.

    d. decrease in toxic effects.

55. Drug use in elderly patients in extended care facilities is which of the following?

    a. Similar to that seen in family practice settings.

    b. Lower than that seen in family practice settings.

    c. Higher than that seen in family practice settings.

    d. Lower in the United States than in Great Britain.

56. Which of the following is among the guidelines for medication use specified by Title 22, in the chapter, Health Facilities and Referral Agencies?

    a. Prn orders are no longer allowed.

    b. Prn orders must be accompanied by appropriate indications for drug use.

    c. Drugs may be used as chemical restraints as long as they are ordered by a physician.

    d. Drugs may be used as chemical restraints if there is limited staff available to care for that patient.

57. OBRA '87 specifies that residents shall be free from which unnecessary drugs?

    a. Drugs given in small amounts.

    b. Drugs given that exhibit expected but tolerated side effects.

    c. Drugs previously given in the hospital.

    d. Drugs given in the absence of a diagnosis.

58. Which of the following is an acceptable indication for antipsychotic drug use in an extended care facility?

    a. Depression

    b. Insomnia

    c. Atypical psychosis

    d. Anxiety

59. Adverse drug reactions are more likely to occur in which of the following patients?

    a. Those who have small physical stature.

    b. Those who take fewer than three medications.

    c. Those who have normal renal and hepatic function.

    d. Those who are less than 65 years old.

60. One type of drug that commonly produces adverse reactions in the elderly is

    a. antimetabolites.

    b. diuretics.

    c. antibiotics.

    d. over-the-counter drugs.

CHAPTER 7

NUTRITIONAL PROBLEMS OF THE ELDERLY

by

Anne Harbord MS, RD

CHAPTER OBJECTIVE

After studying this chapter, the reader will be able to recognize the nutritional problems that are prevalent in the geriatric population.

LEARNING OBJECTIVES

After studying this chapter, the reader will be able to:

1. Identify common parameters used to assess nutritional status.

2. Recognize key components of a nutritional screening program for residents in long-term care facilities.

3. Recognize major factors that indicate a person is at nutritional risk.

4. Specify the indications for use of enteral feeding in the elderly.

5. Indicate the importance of social dining in the nutritional status of an elderly resident in a long-term care facility.

6. Specify the major factors in the prevention of pressure sores in the institutionalized elderly.

7. List diseases that may contribute to nutritional deficiency in the elderly.

8. Specify the proper procedure for administering medications to tube-fed residents.

9. Recognize physiological changes associated with aging that affect nutritional status.

10. Recognize the importance of fluid balance in the health and nutrition of the elderly.

11. Specify the legal implication of tube feeding an elderly resident.

12. List the three types of malnutrition evident in the elderly.

13. List nutrients essential for skin healing.

14. Describe the different types of anemias and how they are diagnosed.

NUTRITIONAL ASSESSMENT

As the fastest growing age group in the United States, the elderly pose an important challenge to the healthcare profession. Quality nutritional care has a significant impact on nutritional status and general well being (Fretwell, 1997; *Nutrition Interventions Manual* (NIM), 1992). The elderly are often at nutritional risk for many reasons, in part related to physical mobility, psychological stress, and the degenerative processes of aging. Nutritional assessment is the first step in providing nutritional care (Fretwell, 1997; NIM, 1992).

An effort by several professional organizations targeting the nutritional health of older Americans has been distributed. This effort, which combined resources of the American Academy of Family Physicians, The American Dietetic Association, and the National Council on the Aging, Inc., is called the Nutrition Screening Initiative. The organizations have formulated several assessment tools and interventions for detecting and correcting nutritional problems in this population (NIM, 1992). Basic questions can be used in screening. *Table 7-1* can be used to assess the warning signs of poor nutritional health that are often overlooked. It is usually self-administered. *Table 7-2* describes a more detailed screening and includes measurement of anthropometric and laboratory values. *Table 7-2* outlines the three levels of screening set forth by the Nutrition Screening Initiative (NIM, 1992). Anthropometrics (measurement of body size, weight, and proportion) should always be done (NIM, 1992). Biochemical indexes and immune testing are easily obtainable for patients who are hospitalized or reside in a skilled nursing facility.

Malnutrition in the elderly is common. Studies by the Nutrition Screening Initiative have estimated that as many as 85% of older Americans are at risk for malnutrition (Jackson, 1997). Three types of protein-calorie malnutrition (PCM) are prevalent in hospitalized patients and skilled nursing facility residents: marasmus (calorie deficiency), hypoalbuminemia (kwashiorkor or protein deficiency), and a mixture of both (Nelson & Franzi, 1992). The prevalence of PCM is 30–65% in hospitalized patients. Estimates of PCM in older adults residing in long-term care facilities vary tremendously, from 10% to 85% (American Dietetic Association (ADA) Position Paper, 1998). Among the elderly, PCM may develop as a result of chronic disease, isolation, poverty, diminished physical or mental function, poor oral health and polypharmacy.

Marasmus results from an inadequate supply of calories. In this type of starvation, skeletal muscle, fat, and glycogen are mobilized for sources of energy; levels of visceral protein remain normal. Immune function usually is not affected by calorie malnutrition. Marasmus or calorie malnutrition may be indicated by weight loss and decreased weight for height.

Hypoalbuminemia is indicated by a decrease in the serum level of albumin, reflecting the depletion of stores of visceral protein. Additionally, the immune response at the cellular level is decreased. In this type of malnutrition, however, muscle mass and weight may be normal or even above normal as a result of obesity or edema. For this reason, malnutrition usually is not suspected. Preliminary signs and symptoms of protein-calorie malnutrition are vague and often overlooked or attributed to other chronic diseases. Signs and symptoms include anorexia, lassitude, irritability, and anxiety. Dehydration as well as protein-calorie malnutrition can cause confusion. This disease is frequently not recognized until hospitalization and if not treated would lead to worsening of malnutrition during hospitalization (Nelson & Franzi, 1992).

A combination of marasmus and hypoalbuminemia is called a *mixed marasmic state*. Changes in body composition, weight loss, laboratory indexes, and anthropometrics can be used to assess moderate and severe PCM. All three malnourished states require an aggressive approach to resolve the condition.

Assessment of weight status is more meaningful if the person's previous weight is known. The change in weight over time expressed as a percentage is a more accurate indicator of nutritional risk than values given in the traditional height-for-weight tables. The change in weight can be calculated as follows:

$$\text{percentage weight change} = \frac{\text{usual weight - current weight}}{\text{usual weight}} \times 100$$

By using *Table 7-2,* the severity of nutritional deficit can be estimated on the basis of weight loss in a specified period.

TABLE 7-1
Nutrition Counseling Checklist

	YES
I have an illness that the doctor has told me needs a special diet.	2
I am supposed to be on a special diet, but I am having trouble following it.	2
I have gained or lost 10 lb. or more without trying in the past 6 months.*	2
I have one or more of these problems: insulin-dependent or adult-onset diabetes, high blood pressure, high blood cholesterol, stroke, gastrointestinal problems, constipation, diarrhea or other bowel problems, osteoporosis, osteomalacia, kidney disease, alcoholism, anemia, or metabolic problems.	**1 point for each problem**
My appetite is poor, and food doesn't taste good to me.	1
I have trouble chewing and swallowing.	1
I have oral health problems.	1
I have medication use problems.	1
I treat my illnesses with vitamin and mineral supplements I have chosen myself.	1
I have many questions about nutrition or need advice about what to eat.	1
I spend less than $30 a week on food.	1
I usually need help shopping for food or cooking.	1
	TOTAL

*Contact a physician if you have lost 10 lb. or more unexpectedly.

If you have a score of 4 or more, contact a dietitian by asking your doctor for a referral or by calling your local hospital, health department, or the American Dietetic Association (1-800-366-1655), or look in the yellow pages, under "Registered Dietitians."

Source: The Nutrition Screening Initiative, 1992.

TABLE 7-2
Nutrition Support Screening Alerts

If an older person indicates that the following questions of level I and II screens are descriptive of his or her condition or life situation, nutritional counseling and support interventions may help solve nutritional problems and improve nutritional status.

DETERMINE Your Nutritional Health Checklist Alerts

I have an illness or condition that made me change the kind and/or amount of food I eat.

Without wanting to, I have lost or gained 10 lb in the last 6 months.

I am not always physically able to shop, cook, and/or feed myself.

Level I Screen Alerts

Lost or gained 10 lb or more in the past 6 months

$$\text{Body Mass Index (BMI)} = \frac{\text{weight (kg)}}{\text{height (cm)}^2} \times 100$$

Body mass index less than 22

Body mass index greater than 27

On a special diet

Difficulty chewing or swallowing

Pain in mouth, teeth, or gums

Usually or always needs assistance with preparing food, shopping for food

Level II Screen Alerts

Lost or gained 10 or more lb in the past 6 months

$$\text{Body Mass Index (BMI)} = \frac{\text{weight (kg)}}{\text{height (cm)}^2} \times 100$$

Body mass index less than 22

Body mass index greater than 27

On a special diet

Difficulty chewing or swallowing

Usually or always needs assistance with preparing food, shopping for food

Pain in mouth, teeth, or gums

Mid-arm muscle circumference less than 10th percentile

Triceps skinfold less than 10th percentile

Triceps skinfold greater than 95th percentile

Serum albumin less than 3.5 g/dl

Serum cholesterol less than 160 mg/dl

Clinical evidence of mental or cognitive impairment

Clinical evidence of depressive illness

Clinical evidence of insulin-dependent diabetics, adult-onset diabetics, heart disease, high blood pressure, stroke, gastrointestinal disease, kidney disease, chronic lung disease, liver disease, osteoporosis, osteomalacia

Source: *Nutrition Interventions Manual for Professionals Caring for Older Americans,* 1992.

Some standard tests may need adjusting to reflect altered body composition and other age-related changes. For example, consider that the "ideal" body weight for persons more than 65 years old may be 10% to 20% greater than the weights listed on basic height/weight tables. A review of data from many studies shows that for older adults, being overweight actually may be more protective than being underweight. Older persons whose weights were no more than 130% of the standard weight for their height had less morbidity and mortality than those whose weights were 20% or more below average. The Nutrition Screening Initiative has made an effort to use multidisciplinary measures for the assessment of nutrition: social services screening, nutritional screening (anthropometric, blood chemistry measures), mental health screening, medication use, oral health, and educational interventions (NIM, 1992). Therefore, standard body/height measures alone may be irrelevant in assessing and intervening nutritionally for the elderly. Detailed information contained in the NIM is beyond the scope of this chapter; however, copies of the manual can be obtained by calling or writing the Nutrition Screening Initiative, 1010 Wisconsin Avenue, N.W., Suite 800, Washington, D.C. 20007; telephone (202) 625-1662.

The laboratory tests most commonly used in routine nutritional assessment include determination of the levels of serum proteins (for protein status); determination of levels of iron, folate, and vitamin B12, (for anemic status); and skin testing with antigens (for immune status).

Visceral protein reserve is an important indicator of nutritional status. A reduction in lean body mass usually indicates that body reserves of protein have been used for energy because of an inadequate intake of dietary protein (Nelson & Franzi, 1992). Lean body mass can be estimated by using laboratory determinations. Determination of serum albumin is probably the most practical to use in an institutional setting. A serum albumin concentration of less than 3.4 g/dl can indicate protein malnutrition and dehydration; levels are decreased also in liver and renal disease.

The decrease in lean body mass seen with protein malnutrition is associated also with poor wound healing and prolonged length of stay in acute care hospitals. Many studies have shown a correlation between decreased serum albumin and increased mortality.

Anemia is a decrease in the number of erythrocytes, or level of hemoglobin or a below-normal hematocrit. Anemia is the most common hematological problem found in the geriatric population. This is most likely due to the nutritional status of the elderly person rather that related to the aging process itself (Chernoff, 1991; Jackson, 1997). Physical indications of anemia in the elderly are headaches, light-headedness, fatigue, lack of energy, sleeplessness, angina pectoris, pallor of mucous membranes and fingernails, tachycardia, functional systolic murmurs, and cardiac enlargement. Severe anemia in the elderly can lead to congestive heart failure. A variety of nutrients are needed for the production of erythrocytes: iron, folic acid, vitamin B12, protein, pyridoxine, ascorbic acid, copper, and perhaps also vitamin E. A deficiency of any of these can cause anemia.

Anemia generally is defined as a hemoglobin level below expected reference ranges (less than 12gm/dL for females and 14gm/dL for males). However, the knowledge of the hemoglobin concentration alone is not enough to distinguish between types of anemia. A mean corpuscular hemoglobin concentration (MCHC, the hemoglobin value divided by the hematocrit value) that is less than 30g/dl indicates hypochromic anemia and a need for increased iron intake. A mean corpuscular volume (MCV) that is more than 95mm^3 indicates that the red blood cells are larger than normal, which suggests a deficiency of either folic acid or vitamin B12. If results of the complete blood count indicate a low hemoglobin and hematocrit and an elevated MCV, then blood levels of folate and vitamin B12 should be measured to determine if a deficiency of either nutrient exists. Iron deficiency anemia is the most common type of anemia in the elderly.

Table 7-3 lists these and other tests used in routine nutritional assessment. Laboratory tests alone are not infallible, and good clinical judgement must be used to interpret results.

PHYSIOLOGICAL CHANGES IN AGING

Many physiological changes that occur with aging may have a negative impact on nutritional status. Decreases in muscle mass or lean body mass with an accompanying increase in body fat are normal changes in body composition caused by aging. There is a 30% muscle mass decrease in elders, resulting in decreased muscular strength, endurance, and bulk. These changes are partially related to nonuse (Nelson & Franzi, 1992). These changes may also be attributed to reduced physical activity, poor diet, reduced body water, and a decrease in metabolically active tissues. Because of the decline in lean body mass (muscle tissue burns more energy than fat tissue), basal energy expenditure (BEE) also decreases, at a rate of about 2% per decade after age 30. This reduction in BEE also reduces the caloric need, making it difficult to obtain an adequate intake of micronutrients (vitamins, minerals) from a lower level of calories. In many cases, nutrient-dense foods must be substituted for so-called empty calories, foods that provide calories but few or no nutrients. Total energy requirements can decline as much as 20% by age 95.

With age, body water and renal function decrease. Dehydration, edema, and ascites associated with illness can alter greatly these normal hydrostatic changes in weight, especially in nutritionally compromised patients. (The effects of these changes are covered further in the section on hydration.) In the elderly, changes in body composition during malnutrition are more drastic because metabolic and excretory capacities are greatly reduced.

Most women begin to lose bone and muscle mass at about age 40 and men at about age 50, partly due to decreased activity levels. Each year after menopause, a woman typically loses 1% of her bone mass (Nelson, 1997). This loss can cause serious clinical problems in the elderly, leading to osteoporosis (reduction in bone density where bones become so porous they easily break) and kyphosis (curvature of the spinal column). A combination of hormone replacement therapy, adequate calcium intake and exercise can minimize accelerated bone loss. Studies in recent years have shown that strength-training halts bone loss and can even restore bone, improves balance, helps prevent bone fractures from osteoporosis and improves flexibility (Nelson & Wernick, 1997). One study published in the Journal of the American Medical Association in 1990, reported that in an 8 week period, frail elderly men and women, ages 86 to 96, who participated in a strength-training study increased their strength by an average of 175% and improved their walking speed and balance by an average of 48% (Nelson, 1997).

As many as 50% of Americans have lost all their teeth by the age of 65 years (ADA Position Paper, 1998). Changes in dentition can be harmful to nutritional status. Lack of teeth or poor oral health reduces chewing ability and limits food selection. Poor dentition or use of dentures can also affect the ability to perceive food flavor. Declining senses of taste, smell, and vision can further reduce dietary intake. Visual impairment can cause an older adult to have a diminished appreciation for the color of foods or have a decreased ability to

TABLE 7-3

Laboratory Analyses Used in Routine Nutritional Assessment

Area of Concern	Consider Deficiency of	Comments
Serum proteins Albumin decreased	Protein	Long half-life (14–20 days), slow to change during malnutrition and repletion; decrease in liver disease and nephrosis
Transferrin (iron transport protein) decreased	Protein	Shorter half-life than albumin (7–8 days); prevalence of iron deficiency limits usefulness in diagnosing PCM (increase in iron deficiency)
Prealbumin decreased	Protein	Half-life 2–3 days; decrease in trauma, inflammation
Hematologic values Anemia Normocytic (normal MCV, MCHC)	Protein	
Microcytic (decreased MCV, MCHC, MCH)	Iron, copper	
Macrocytic (increased MCV)	Folate, vitamin B_{12}	
Total lymphocyte count (number of WBC times percent of lymphocytes)	Protein	Decrease from severe debilitating disease (e.g., cancer, renal disease)
Urinary Values Creatinine-height index (CHI), decreased	Protein (reflects lean body mass)	Expected creatinine excretion: 20 mg/kg body weight for children, 17 mg/kg for women, and 23 mg/kg for men; CHI expressed as percentage of expected value. Problems: difficult to collect accurate 24-hr urine, wide variation in day-to-day creatinine excretion
Nitrogen balance*	Protein	Used in evaluation of nutritional therapy; negative values occur when more nitrogen is lost than is consumed (inadequate intake or physiological stress); positive values occur when more is consumed than lost (e.g., during nutritional repletion). Problems: difficult to collect accurate 24-hr urine; retention of nitrogen does not necessarily mean that it is being used for anabolism.
Skin testing**	Protein	Indicator of immune function; response may be impaired in diabetic patients and the elderly, use of corticosteroids or general anesthetics, trauma, elevated blood urea nitrogen.

*Equation for calculation of nitrogen balance is (24-hr protein intake [in grams] - 6.25) - (24-hr urine urea nitrogen [in grams] + 4 g).

**Skin testing involves intradermal injection of three to five antigens, often including antigens for *Candida,* tricophytin (a fungus), purified protein derivative (tuberculosis), and antigens for mumps. Response ("reactivity") is evaluated at 24, 48, and 72 hr after injection. Induration (and sometimes erythema) of greater than 10 mm diameter is considered a positive reaction.

Source: Moore, M. C. *Pocket guide to nutrition and diet therapy.* St. Louis: Mosby, 1988.

recognize foods. With a decrease in the ability to smell, the role of aroma in stimulating appetite is diminished. The loss of taste perception may alter the flavor of foods. Dysphagia symptoms, which have been estimated to occur in 40% to 60% of older adults in long-term care facilities, may contribute to decreased oral intake and enjoyment of eating (ADA Position Paper, 1998). Foods that are soft, moist, and easy to chew may be beneficial because of the decrease in saliva and changes in esophageal function.

With advancing age, the muscle tone and motor function of the large bowel decline. Constipation is a common complaint. Factors that increase the risk for constipation include diets low in fiber, inadequate fluid intake, decreased physical activity, stress, hemorrhoids, laxative abuse, and drug therapies. The goal of nutrition therapy is to avoid impaction and reduce a dependence on laxatives by promoting a normal bowel routine. For atonic constipation, dietary fiber from a variety of sources and fluids should be increased. For spastic constipation, fiber should be decreased during painful episodes, followed by a gradual increase in soluble and insoluble fiber and fluids (Jackson, 1997). Exercise within individual limitations also may be helpful in treating constipation. Mineral oil, sodium-containing laxatives and long-term use of laxatives may have negative effects on bowel function and nutritional status (Jackson, 1997).

Certain immune cell functions decrease with age. This decrease is caused in part by nutritional deficiencies over time. Research has indicated that zinc supplementation improves immune response in persons who are deficient in zinc or who are diabetic.

A decrease in immune function also has been associated with certain diseases of aging, namely arthritis, cancer, and vascular injury. A pronounced increase in susceptibility to infectious disease has been associated with reduced immune cell function.

HYDRATION

Fluid intake is frequently overlooked in the diets of the elderly. Water is the medium in which all the body's various metabolic activities take place, and is an essential structural component of every cell. Digestion, absorption of nutrients, circulation (blood is 80% water), and excretion (urine is 97% water) all rely on the body's water component. Water is essential in the regulation of body temperature and in the lubrication of joints and abdominal viscera.

Approximately two thirds of the body's weight is water. The specific amount varies with age and with the amount of body fat present. The amount of water tends to decrease as persons grow older. Data indicate that total body water decreases to about 60% of total body mass in adults older than 65 years (Chidester and Spangler, 1997). Fat tissue contains little or no water. Thus, a person with a large amount of body fat might be expected to have somewhat less body water.

The decrease in body water in the elderly makes them more susceptible to dehydration (Chidester and Spangler, 1997). Dehydration may refer to any one of three conditions where fluid intake does not equal fluid output. Hypertonic dehydration: body water losses > sodium losses, such as with a high fever. Isotonic dehydration: body water losses = sodium losses, such as in extreme diarrhea or vomiting. Hypotonic dehydration: body sodium losses > water losses, such as when using diuretics and/or sodium restricted diets (Welch, 1998).

Many elderly persons become dehydrated for a combination of reasons. The activity of the hypothalamus, which stimulates thirst, declines with age. As a result, elderly persons may fail to drink adequate amounts of fluids. In many institutions, water is not routinely placed on the table at mealtimes. Even though water is available at the bedside, bedridden residents may be unable to drink without assistance or they may be confused or severely depressed and forget to drink. Perhaps the most significant reason for decrease in fluid consumption is the decrease in bladder control that is a part of aging. Persons may restrict their fluid intake intentionally in an effort to decrease the frequency of urination. Nocturia also may be a consideration. In this case, drinking more fluids earlier in the day may prevent frequent urination at night.

Infections, especially pneumonia and urinary tract infections, can contribute to dehydration because of accompanying fever. Every degree of fever increases basal water needs by 10% (Welch, 1998).

The consumption of alcohol and many therapeutic agents, such as diuretic medications and cardiac glycosides, can increase the rate of loss of body water. Overexertion as a result of activity or exercise can increase fluid losses. The elderly are also at great risk during exposure to extreme heat or cold. The reduction in body water makes it more difficult to regulate body temperature. It is reported that two thirds of the victims of heat stroke are more than 60 years old. Enteral nutrition support with a high protein tube feeding may also cause dehydration if extra fluids are not provided.

Signs of dehydration include sunken eyes, dry tongue, dry skin and weight loss. Dehydrated skin is loose and lacks elasticity. In the elderly, nausea, constipation, diarrhea, vomiting, fever, infection, hypotension, decrease in appetite, decreased urinary output and dizziness on sitting or standing may also be associated with dehydration. Dehydration may cause confusion, which in an elderly person might be mistaken for chronic dementia.

Assessing fluid status is essential in preventing and reducing incidents of dehydration in the elderly. Besides physical assessment of the resident, laboratory data, if available, may be useful in determining fluid status. This data includes: serum sodium (>145 mmol/L), serum urea nitrogen/creatinine ratio (>25), serum osmolality (>300 mOsm/L), decreased volume of concentrated urine (30–40 ml/Hr) and urine specific gravity (>1.010) (Welch, 1998).

In the past, fluid has been severely restricted in several situations: cardiac or renal failure (CHF), pulmonary edema, and cataract surgery. The trend now, however, is to allow normal consumption of fluid along with the use of diuretics. This reduces the possibility of dehydration.

Calculating fluid needs should be a standardized part of the nutritional assessment process. The literature suggests several methods for determining fluid recommendations for the elderly with an average goal of 1,500 to 2,500 ml per day. A 1997 study of forty nursing home residents calculated recommended fluid intake based on three formulas:

1. 30 ml fluid per kilogram (kg) actual body weight

2. 1 ml fluid per kilocalorie (kcal) energy consumed

3. 100 ml fluid per kg for the first 10 kg actual body weight, 50 ml fluid per kg for the next 10 kg actual body weight, and 15 ml fluid per kg for the remaining kilograms actual body weight (Chidester and Spangler, 1997).

The results of the study indicated that when formulas 1 and 2 were used, the residents received adequate or more than adequate fluid based on the calculations. However, if the resident was underweight or had a low caloric intake, the fluid recommendations were unrealistically low when compared to a standard of a minimum of 1,500 ml for most elderly persons. Formula 3 provided adjustment for extreme differences in body weight.

Calculations using this formula indicated that residents in the study had inadequate fluid intake. The authors concluded that since low caloric intake and underweight status is common among skilled nursing facility residents, formula 3 may be the most accurate at establishing fluid recommendations for this population (Chidester & Spangler, 1997; Welch, 1998).

DISEASES THAT AFFECT NUTRITIONAL STATUS

Most health care problems in the elderly who are ill are chronic conditions. Arthritis, diabetes, hypertension, and heart conditions are the most prevalent. For older adults residing in long-term care facilities, diabetes, congestive heart failure, chronic obstructive pulmonary disease, dysphagia, depression and hypertension are common medical diagnoses. Seventy percent have some organic brain disorder accompanied by dementia. Confusion affects 44% of all nursing home residents. Sixty-six percent of elderly people suffer from anorexia and involuntary weight loss prior to admission to a skilled nursing facility (ADA Position Paper, 1998).

Coronary heart disease remains the leading cause of death in the US for both men and women and it accounts for nearly half of the total mortality in those age 65 and greater (Smith and Crumpacker, 1997, Nelson et al., 1994). The heart itself requires a supply of nutrients to function properly. The heart is fed by blood flow through the right and left coronary arteries. Over time, cholesterol and other lipid material may adhere to and accumulate on the arteries that feed the heart muscle. This process results in the narrowing of the artery and the subsequent loss of elasticity and eventually may lead to complete blockage. If the heart muscle is deprived of sufficient oxygen and nutrients, permanent damage may occur.

A number of risk factors are associated with an increased susceptibility to coronary disease. These risk factors include genetic predisposition (male sex); certain endocrine and pathological disease states, such as hypertension and hyperglycemia (diabetes); environmental (e.g., sedentary living and psychosocial tensions); smoking; hypercholesterolemia (elevated levels of serum cholesterol); obesity; and hypertriglyceridemia (elevated levels of serum triglycerides).

Nutritional approaches in the prevention of heart disease are controversial. Researchers are divided, although correlative evidence indicates that high intakes of cholesterol and dietary fat may be harmful. Research has proposed that cessation of smoking and control of blood pressure have a much greater effect on longevity than does a reduction in the level of serum cholesterol.

Epidemiologic data indicates that elevated serum cholesterol is less of a risk factor for coronary heart disease as age increases above 44 years, and almost disappears after the age of 65 years (ADA Position Paper, 1998).

For most persons, a varied diet is recommended. This should include protein from various sources, complex carbohydrates, fiber, and fat in moderation from both vegetable and animal sources. The diet should be sufficient in vitamins and minerals but restricted in total calories to prevent an increase in weight. Exercise is also helpful both in control of blood pressure and in a lifelong weight control program.

With advancing age, blood pressure tends to increase, placing older patients at higher risk for hypertension. Approximately two thirds of all Americans more than 65 years old have systolic blood pressure greater than 140mm Hg and/or diastolic pressures greater than 90mm Hg. Hypertension is an important risk factor for morbidity from cardiovascular and cerebrovascular disease.

The success of dietary approaches in the management of hypertension is difficult to assess in the elderly. Intake of nutrients such as sodium, potassium, calcium, and magnesium affects blood pressure. Calorie restriction also has been associated with reduced blood pressure. Because kidney function is decreased in the elderly, a reduction in salt intake may be more beneficial than in younger persons. On the basis of data from studies, the current recommendation is to initiate only moderate reductions in sodium intake, to 4–6g/day. The average sodium intake in the United States is 6g/day or more.

Potassium intake has an inverse relationship with blood pressure. The antihypertensive effect of potassium in humans appears to be related to a decrease in the amount of sodium usually excreted in the urine. However, the risks of hyperkalemia (potassium excess) may be a drawback to the use of potassium in control of hypertension in the elderly. Studies that support the benefit in humans of using potassium for this purpose are lacking.

Interest in the use of dietary calcium to prevent and treat hypertension has increased. Evidence exists that a low intake of calcium predisposes to hypertension. Numerous studies in humans have been reported. A decrease in blood pressure has been detected in about two thirds of these trials. Most nutritional surveys of the elderly in North America have shown that a deficient intake of dietary calcium is more pronounced in women than in men. The amount of calcium needed to cause a decrease in blood pressure is well within the recommended daily allowance for calcium (RDA Ages 51+ = 800–1200mg/day). It is legitimate to encourage this level of calcium intake.

Weight reduction is considered to be the single most effective nonpharmacological approach to the control of hypertension. Because no research studies have been done on elderly subjects, the safety of this nondrug method of blood pressure control needs to be studied further.

Finally, it is difficult to quantify an acceptable level of alcohol use for hypertensive persons. During initial treatment, abstinence from alcohol may be warranted to determine its effect on blood pressure levels. The Joint National Committee on Detection, Evaluation, and Treatment of High Blood Pressure recommends alcohol consumption in moderation (no more than 1 fluid ounce of alcohol daily, which is equivalent to 2 ounces of 100-proof spirits, 8 ounces of wine or 24 ounces of beer). The caloric content of alcohol should also be considered, especially for overweight individuals with hypertension who need to lose weight (Nelson, et al., 1994). The prevalence of hidden alcoholism in the elderly is high. Because of the relationship between alcohol and blood pressure, and because drinking also can interfere with pharmacological therapy, consumption of alcohol should be evaluated carefully, and excess intake should be discouraged in elderly persons who are hypertensive.

Diabetes mellitus is very much a disease of aging, with a prevalence of nearly 20% in persons who are more than 65 years old. Impaired glucose tolerance without actual diabetes is found in an even greater proportion of the population. Elevated levels of blood glucose have been associated with an increased prevalence of atherosclerotic heart disease and a poor prognosis after ischemic stroke. One major component in the development of glucose intolerance is insulin resistance, which has been well documented in the elderly.

The normalization of blood glucose and lipids is the primary goal of nutrition therapy for type 2 diabetes. This can be accomplished through avoiding too much fat, improving overall food choices, reducing caloric intake, eating smaller meals and snacks throughout the day and increasing physical activity. Weight loss of the first 10 to 20 pounds is the most beneficial in improving blood glucose levels (Schafer, R, et al., 1997). If insulin is required, an individualized meal plan should be developed first and then insulin should be coordinated with the individual's usual eating and exercise patterns.

In the long-term care setting, consistency in carbohydrate intake at meals and snacks, consistent portion sizes and routine mealtimes can achieve good glycemic control in elderly residents. Sucrose-containing foods can be incorporated into the diet as part of the total carbohydrate intake. With the greater incidence of malnutrition in institutionalized settings, restricting foods to control blood glucose levels is not indicated. Older adults with diabetes should have their blood glucose levels monitored to evaluate the effectiveness of the dietary interventions (Schafer, R, et al., 1997, ADA Position Paper, 1998, American Diabetes Association Position Statement, 1997).

NUTRITIONAL CONSIDERATIONS IN DRUG THERAPY

Drug therapy is part of the treatment of most diseases. Drugs can affect a person's nutritional status by altering food intake, absorption, metabolism, and excretion of nutrients. Conversely, food intake can alter the absorption, metabolism, and excretion of certain drugs (Nelson, et al., 1994). Food and drug interactions are more likely in elderly patients because of organ deterioration, underlying chronic diseases, restricted dietary regimens, an already compromised nutritional state, and other factors related to aging. An average of 8 medications per day are taken by residents residing in long-term care facilities. Twenty-three (23) of the more frequently used medications are known to reduce food intake, and can cause nausea, anorexia, vomiting, food aversions, somnolence, and disinterest in food (ADA Position Paper, 1998).

Some of the specific effects of drugs on nutritional status are as follows:

• Alteration of food intake caused by changes in appetite, changes in the senses of smell and taste, or nausea and vomiting

• Alteration of nutrient absorption caused by changes in gastrointestinal pH or motility, reduction of bile acid activity, formation of drug-nutrient complexes, inactivation of the nutrient transport mechanisms in the bowel, or GI mucosal damage;

• Gastrointestinal irritation with blood loss

• Alteration in the metabolism and excretion of nutrients

Because of the extensive number of drugs and foods, most interactions between specific drugs are not discussed here. Some general guidelines, however, are addressed.

If a particular drug appears to be affecting a patient's appetite, the physician may be able to choose another drug that has less pronounced effects. Occasional interruption of therapy may be beneficial in extreme cases. Appetite-stimulating drugs are used sometimes when other drugs suppress appetite.

Chronic use of laxatives, antacids, anticonvulsants and lipid-lowering medications can increase the requirements for many vitamins and minerals. A daily multivitamin/mineral supplement that provides 100% of the US RDA is recommended for residents consuming these drugs (Gallagher-Allred, 1993).

Drugs that may cause malabsorption or increased excretion of nutrients deserve special attention. The diet should include ample sources of these nutrients in order to compensate for losses. For example, cardiac glycosides can cause anorexia and increase potassium requirements, especially when given with potassium-depleting diuretics or corticosteroids (Gallagher-Allred, 1993). Residents taking these drugs need several daily servings of foods high in potassium: meats; dairy products; and fresh fruits and vegetables such as oranges, bananas, melons, tomatoes, squash, carrots, and deep-green leafy vegetables. If dietary intake is inadequate, then supplements can be given.

Psychotropic drugs can cause taste alterations and dry mouth which leads to decreased appetite and food intake. Residents should be monitored for these side effects and nutritional interventions should be implemented when necessary.

Analgesics and non-steroidal anti-inflammatory drugs can cause gastric pain, nausea, vomiting and loss of iron if bleeding occurs. These medications should be taken with meals. Steroids can also cause abdominal bleeding, altered glucose metabolism, increased appetite and weight gain (Gallagher-Allred, 1993).

When drug absorption is affected by food intake, the drug routinely should be taken before or after mealtimes so the stomach is empty and the blood level of the drug remains fairly constant. When absorption is stimulated by food intake, the drug should be taken with a meal or snack. When absorption is decreased by food intake, it is best if the drug is taken at least 1 hr before or 2 hr after eating or when receiving intermittent tube feeding. When continuous feedings are being used, it is best if the feedings can be stopped 2 hr before and for 2 hr after administration of the drug. When pauses are not feasible, drug levels should be monitored carefully. Drugs whose absorption is inhibited by food should never be mixed with the tube feeding.

Whenever questions arise concerning the appropriate method of administering a medication, the pharmacist and physician should be contacted. It generally is not justified to assume that nutrient supplementation is needed because of drug therapy alone. Laboratory data are needed to verify possible changes in nutritional status. A nutritious diet will help improve the health of the elderly for whom drugs are prescribed.

NUTRITION AND THE CARE OF PRESSURE SORES

A person's nutritional status has a direct effect on the likelihood of a pressure sore developing. Likewise, the progress of healing is directly related to previous and current nutritional intake. It has been estimated that pressure sores develop in 5–10% of all hospitalized patients and approximately 60,000 persons die each year from associated complications (Jackson, 1997). In long-term care facilities, 50% of the pressure sores reported occur in residents over the age of 70 years and are associated with a fourfold increased risk of death (ADA Position Paper, 1998). From a nursing standpoint, immobility is the most important risk factor in the development of pressure ulcers.

The first issue of importance in the process of skin healing is weight status. Underweight patients are at risk simply because they lack the body fat to provide cushioning over the bony prominences. A generalized approach to weight gain for those who are under their optimal weight is appropriate. Adequate calories must be present in order for the protein ingested by the body to be used in tissue healing. Caloric intake of 2200 to 3500 kcal/day may be indicated (Jackson, 1997). Likewise, overweight patients are at risk because the additional weight adds to the pressure on vulnerable parts of the body. Overweight patients also place an added burden on the nursing staff in that repositioning requires additional effort. Infrequent repositioning contributes to the pressure areas. If obesity is a concern, an effort must be made to provide adequate calories for skin healing while avoiding excessive weight gain.

Protein intake is directly related to the progress of skin healing. Protein is an essential element of body tissues. It must be consumed in an adequate amount on a daily basis in order to maintain tissue quality. Lack of protein leads to hypoalbuminemia, which also has been correlated with a greater prevalence of pressure sores, in part because of its effect on the immune system and the resultant decreased ability to fight infection. As noted previously, reduced stores of body protein lead to a variety of nutritional problems. It may be necessary to include additional protein in the form of lean meats and poultry, dairy products, and, perhaps, dietary supplements high in protein in order to provide adequate amounts for tissue synthesis. Fortified milk (whole milk with non-fat dry milk powder added to it) can be used to increase protein without increasing the volume of food. Recommendations of 75–100 grams/day may be indicated to replace protein losses from the wound and to promote healing, especially when the pressure sore is a stage III or IV (Jackson, 1997).

Vitamin C and zinc also are known for their essential roles in wound healing. Vitamin C is the intracellular "cement" that supports the collagen in the capillaries and various connective tissues. Stress conditions such as infections and wound healing cause increased loss of vitamin C stores in the body. Vitamin C-rich foods such as juices and fruits or, perhaps, an oral supplement, should be provided in order to meet additional needs for skin healing. A supplement of 100–200mg/day may increase wound healing and assist the body in resisting infection (Jackson, 1997).

Zinc is the predominant mineral involved in skin healing. Twenty percent of the body's stores of zinc are found in the skin. A high-protein diet generally has sufficient quantities of zinc. Some studies suggest supplementation of 15-25mg zinc/day if the individual is clinically deficient. However, other studies have shown little or no effect from zinc supplementation in the treatment of pressure sores (Jackson, 1997).

Anemia also may be detrimental to healing of wounds and pressure sores. Low levels of hemoglobin mean less oxygen in the bloodstream and therefore less oxygen delivered to body tissues. If anemia is present, efforts should be made to resolve it to help skin healing.

Finally, fluid intake is an essential component of the treatment of pressure sores. Additional fluid is required for metabolism of the higher protein diets usually prescribed. As mentioned earlier, fluid is necessary to carry nutrients to and from the cells and in the control of body temperature. Fluids can be given with or between meals in the form of beverages, gelatin, or soups. It may be advisable to include additional juices between meals in order to encourage adequate fluid intake, as well as vitamin C.

Treatment of pressure ulcers must be interdisciplinary to be successful. The best approach to treatment is prevention, and nutritional care has an essential role in good skin health.

RESTORATIVE FEEDING

The philosophy of an overall restorative nursing approach to care of patients in long-term-care facilities is that the more a person can do for himself or herself, the more content that person will be. As other choices are taken away from aging patients or residents, their ability to feed themselves becomes of great importance. A good mealtime program addresses improving psychological and physical functioning in order to meet nutritional needs. The primary goals of a restorative feeding program are to increase the patient's or resident's level of independence and to improve or maintain his or her nutritional and health status.

Mealtime is a social event. Throughout our lives, specific accomplishments and events almost always are accompanied by the sharing of food. In the hospital or nursing home, the challenge of providing adequate nutrition is met more easily by using a dining program. Persons tend to eat better when they are in a social environment.

A restorative feeding program involves a variety of team members: the nursing component, an occupational therapist, a speech therapist, the dietitian, and others who may assist in maintaining the dining room facilities and in transporting residents to and from the dining room.

The facility must be evaluated to determine obstacles in both the physical plant and the attitudes of the staff in allowing residents to do more for themselves. Some questions to address include the following:

- Are the residents treated with respect?

- Is staffing adequate to meet the residents' needs?

- Are residents allowed to feed themselves, if able, or are they simply fed to expedite feeding?

- Is adaptive equipment available for those who need it?

- Is the dining room large enough to accommodate those who wish to eat there? If not, are two seatings provided?

- Are nutritional needs being met? Are portion sizes adequate? Are the food temperatures appropriate?

- Are residents appropriately dressed and well groomed?

These and other questions may help in problem solving.

Various levels of dining may be needed to accommodate all residents. Those who are able to feed themselves independently may prefer to eat in a private dining room away from those who are "messy" eaters. For the former group, music, select menus, or even family-style dining may be offered. It is also likely that some residents will prefer to eat by themselves in their rooms, although the size of this group usually decreases when an aggressive dining program is developed.

Those residents who require assistance or are totally dependent in eating fare better if they are grouped together, allowing the nursing staff to use its time more efficiently. One-on-one feeding in patients' rooms is much more time-consuming and does not provide the added stimulus of the social setting. Residents with like needs should be grouped together to best meet their needs.

An important component of any dining program is the involvement of the activities coordinator. Perhaps entertainment could be scheduled before meals to encourage greater participation. Music can be a pleasant backdrop to any meal.

The development of a dining program can greatly improve the overall attitudes of staff members and residents alike. Nutritional status generally improves when an emphasis is placed on dining.

ENTERAL AND PARENTERAL SUPPORT IN LONG-TERM CARE

When a person has an intact gastrointestinal tract but is unable to ingest food, tube feeding provides a practical alternative for oral nutrition. Enteral feeding relies on the normal physiological actions of digestion and absorption. It is safe and avoids complications that are common in total parenteral nutrition. Enteral therapy is convenient and requires clean technique instead of sterile technique. With the advent of closed systems, problems of infection control are nearly eliminated. In the long-term care setting, tube feedings continue to be a commonly used method of supplying nutrients to elderly residents. Several considerations, however, will affect the tolerance of enteral feeding and its success.

Some of these include the following: the patient's ability or lack of ability to ingest food normally, the patient's digestive capacities, and other physical and mental problems. Persons who recently have had head or neck surgery or who have cancer or neurological disorders such as a cerebrovascular accident are examples of those who are appropriate candidates for enteral feeding by tube. In some cases, tube feeding is used as an adjunct to oral feeding. In that situation, the team members will need to work closely to ensure that nutrient needs are met and to establish a time frame for oral feeding to be achieved. So-called weaning programs are an essential component of any rehabilitation-oriented facility.

Contraindications for the use of enteral feeding include intractable vomiting, intestinal obstruction, severe intractable diarrhea, and hemorrhaging in the upper part of the gastrointestinal tract. Also, persons who are at a high risk for respiratory aspiration are not good candidates for enteral therapy.

The route for tube feeding depends on three factors: the length of time the tube feeding will be needed, the condition of the gastrointestinal tract and the potential for aspiration (Nelson, et al., 1994). A nasogastric tube is preferred when feeding will be short-term and an oral diet will resume. When feeding is anticipated to be long-term, a gastrostomy can be placed surgically or a percutaneous endoscopic placement of a gastrostomy (PEG tube) can be performed that requires minimal sedation. These tubes provide increased comfort and are the best alternative for alert, ambulatory residents needing long-term enteral nutrition support. When gastric feeding is contraindicated or the individual is at increased risk for aspiration, a percutaneous endoscopic jejunostomy tube can be placed directly into the jejunum or through an existing gastrostomy (Nelson, et al., 1994).

Mechanical, metabolic, and gastrointestinal complications can evolve as a result of tube feeding therapy. Mechanical problems are associated with the type of tube used and the position of the tube. Examples of mechanical complications include: obstruction or dislocation of a nasogastric tube, reflux of gastric contents that can lead to aspiration pneumonia and leakage of a gastrostomy or jejunostomy tube that can lead to skin irritation or erosion (Nelson, et al., 1994). Tubes with small lumen are now used almost exclusively because of the greater comfort they provide the individual. These also can be more prone to clogging. Adequate water must be used frequently to flush the tube as well as before and after medications. When the tube becomes obstructed, it usually requires removal of the tube and reinsertion of a new one. Frequent replacement of the tube can cause irritation and breakdown of the nasal mucosa.

Gastrointestinal complications may include: delayed gastric emptying, nausea, vomiting, abdominal pain, malabsorption, diarrhea and constipation. These problems are usually related to the rate and/or the concentration of the enteral formula being administered (Nelson, et al., 1994). Aspiration pneumonia occurs frequently in the institutionalized elderly and is one of the most frequent reasons for transfer to an acute care facility. The elderly have a high risk for aspiration because of a reduced gastric-emptying rate: foodstuffs stay in the stomach longer before digestion. The lower esophageal sphincter may also be weak and allow gastric contents to reflux into the esophagus. If feedings are given as a bolus, then the amount remaining in the stomach should be measured before the scheduled feeding is administered. If the amount is more than 100ml, the feeding should be held for 1 hr and the residual amount rechecked. If feedings are being given continuously, the residual amounts are not measured. In this case, it is important to observe the patient for abdominal distension and monitor for complaints of "fullness." To avoid reflux of gastric contents, elevate the head of the bed to greater than a 45° angle and feed for a duration of 1 hr.

Fluid and electrolyte disturbances are particularly dangerous to older adults. Dehydration can result from serious diarrhea, excessive protein intake, or osmotic diuresis. Dehydration, hypernatremia, hyperchloremia, and azotemia—tube-feeding syndrome—may result from excessive protein intake accompanied by inadequate fluid intake. Signs include confusion and decreasing levels of consciousness. This syndrome can be prevented by monitoring levels of serum electrolytes and blood urea nitrogen and watching for signs of dehydration (rapid weight loss, high specific gravity of urine, and elevation of such routine laboratory values as hematocrit). Monitoring tube-fed patients for glucosuria is also essential. Glucosuria can lead to osmotic diuresis and eventually hyperosmolar, hyperglycemic, nonketotic dehydration.

Some electrolyte disturbances that may occur include hypernatremia, hyponatremia, hyperkalemia, hypokalemia, and hypophosphatemia. Hypernatremia is usually indicative of dehydration. Hyponatremia is frequently not a true hyponatremia but instead a dilutional hyponatremia reflecting a fluid overload. True hyponatremia is not usually related to dietary intake but may be a reflection of renal disease, excessive use of diuretics, vomiting, diarrhea, or fistula drainage. In true hyponatremia, weight loss occurs, whereas dilutional hyponatremia is accompanied by weight gain. Catabolism may result in hyperkalemia as body cells are broken down. However, hypokalemia may occur during nutritional repletion if insufficient amounts of potassium are available for anabolism, the building of new body tissue. Hypophosphatemia is also a possibility during refeeding of a severely depleted patient. The body needs increased phosphorus to meet the demands for tissue synthesis.

The most frequent complications are largely preventable by careful routine monitoring. When tube feeding is started or when the feeding schedule is changed in diabetic patients, glucose levels should be checked daily and diabetic therapy adjusted until blood glucose levels are controlled. A sliding-scale insulin regimen may be used. When tube feeding is started in nondiabetic patients, blood glucose levels should be checked initially, after the feeding regimen is established and then on a periodic basis.

Accurate recording of intake and output is essential for monitoring fluid balance. Fluid intake consists of fluid taken by mouth, intravenous fluids, and the tube feeding formula and water given via the tube. Output consists of the fluid lost through the urine and feces and the insensible loss from perspiration and water evaporation from the lungs. Additional water losses may occur through draining wounds or fistulas. Fluid intake should be approximately equal to fluid output. Fluid balance is essential for normal bodily functioning because water is a vital component of every body cell. Inadequate fluid intake is often the cause of constipation associated with tube feeding. Fluid requirements usually are estimated by assuming that the patient needs 30ml of water for each kilogram of body weight. This may be adjusted upward in the case of fever, pressure ulcers, or a history of dehydration. The total water given may be restricted in the presence of cardiac insufficiency, pulmonary disease, or decline in renal function. Nursing monitoring for signs and symptoms of edema or dehydration is an important part of tube feeding therapy.

Diarrhea is the most common complication of tube feedings. Diarrhea can result when one or a combination of factors is present, including bacterial contamination, inappropriate feeding technique, lactose intolerance, low-levels of serum albumin, or concurrent drug therapy. Diarrhea may be a sign of fecal impaction.

Constipation is also a problem in patients maintained on long-term tube feeding. Many commercially available feeding solutions are designed to be low in residue, so decreased frequency of bowel movements is to be expected. If constipation is a problem, use of a formula that contains fiber may be indicated. However, fiber should be introduced gradually into the diet, and adequate water must be given to avoid impaction.

Other gastrointestinal upsets during tube feeding include nausea, abdominal cramps, and distension. Generally, these problems are avoided when an appropriate volume of feeding is started and increased gradually as needed and tolerated. If the patient experiences nausea, the feeding should be stopped and the amount of formula remaining in the stomach should be checked. Nausea can be relieved by stopping the feeding for 1 hr or by slowing the rate. If gastric distension is the cause of the nausea, ambulation may help.

Feedings should be discontinued if vomiting occurs or if decreased gastric motility or obstruction is suspected. The presence of more than 150ml of formula in the gastric contents probably indicates delayed gastric emptying. Possible causes should be evaluated.

Most patients tolerate an isotonic (osmolarity similar to that of the gastrointestinal tract, approximately 300 mOsm) formula well. Dilution of the formula to half-strength is not recommended. When an isotonic formula is diluted, diarrhea and intolerance to the feeding can result.

In the elderly, lactose intolerance is common. It is therefore wise to avoid formulas that contain milk or milk products. Most standard and calorie-dense formulas are lactose-free to avoid potential problems from malabsorption. They are low in residue and electrolytes, and flow easily through small-bore feeding tubes.

Medications administered through the feeding tube may cause intolerance to the feeding or the feeding may interfere with the effectiveness of the drug. Certain medications can change the osmolality or pH of the feeding and may cause gastrointestinal intolerance or curdling, with resultant tube clogging. In addition, many drugs are known gastrointestinal irritants.

Guidelines regarding suitability of certain medications for enteral administration are obtainable from any pharmacy. In general, it is wise to use the liquid form of a drug whenever available. Certain solid oral dosage forms can be thoroughly crushed, dissolved in a suitable diluent, and administered via the feeding tube with a water flush before and after administration. Enteric-coated, slow-release, and sublinguial forms of drugs should never be given via the tube. The effectiveness of a medication can be enhanced or diminished when administered with a tube feeding, and blood levels of medications should be monitored when indicated.

Special care should be taken to satisfy the psychological and social needs of individuals receiving enteral feeding. This is especially important for patients in a hospital or residents in a skilled nursing facility who require long-term tube feeding. These residents are denied the pleasures of eating and socializing with others. Although the nutrition needs of the resident may be met, the "food" no longer looks, tastes, or smells familiar. Reassessment should be done periodically to determine if the resident is a candidate for weaning to oral feeding.

Many factors must be considered if a weaning program is to be successful. Members of the healthcare team who should be involved include speech or occupational therapists, the dietitian, rehabilitation nurses, and the nursing assistants. Nutritional needs of the patient or resident must be met during a trial feeding program.

Feedings administered immediately before a meal will interfere with appetite and reduce oral intake. Feedings given after a meal may result in gastric distension and create the potential for aspiration. An individual protocol may include a nocturnal feeding, for example, from 8 p.m. to 6 a.m., to allow the resident to be up during the day for activities. Appetite and interest in meals likely will improve.

Tube feeding is a feasible alternative method for nutrition when oral feeding is restricted or contraindicated. However, many adverse responses are possible, and the patient should be observed and monitored. Failure to do so can be costly to both the institution and the resident.

Total parenteral nutrition (TPN) is the alternative method of feeding for those patients who can neither accept nor absorb nutrients taken enterally. Examples of such patients include those with impaired digestive function (e.g., bowel inflammation, bowel obstruction, or Crohn's disease) and those with malnutrition associated with chemotherapy, cancer, stress, or trauma. These types of patients are often admitted to skilled nursing facilities after their medical conditions have stabilized.

To provide adequately for residents who are receiving TPN, the long-term care facility should have 24-hr staffing with registered nurses, established policies and written procedures for TPN therapy, and an ongoing staff education program. Adequate refrigerated storage facilities for solutions are an additional requirement.

Two routes are used for TPN: peripheral vein and central vein. The first route is used short term for patients with mild-to-moderate nutritional deficiencies and for those at risk for such deficiencies. The central route is used for those who require therapy for longer than 5–7 days; more than 2400 calories/day can be given via this route. The hypercaloric solutions are delivered through a silicone catheter directly into the subclavian vein running into the superior vena cava and into the right atrium. The potential for infection is great, and

meticulous infection control procedures must be followed.

Components of the TPN solution include energy sources; dextrose and fat emulsions are the principal calorie sources. Nitrogen is supplied in the form of amino acids to meet the patient's protein needs. Vitamins, electrolytes, and trace elements are added to meet basic needs and replace losses. Some patients require insulin to maintain normal levels of blood glucose when they are receiving highly concentrated dextrose solutions. Heparin also may be added to prevent clotting in the subclavian catheter and in the central line itself.

When patients begin taking food by mouth or tube, TPN can be stopped gradually. However, as with the enteral weaning program, provisions must be made to meet nutritional needs during this tapering process. The dietitian is involved and frequently assesses nutrient intake to determine its adequacy.

TPN is associated with many complications, and strict protocols for their prevention are required. Pneumothorax may occur during placement of the central line; the placement of the catheter usually is confirmed by obtaining a radiograph before the infusion is started. Air embolism is a constant risk if the line is interrupted or accidentally disconnected. Strict aseptic technique is essential to prevent infections. Metabolic problems similar to those associated with enteral therapy may occur, particularly in nutritionally depleted geriatric patients. When hyperglycemia or hypoglycemia occurs, the concentration of the formula must be adjusted, with the possible use of insulin to control levels of blood glucose. In prolonged therapy, deficiencies in essential fatty acids may occur if a fat emulsion is not given periodically, usually two to three times a week.

TPN therapy can be provided in a long-term care facility, but education and training must be ongoing to prepare staff members and to provide the team approach essential to make TPN successful. When able, residents should be encouraged to take an active role in their nutritional care. Physical therapy and occupational therapy can be used to help the patients cope with their treatment and to provide the skills necessary to wean them from therapy.

ETHICAL CONSIDERATIONS OF FEEDING

In addition to the psychosocial factors discussed, ethical considerations play a role in the provision of nutritional care. Each institution needs to clarify its policies for dealing with ethical issues and concerns related to feeding. A bioethics committee should be formed to deal with the questions that arise. The medical director, the physician, the director of nursing, the administrator, clergy, the ombudsman or state representative, the patient, and the patient's family members all should be involved in the decision-making process.

Life-sustaining procedures are any therapy or intervention that uses mechanical or other artificial means to sustain, restore, or supplant a vital function that, when applied to a qualified patient, would serve only to prolong artificially the moment of death. Life-support therapies should not include the administration of medication or any procedure deemed necessary to alleviate pain. Enteral and TPN therapies are considered to be life-sustaining when the patient is unable to take adequate nutrition by conventional means.

Generally, in decisions involving life-and-death situations, three areas come in to play: informed consent, the patient's competency, and the role of surrogate decision-makers.

According to guidelines issued by the California Association of Health Facilities, informed consent is the process through which decisions on medical treatment are made (1989). The physician provides the patient with a full explanation of diagnosis and treatment, the patient participates in establishing the goal of treatment. The patient's permission is obtained before treatment.

A patient is deemed competent if he or she has the ability to understand the nature and consequences of that to which he or she is asked to consent. Mental incompetency is not limited to those who legally have been declared incompetent. It includes those who, in the opinion of the attending physician, are either permanently (e.g., mentally deficient, senile) or temporarily (e.g., head injury, alcohol or drug abuse) incapable of giving consent. In some cases, it is necessary to have a psychologist evaluate the person to determine competency. In most cases, a competent patient has the right to refuse treatment after considering countervailing interests of the state and some rights of third parties who may be dependent on the person refusing treatment. Decision-making capacity (competency) is defined as the ability to (1) comprehend information relevant to the decision (2) deliberate about the choices in accordance with personal values and goals and (3) communicate (verbally or nonverbally) with caregivers (Hastings Center, 1987).

A surrogate decision-maker is a person designated by the patient, a court-appointed person, or the patient's closest available relative. The surrogate should be guided by the patient's own desires and feelings to the extent they were expressed before the patient became incompetent or by the patient's best interest.

The Self-Determination Act of 1990 mandates that healthcare facilities inform patients about living wills and/or durable powers of attorney for health care. The process is simple and requires no legal assistance. The Self-Determination Act is further discussed in chapter 9.

Granting durable power of attorney for health care is the preferred method for patients to establish their wishes in advance. A power of attorney enables patients to grant decision-making authority about health-related matters to someone they trust in the event they become incompetent.

In the case in which no surrogate has been designated or a conflict arises in the question of life support, the bioethics committee can be used to evaluate and perhaps comply with a family's request to withhold or to provide enteral therapy. If this fails, judicial direction may be sought by the facility.

Because a large percentage of patients in the long-term care environment are on nutritional support, current and future legal cases will have a profound bearing on policies and procedures within skilled nursing facilities. Although it is not advisable for a facility to solicit a decision on whether a patient wishes to be given life-sustaining proce-

dures in the event they are needed, the facility should advise on the process of obtaining the appropriate legal document. Documentation of these wishes must be done according to state guidelines and then be kept available to the staff members who provide care to that resident.

Because of the prospective payment system based on diagnosis-related groups, residents admitted to skilled nursing facilities are sicker and require more advanced medical technologies. It is clear that the changing environment of long-term care demands a formulation of bioethical procedures. Each facility must develop a policy on the withholding or withdrawing of life-sustaining procedures, adhering to both state mandates and the wishes of the resident.

EXAM QUESTIONS

CHAPTER 7
Questions 61–70

61. Which of the following types of medication can be crushed and administered through an enteral feeding tube?

    a. Compressed tablets

    b. Enteric-coated tablets

    c. Slow-release compounds

    d. Sublingual tablets

62. The primary goal of a feeding program is to

    a. increase the patient's level of independence.

    b. simplify feeding for the nursing staff.

    c. shorten the length of feeding time.

    d. meet regulatory requirements.

63. The primary goal in the treatment of type 2 diabetes mellitus is

    a frequent exercise.

    b. normalization of blood glucose and lipids.

    c. elimination of the need for insulin.

    d. achievement and maintenance of normal weight.

64. Which of the following is the best way to prevent osteoporosis?

    a. Ensure adequate fluid intake.

    b. Engage in moderate, routine endurance exercise throughout one's lifetime.

    c. Eat a variety of foods.

    d. Maintain normal weight for height and age.

65. The item frequently overlooked in the diets of the elderly is

    a. protein.

    b. vitamins.

    c. water.

    d. carbohydrate.

66. The recommendation for the amount of daily fluid consumption by elderly individuals is:

    a. 500 to 1,000 cc per day.

    b. 1,000 to 1,500 cc per day.

    c. 1,200 to 1,500 cc per day.

    d. 1,500 to 2,500 cc per day.

67. Which of the following is most important in the prevention of pressure ulcers?

    a. Independence in feeding

    b. Vitamin C intake

    c. Frequent repositioning

    d. Low body weight

68. What is the most frequently used enteral feeding product in the elderly?

    a. Hyperosmolar formula

    b. Isotonic, lactose-free formula

    c. Blenderized food

    d. Carnation Instant Breakfast

69. Total body water decreases to what percentage of total body mass in older adults more than 65 year of age?

    a. 70%

    b. 50%

    c. 65%

    d. 60%

70. Which of the following laboratory tests is the best measure of protein status?

    a. Serum albumin levels

    b. Serum transferrin levels

    c. Mean corpuscular volume

    d. Hemoglobin levels

CHAPTER 8

DEMENTIA

by

Doris Bower RN, ANP, & Kim Butrum RN, MS, GNP

CHAPTER OBJECTIVE

After studying this chapter, the reader will comprehend that dementia is a disease and not a part of normal aging. The reader also will be able to develop a comprehensive care plan for a patient with Alzheimer's disease.

LEARNING OBJECTIVES

After studying this chapter, the reader will be able to:

1. Specify risk factors for Alzheimer's disease and vascular dementia.

2. Recognize pathological changes in the brain that are the hallmark of Alzheimer's disease.

3. Indicate changes in activities of daily living, function, and mental status that occur in Alzheimer's disease.

4. Specify the four steps in assessing psychotropic medication need in the management of problem behaviors.

5. Define *catastrophic reaction*.

6. Indicate the key concept in providing a therapeutic milieu for patients with Alzheimer's disease.

7. Recognize appropriate techniques to enhance communication with cognitively impaired patients.

8. Differentiate between the two behavioral techniques used to manage functional incontinence in demented patients.

9. Recognize the usual side-effect profiles of the psychotropic medications, that is, neuroleptics, antidepressants, and sedative-hypnotics.

10. Specify resources and legal issues involving the demented patients and their caregivers.

INTRODUCTION

Epidemiology

It has been called the "graying of America." Thanks to improved living conditions and modern medicine, we are all living longer. The number of persons in the United States over age 65 changed from 3.1 million in 1900 to 31.1 million in 1990, a tenfold increase. According to the U.S. Bureau of the Census, the number of persons 65 years and over could more than double by 2050, to nearly 69 million. About 1 in 8 Americans were elderly in 1990, but by the year 2030, that figure will rise to about 1 in 5 (U.S. Bureau of the Census, 1996). In the community-dwelling population over age 65, the prevalence of dementia ranges from 10% to 50%. More than 50% of nursing home patients have a dementing illness. The most common causes of dementia are Alzheimer's disease and strokes, accounting for 66% of the cases (Fretwell, 1997). Unless cures or a means of prevention are found, the number of cases is expected to rise along with life expectancy and the increased duration of illness.

Definition

Is dementia part of normal aging? Our thought processes and reflexes do slow down as we get older. It takes longer to learn new material, and there may be some forgetfulness looking for keys, glasses. But this is not dementia. Dementia is a loss of intellectual abilities of sufficient severity to interfere with occupational or social functioning.

Although loss of recent memory is the outstanding feature, the term dementia implies global impairment of mental functions. The signs and symptoms can include (1) impairment in abstract thinking; (2) impaired judgment; and (3) disturbances of higher cortical function, such as aphasia (disorder of language) and apraxia (inability to carry out motor activities despite intact comprehension and motor function, that is, difficulty in using objects correctly, such as brushing one's hair or dressing). Agnosia, loss of perception powers (visual, auditory, tactile) may occur with failure to recognize or identify objects despite intact sensory function. Personality changes may also occur; the clinical picture is sometimes complicated by the presence of significant depressive features or delusions (American Psychiatric Association [APA], 1994).

Dementia is different from mental retardation because it indicates a loss of previous abilities. Dementia differs from delirium because delirium is associated with diminished attention or temporary confusion. Delirium implies a transient loss of mental abilities. In dementia, the person is alert and the signs and symptoms are relatively stable. However, delirium and dementia may coexist (APA, 1994).

Primary degenerative dementia of the Alzheimer's type is the most common form of dementia, found in 50–60% of all cases (Burns,

Howard & Pettit, 1995; Berkow, et al., 1995). Other degenerative diseases causing dementia include Pick's disease, Huntington's chorea, Parkinson's disease (not all cases), and amyotrophic lateral sclerosis (not all cases). Age is a risk factor, with prevalence of disease increasing with age. For example, at age 70, the probability of becoming demented is approximately 1.2%; at age 80, the probability is 5.2% (Burns et al., 1995).

Other risk factors for Alzheimer's disease include family history in some cases. Also, patients with Down's syndrome who survive past age 40 often have similar pathological changes in the brain as patients with Alzheimer's disease have a greater risk (Burns et al, 1995). The risk of Alzheimer's disease developing is increased fourfold to fivefold among first-degree relatives of Alzheimer's probands. The occurrence of many cases of Alzheimer's disease in several generations is consistent with autosomal dominant inheritance; however, most cases occur sporadically. Down's syndrome patients who survive past the age of 40 almost invariably have plaques, tangles, and a loss of choline acetyltransferase in the neocortex and hippocampus, with the same distribution as that in typical patients with Alzheimer's disease. They also have the same abnormal amyloid protein. This protein, found on chromosome 21 (called trisomy 21), is found in the cells of patients with Down's syndrome and has been established as a marker for this disease. It may also be a marker for familial Alzheimer's disease. It should be noted that although at this time there is a small percentage of families in which Alzheimer's disease appears to have an autosomal dominant inheritance, in the larger population of Alzheimer's patients, there is no genetic connection. At this time, there is no blood test or skin biopsy that will tell us if a person does indeed have Alzheimer's disease. The only way to establish that diagnosis is by brain biopsy, and because there is no cure available, the risk of biopsy is not warranted.

Head injury with loss of consciousness is a risk factor for Alzheimer's disease. Systemic diseases such as hypothyroidism and vitamin B12 deficiency may also cause dementia. Thus it is important to get a thorough history to preclude a patient's being labeled with Alzheimer's disease when in fact the patient may have something that is treatable or reversible.

Dementia caused by disease of the blood vessels (vascular or multi-infarct dementia) accounts for the second largest number of cases, 15%. This includes lacunes (smaller infarcts) and cerebral embolic disease (fat, air thrombus fragments). Risk factors for multi-infarct dementia include cardiac arrhythmias, hypertension, cardiovascular disease, rheumatic heart disease, stroke, and transient ischemic attacks. A combination of Alzheimer's disease and multi-infarct disease is found in 0.6% of demented patients (Terry, 1988).

Table 8-1 shows diseases that are manifested as dementia; some are treatable, and others are irreversible. These include dementia due to anoxia, trauma, and infections. *Table 8-2* gives reversible causes of dementia. Diseases that can simulate dementia are psychiatric disorders, mainly depression, anxiety, psychosis, and sensory deprivation. Drug-induced dementias can be caused by medications that affect the central nervous system, namely tranquilizers, antihypertensives, and drugs with anticholinergic side effects (Terry, 1988).

PATHOLOGY OF ALZHEIMER'S DISEASE

The first case of Alzheimer's disease was described by the German physician, Alois Alzheimer, in 1906, when a 55-year-old woman with progressive dementia was found at autopsy to have senile plaques and neurofibrillary tangles. These physical changes in the brain have been recognized since as the hallmark of Alzheimer's disease. On electron microscopy, the neurofibrillary tangles consist of double helical twisted tubes; the senile plaques consist of a degenerated amyloid center and surrounding neurofibrillary tangles. Similar but less abundant senile plaques and neurofibrillary tangles may be seen in healthy elderly persons and in some other disease entities (Burns et al., 1995). *Figures 8-1–8-6* illustrate the pathologic changes that occur in Alzheimer's disease (Gwyther, 1985).

Also in Alzheimer's disease, recent studies have shown that there is a reduction of choline acetyltransferase in the brain, a 50–90% decrease; somatostatin may also be decreased, frequently as much as 50% (Burns et al., 1995). Choline and somatostatin are neurotransmitters that act as messengers between neurons. Neurotransmitter loss appears to be a consequence rather than a cause of the disease; as various cells die, they lose their ability to produce normal quantities of neurotransmitter compounds. Certain drug studies have been aimed at increasing the availability of acetylcholine in the brain.

Early onset of familial Alzheimer's disease has been linked with genes on chromosomes 14 and 21 (Mullan, Crawford, & Axelman, 1992). Researchers believe later onset familial Alzheimer's disease may be linked to a gene on chromosome 19 (Strittmatter et al., 1993).

Recent research studies in Alzheimer's disease have concentrated on the areas of biochemistry and anatomy, methods of diagnosis, genetics, viral disorders, pharmacology, and physiology. Also, studies have looked at memory, language, and perception as they relate to Alzheimer's. Nutrition and vitamin therapy have been scrutinized as well. Work with neurotransmitters and drug therapy have shown progress using various substances such as Vitamin E at post-synaptic receptor sites (Ebersole & Hess, 1998). Recent studies have demonstrated how beta and tau amyloid proteins relate to early

TABLE 8-1
Diseases Presenting as Dementia

Alzheimer disease
　　With or without vascular disease
　　With or without Parkinson disease
　　With or without other dementing diseases
Other irreversible dementias
Degenerative diseases
　　Pick disease
　　Huntington disease
　　Progressive supranuclear palsy
　　Parkinson disease
　　Cerebellar degenerations
　　Amyotrophic lateral sclerosis (ALS)
　　Parkinson—ALS—dementia complex of Guam
　　　　and New Guinea
　　Rare genetic and metabolic diseases
　　　　(Hallervorden-Spatz, Kuf, Wilson, late-
　　　　onset metachromatic leukodystrophy,
　　　　adrenoleukodystrophy)
Vascular dementias
　　Multi-infarct dementia
　　Cortical microinfarcts
　　Lacunar dementia
　　Binswanger disease
　　Cerebral embolism by fat or air
Anoxic dementia
　　Cardiac arrest
　　Cardiac failure (severe)
　　Carbon monoxide
Traumatic
　　Dementia pugilistica (boxer's dementia)
　　Head injuries (open or closed)
Infections
　　Acquired immunodeficiency syndrome (AIDS)
　　AIDS dementia
　　Opportunistic infections
　　Creutzfeldt-Jakob disease (subacute spongiform
　　　　encephalopathy)

　　Progressive multifocal leukoencephalopathy
　　Postencephalitic dementia
　　Behçet syndrome
Treatable dementias
Infections
　　Herpes encephalitis
　　Fungal meningitis or encephalitis
　　Bacterial meningitis or encephalitis
　　Parasitic encephalitis
　　Brain abscess
　　Neurosyphilis (general paresis)
Normal-pressure hydrocephalus (communicating
　　hydrocephalus of adults)
Space-occupying lesions
　　Chronic or acute subdural hematoma
　　Primary brain tumor
　　Metastatic tumors (carcinoma, leukemia, lym-
　　　　phoma, sarcoma)
Multiple sclerosis (some cases)
Autoimmune disorders
　　Disseminated lupus erythematosus
　　Vasculitis
Toxic dementia
　　Alcohol dementia
　　Metallic poisons (e.g., lead, mercury, arsenic,
　　　　manganese)
　　Organic poisons (e.g., solvents, some
　　　　insecticides)
Other disorders
　　Epilepsy
　　Concentration camp syndrome
　　Whipple disease
　　Heat stroke

Note: Many of these disorders produce dementia in
　　a small percentage of patients (e.g., epilepsy,
　　tumors).

Source: Advances in Diagnosis of Dementia

TABLE 8-2
Reversible Causes of Dementia

Psychiatric disorders
    Depression
    Sensory deprivation
    Other psychoses

Drugs
    Sedatives
    Hypnotics
    Antianxiety agents
    Antidepressants
    Antiarrhythmics
    Antihypertensives
    Anticonvulsants
    Digitalis and derivatives
    Drugs with anticholinergic side effects
    Other (mechanism unknown)

Nutritional disorders
    Pellagra (vitamin B_6 deficiency)
    Thiamine deficiency (Wernicke syndrome,
        acute phase treatable)

Cobalamin (vitamin B_{12}) deficiency or perni-
    cious anemia
Folate deficiency
Marchiafava-Bignami disease

Metabolic disorders
    Hyper-and hypothyroidism (thyroid hormones)
    Hypercalcemia (calcium)
    Hyper-and hyponatremia (sodium)
    Hypoglycemia (glucose)
    Hyperlipidemia (lipids)
    Hypercapnia (carbon dioxide)
    Kidney failure
    Liver failure
    Cushing syndrome
    Addison disease
    Hypopituitarism
    Remote effect of carcinoma

Note: Most of these disorders produce dementia in
only a small percentage of cases.

Source: Advances in Diagnosis of Dementia

---

and late onset Alzheimer's. Studies in 1997 suggested a link between herpes simplex virus and the formation of neurofibrillary tangles and plaque seen in Alzheimer's disease (LaVoie, 1997). In 1996 Ying developed a theory related to a harmful network of factors that may form the key components of Alzheimer's. These include free radical damage, abnormalities of calcium homeostasis, and alterations in amyloid precursor protein metabolism. Although there are promising theories and research, no consensus has been reached to explain the complex set of symptoms for families and individuals affected by Alzheimer's (Ebersole & Hess, 1998).

EVALUATION OF DEMENTIA: MAKING THE DIAGNOSIS

History of Onset

Again, as in other diseases, getting an accurate history will be essential in making a diagnosis of dementia. The history should be obtained without the patient present, so the informant will be free to express the patient's deficits and behavior without embarrassment to the patient. The history of onset is of utmost importance: Was it gradual, insidious, and progressive, which is typical of Alzheimer's disease, or was it abrupt, with a stepwise progression of signs and symptoms, which would be typical of multi-infarct

FIGURE 8-1. Normal human brain.

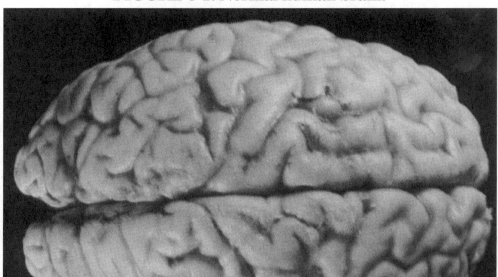

FIGURE 8-2. Brain of patient with Alzheimer's disease. Note atrophic surface area lost by decrease in gyri and deeper, wider sulci.

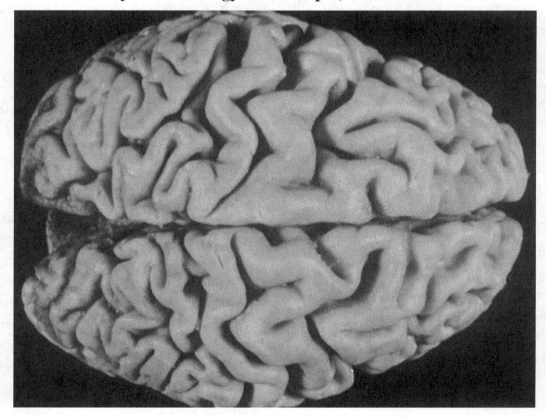

Slides courtesy of Duke University Medical Center, Durham, NC.

FIGURE 8-3. Normal brain section.

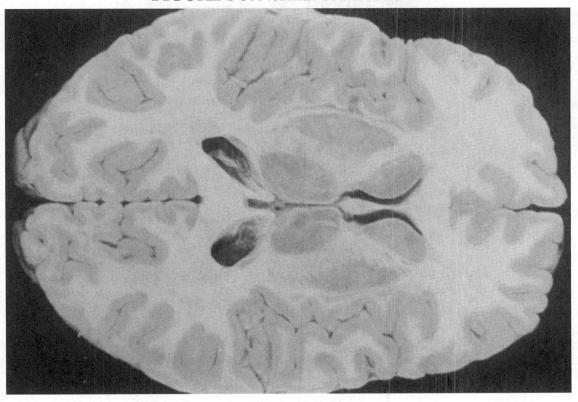

FIGURE 8-4.
Brain section of patient with Alzheimer's disease showing enlarged ventricles.

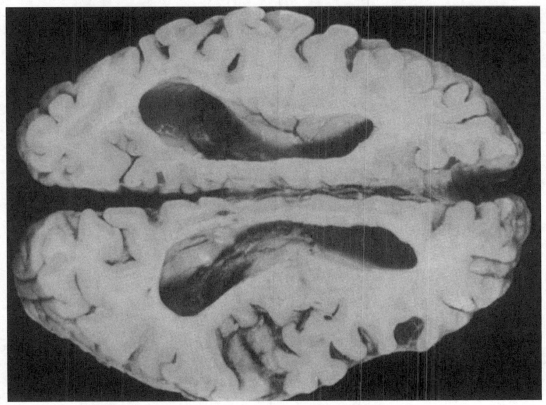

Slides courtesy of Duke University Medical Center, Durham, NC.

FIGURE 8-5. Normal neurons.

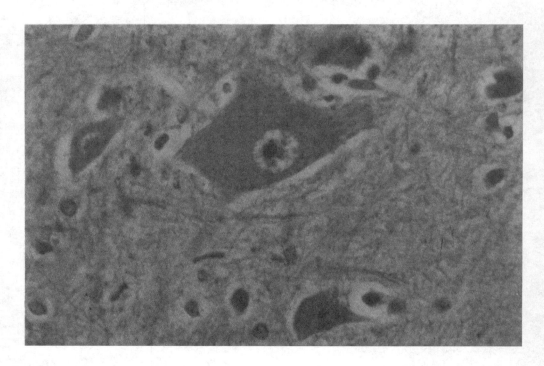

FIGURE 8-6. Abnormal neurons. Inside are neurofibers in paired helixes.

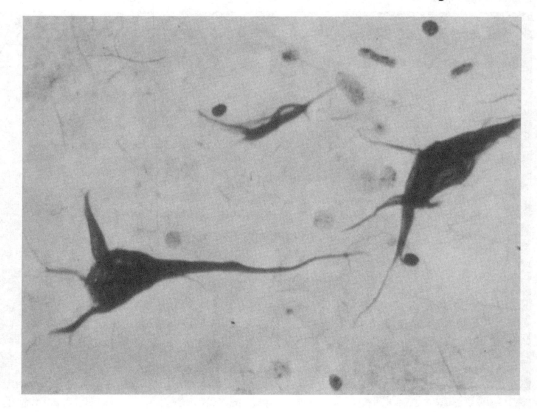

Slides courtesy of Duke University Medical Center, Durham, NC.

or vascular dementia? Was there a decline in day-to-day intellectual functioning such as remembering appointments, or managing finances? Has there been a change in activities of daily living, with the patient needing help bathing, dressing, toileting, or grooming? Does the patient have word-finding problems? Does the patient wander? Has the patient gotten lost? Each person is different, so the onset of signs and symptoms varies accordingly.

Medical History

The medical history is helpful in making the diagnosis in dementia because certain diseases may predispose patients to vascular or multi-infarct dementia. A history of hypertension may point to strokes. Has there been an incident of a transient ischemic attack (TIA) or a stroke? Does the patient manifest signs of a stroke, weakness on one side of the body or facial drooping? Is there evidence of cardiovascular disease such as bruits, murmurs, arrhythmias? Patients with a history of rheumatic heart disease and arrhythmias are more at risk for multi-infarct disease because of emboli that may be discharged to the brain. Is there a history of diabetes? Diabetic patients are more prone to cardiovascular disease and will be more at risk for multi-infarct dementia. Systemic diseases such as hypothyroidism and vitamin B$_{12}$ deficiency may also cause dementia. Obtaining a thorough medical history is essential in making a differential diagnosis.

Current medications should be reviewed for possibly contributing to deficits, namely beta-blockers, tranquilizers, antipsychotic medications, antihypertensive medications, and over-the-counter drugs such as antihistamines. Polypharmacy is not uncommon in older patients, and all medications should be assessed. Have the caregiver bring in all medications so you can check the dosages and dates (Ives, 1997).

Nutritional status should also be checked. Is the patient eating an adequate diet? Does he or she have a low income and seem unable to afford basic needs? A diet deficient in calories, vitamins, iron, and other minerals can contribute to a confused mental state. Is the patient unable to shop for himself or herself? A home visit is useful to assess what food supplies are available. Also the patient may have poorly-fitting dentures or sensory losses that discourage eating or inhibit food preparation. Is the patient able to cook? Perhaps the patient is now alone because of the death of a spouse who formerly did the cooking and is unable to manage in the kitchen. Asking the patient or the patient's caregiver to keep a food-intake diary and bring it in for evaluation is helpful.

A history of alcohol abuse may indicate that the memory problems are due to excessive alcohol consumption rather than Alzheimer's disease. In these patients, memory is the most affected of cognitive functions; it may be accompanied by frontal lobe dysfunction with loss of inhibitions. The prognosis for this patient is different, so this knowledge will be helpful to the family.

Family history should be examined to determine if other members had or have Alzheimer's disease and whether there is a history of Down's syndrome. Also, it should be ascertained whether there is a family history of alcohol abuse and affective disorder (major depression), as these tend to run in families also.

Examination of the Patient

Because social skills may be maintained by demented patients, it is important that an in-depth mental status test be done. You may not realize how impaired a patient is until you start asking specific questions that assess the patient's orientation and memory. Some physicians might shrug off the patient's impairment as normal aging because the patient presents himself or herself in an intact manner. It is not until one has checked the mental status that a judgment can be made as to the degree of impairment. It is helpful in planning a patient's care.

TABLE 8-3
Six-Item Orientation Memory Concentration Test

	Error	Score	Weighted Score
1. What year is it now?	1	×4	_____
2. What month is it now?	1	×3	_____
Give memory phrase: "Repeat this phrase after me: John Brown, 42 Market St., Chicago." (Repeat twice)			
3. About what time is it? (within an hour)	1	×3	_____
4 Count backward 20 to 1.	2	×2	_____
5. Say the months in reverse order.	2	×2	_____
6. Repeat the memory phrase.	5	×2	_____

Score 1 for each incorrect response. Maximum weighted score: 28.
Scoring: 0–10 indicates mild impairment.
10–20 indicates moderate impairment.
20–28 indicates severe impairment.

Source: Katzman, R. & Terry, R.D. (1983). *The neurology of aging.* Philadelphia: F.A. Davis.

The Six-Item Orientation Memory Concentration Test is short and will give an indication of the level of impairment (Katzman, & Terry, 1983) *(Table 8-3).*

Physical and Neurological Examination

The physical examination should focus on the cardiovascular system to rule out multi-infarct dementia. Check for the presence of heart murmurs, bruits, arrhythmias, and hypertension. The neurological examination should focus on the mental status of the patient, level of consciousness, symmetry of coordination and reflexes, movement disorders (e.g., tremor of Parkinson's disease or gait disorder), motor function, and sensory perception. It is important to ascertain whether hearing and/or vision are impaired, as deficits in these areas could be contributing to the patient's confusion.

Psychometric testing may be ordered to learn more about the patient. Sophisticated neuropsychological tests are used to assess attention, abstraction, problem-solving, motor, verbal, perceptual/constructional, memory, and orientation skills. The results of these tests are helpful in making a differential diagnosis; they map out the different areas of the brain and indicate where deficits may originate.

The Hachinski Ischemia Score is a useful tool for summarizing key clinical characteristics for making a differential diagnosis between Alzheimer's disease and multi-infarct dementia (Rosen et al., 1980) *(Table 8-4).*

Diagnostic Tests

Laboratory tests used in the evaluation of dementia include blood tests, urinalysis, electrocardiography (ECG), electroencephalography (EEG), and computed tomography (CT) or magnetic resonance imaging (MRI). The complete blood cell count will measure anemia, infection; the sedimentation rate will be helpful to rule out temporal arteritis or tumors that may underlie the problem. Blood chemistry tests indicate pulmonary, renal, and endocrine function. If a person is confused, it

---

TABLE 8-4
Rosen Modified Hachinski Ischemic Score

Characteristic	Point Score
Abrupt onset	2
Stepwise deterioration	1
Somatic complaints	1
Emotional incontinence	1
History of hypertension	1
History of strokes	2
Focal neurological symptoms	2
Focal neurological signs	2

A score of 4 or more is consistent with multi-infarct dementia.

Source: Rosen, W. et. al., (1980). Pathological verification of ischemia score in differentiation of dementia. *Annals of Neurology, 7,* 486–488.

---

may be secondary to electrolyte imbalance and not organic damage. Measurements of the levels of T4 and thyroid-stimulating hormone are important to rule out thyroid dysfunction, as low thyroid function can cause mental slowness. Vitamin B12 and folate tests are ordered to rule out pernicious anemia and folate deficiency. Serological tests are done for syphilis. Urinalysis is used to screen for infection, kidney disease; where indicated, screening for heavy metals may be done for environmental or occupational exposure. If there is a condition that is treatable, in some cases the dementia may be reversed.

ECG is done to ascertain whether there is an arrhythmia or history of a myocardial infarct. Persons with atrial fibrillation are at increased risk for embolism, which could cause multi-infarct dementia. Myocardial infarct has been named as a risk factor for Alzheimer's disease. EEG is sometimes done to rule out a focal process, such as a tumor or epilepsy.

It is imperative that CT or MRI be done to provide a picture of the brain. Atrophy or shrinkage is the hallmark of Alzheimer's disease. Increased ventricle size may point to normal-pressure hydrocephalus (NPH); early indications are unsteady gait and urinary incontinence. Normal pressure hydrocephalus, if diagnosed early, may respond to surgical shunting. Multi-infarct or vascular dementia will show radiolucencies and infarcts on imaging. (See pictures of normal brain and brain of patient with Alzheimer's disease, *Figures 8-1* through *8-4*; Gwyther, 1985).

The importance of a comprehensive workup early in the course of the disease cannot be overemphasized, for once patients have been labeled demented, they may never again be evaluated.

Tables 8-5 and *8-6* list the APA diagnostic criteria (1994) for Alzheimer's disease and vascular dementia.

Checking for Depression

A psychiatric evaluation may be useful to rule out depression. The patient may be so depressed that he or she does not concentrate and therefore cannot remember. Older persons often suffer many losses: loss of a spouse, loss of a job and earning power with retirement, loss of health, perhaps loss of a driver's license because of impaired vision or hearing. Coping mechanisms may be inadequate to deal with these losses and depression follows. Depressive disorders are currently the most com-

---

TABLE 8-5
Diagnostic Criteria for Dementia of the Alzheimer's Type

A. The development of multiple cognitive deficits manifested by both
    1. memory impairment (impaired ability to learn new information or to recall previously learned information)
    2. one (or more) of the following cognitive disturbances:
        a. aphasia (language disturbance)
        b. apraxia (impaired ability to carry out motor activities despite intact motor function)
        c. agnosia (failure to recognize or identify objects despite intact sensory function)
        d. disturbance in executive functioning (i.e. planning, organizing, sequencing, abstracting)
B. The cognitive deficits in Criteria A1 and A2 each cause significant impairment in social or occupational functioning and represent a significant decline from a previous level of functioning.
C. The course is characterized by gradual onset and continuing cognitive decline.
D. The cognitive deficits in Criteria A1 and A2 are not due to any of the following:
    1. other central nervous system conditions that cause progressive deficits in memory and cognition (e.g. cerebrovascular disease, Parkinson's disease, Huntington's disease, subdural hematoma, normal-pressure hydrocephalus, brain tumor).
    2. systemic conditions that are know to cause dementia (e.g. hypothyroidism, vitamin B12 or folic acid deficiency, niacin deficiency, hypercalcemia, neurosyphilis, HIV infection)
    3. substance-induced conditions
E. The deficits do not occur exclusively during the course of a delirium.
F. The disturbance is not better accounted for by another Axis I disorder (e.g., Major Depressive Disorder, Schizophrenia).

Reprinted with permission from (DSM-IV) *Diagnostic and statistical manual of mental disorders (4th ed.).* Washington, DC, American Psychiatric Association, 1994.

---

mon psychopathological syndrome afflicting the elderly (Barraclough, 1997).

For Mrs. McC., age 48, Alzheimer's disease was diagnosed after she experienced difficulties performing her office job; she was forgetful about appointments, was slow, and made errors. She had a family history of Alzheimer's disease. When she approached her physician about her problems, he told her that she had early Alzheimer's disease. She was then referred to a research program studying dementia, where it was found that she had depression, not dementia. With antidepressant therapy, she is back on the job, functioning at a high level, and needless to say relieved that she does not have Alzheimer's disease.

THE STAGES OF ALZHEIMER'S DISEASE

When we picture a patient with Alzheimer's disease, the mind may conjure up an image of a person completely "out of it," babbling incoherently, restless, agitated, or withdrawn and totally incapable of caring for himself or herself. This picture is the stereotypic image of the so-called senile patient, a person with dementia. Is this accurate to the diagnosis of Alzheimer's disease? Or are there other pictures that might more accurately portray the disease? The truth is that there are as many different pictures as there are patients with the illness. It is not like measles or mumps, with predictable signs, symp-

---

TABLE 8-6
Diagnostic Criteria for Vascular Dementia

A. The development of multiple cognitive deficits manifested by both
   1. memory impairment (impaired ability to learn new information or to recall previously learned information)
   2. one (or more) of the following cognitive disturbances.
      a. aphasia (language disturbance)
      b. apraxia (impaired ability to carry out motor activities despite intact motor function)
      c. agnosia (failure to recognize or identify objects despite intact sensory function)
      d. disturbance in executive functioning (i.e. planning, organizing, sequencing, abstracting)
B. The cognitive deficits in Criteria A1 and A2 each cause significant impairment in social or occupational functioning and represent a significant decline from a previous level of functioning.
C. Focal neurological signs and symptoms (e.g. exaggeration of deep tendon reflexes, extensor plantar response, pseudobulbar palsy, gait abnormalities, weakness of an extremity) or laboratory evidence indicative of cerebrovascular disease (e.g. multiple infarctions involving cortex and underlying white matter) that are judged to be etiologically related to the disturbance.
D. The deficits do not occur exclusively during the course of a delirium.

Reprinted with permission from (DSM-IV) *Diagnostic and statistical manual of mental disorders (4th ed.).* Washington, DC, American Psychiatric Association, 1994.

---

toms, and outcome. Each patient has a unique "data base," so consequently Alzheimer's disease strikes each person in a different manner. True, the brain in Alzheimer's disease will show loss of neurons and atrophy in all cases. However, in some patients, that loss may first be manifested as problems with speech, such as word-finding problems, difficulty in expression. Another person may have visual or spatial difficulties such as problems using the stove or dressing. Still another may have difficulties with calculations but have totally intact speech and motor skills. Each person is different in the manner in which the disease manifests itself.

It is important to always remember that the disease is different in each person. Second, there are definite stages of Alzheimer's disease. The course is gradually progressive, and the stages may overlap. In rare cases, the disease progresses very rapidly to a terminal conclusion within a year or less, but that is unusual. The first stage is one of mild impairment, usually lasting 2–4 years, leading up to and including the diagnosis. The second stage is one of moderate impairment and may last 2–10

years after the diagnosis; this is the longest stage. The third stage is one of severe impairment; it is terminal and lasts 1–3 years, with the patient dying from complications such as pneumonia and urinary tract infection (Scharre & Cummings, 1998).

The onset of Alzheimer's disease is insidious and may creep up so gradually that it may be sometime before one realizes there is a problem. Older persons in whom the disease is more prevalent often live highly structured lives and are able to function without noticeable decline in their intellectual abilities. Quite often, the first thing that might be noticed is repetitive questions asking for the same information given perhaps 5 or 15 min earlier and promptly forgetting the answer. Failure to keep appointments is another early sign. Difficulty in cooking may also be an early indication of dementia. Mrs. J. was an excellent cook; now she takes forever to prepare a simple meal and then may forget a course. Burned pots may be a frequent occurrence (Gwyther, 1985).

Word-finding problems may present early or later on in the course of the disease; this may include forgetting the names of objects (anomia). There may be problems with the checkbook, forgetting to pay bills, paying bills twice, difficulty with calculations and balancing the checkbook. Mrs. B., a former bank teller, is unable to do simple addition or subtraction but still maintains her social skills and is able to do all other activities of daily living without help. Poor judgment may also be the first indicator that something is wrong: Mr. W. withdrew his money from the bank to invest in trust deeds he had seen advertised and consequently was defrauded of his savings. Mrs. Z., who formerly had taught bridge, is unable to play; she has forgotten the rules of the game and cannot remember cards that were played.

Quite often, apathy occurs with the onset of memory problems, a loss of interest in things previously enjoyed or less social involvement. Perhaps the person with memory problems realizes he or she is having difficulties and wishes to protect himself or herself from embarrassing situations. With this may come mood and personality changes, anxiety, irritability, and withdrawal.

In a mildly impaired person, dementia is often not diagnosed until the family realizes the problem is more than benign forgetfulness. Remember, the definition of dementia calls for impairment not only in memory but also in some other area of cognition such as judgment, abstract thinking, aphasia (speech), apraxia (motor skills), and/or agnosia (sensory loss in spite of an intact sensory system). In a person with memory loss only, the diagnosis is an amnestic syndrome; this may not be progressive (APA, 1994).

In an Alzheimer's patient, as the loss of neurons increases, the disease progresses to the second or moderately impaired stage. This is the longest stage, lasting from 2–10 years. In this stage, the person becomes more confused and disoriented. He or she will increasingly need help with activities of daily living, help with dressing, grooming,

and bathing. Mrs. R. was previously fastidious about her appearance. Now she has to be reminded to bathe and change her clothes and feels insulted when asked to do so. She may have decreased motor skills and be unable to button her blouse. She may put her underclothes on top of her slacks. She may go to bed in her street clothes. Her grooming suffers, and she needs reminding to brush her teeth, file her nails, comb her hair. She may not be incontinent, but she may forget to wipe herself after urinating or defecating. Bladder infections are quite common at this stage of illness.

The moderately impaired patient may experience increasing difficulty with motor activities and visual and perceptual problems. He or she may have trouble getting into a chair, climbing up steps, cutting up food. Wandering and pacing are common as the patient becomes more demented. Mrs. V. spends much of the day looking for her deceased mother. Restlessness and agitation often increase in the late afternoon and at night; this behavior is called *sundowning.* Auditory and/or visual hallucinations may occur; however, these may be illusions rather than real hallucinations due to misinterpreted visual or auditory stimuli. Suspicions and delusions often occur. Mrs. E. hides her jewelry in a safe place; she is convinced the neighbor next door is watching her and will steal her valuables if she does not hide them. When she cannot find the well-hidden jewelry, she accuses this neighbor or someone else of taking her things. Word-finding problems may increase along with difficulty in reading and writing. Repetitive statements and movements increase. Lack of recognition of family members may occur; the husband may tell his spouse he is waiting for his wife to come home.

Again, no two patients are alike. Some patients may need close supervision right from the onset of memory loss, as they may be a danger to themselves or to others.

In the terminal stage, patients are unable to recognize family or even themselves in the mirror. They are unable to communicate with words. There is urinary and fecal incontinence. There is weight loss even with a good diet. There is increased difficulty with swallowing; the patient may forget how to chew, forget that he or she has food in his mouth, forget to swallow. Aspiration is common. The patient is now completely dependent on others for self-care, feeding, dressing, bathing, and toileting. Skin breakdown and urinary tract infections, dehydration, and electrolyte imbalance are all sequelae of impaired skills in activities of daily living. Myoclonic jerks and seizures may occur. It is during this period that institutionalization often takes place (Gwyther, 1985; Stolley & Buckwalter, 1992).

TREATMENT OPTIONS

Unfortunately there is no treatment at this time for Alzheimer's disease. Consequently, care is supportive and should take into account the patient's changing level of performance.

Acetylcholinesterase inhibitors are currently the only approved drugs for the treatment of Alzheimer's disease. Tacrine (Cognex) and donepezil (Aricept) have demonstrated effectiveness in improving cognitive deficits (Scharre & Cummings, 1998). When treated in the early or middle stages of the disease, individuals show modest growth in cognitive abilities and functional activities. Common adverse side effects are nausea, vomiting and diarrhea.

Dementia secondary to HBP, if diagnosed early, may respond to a shunting procedure to reduce intracranial pressure. Multi-infarct dementia has no specific treatment. The best treatment may be prevention of further infarcts with long-term control of hypertension.

Other dementias such as endocrine/metabolic disorders and vitamin deficiencies (B12, folate) can be treated with possible arrest of cognitive impairment if treatment is initiated early in the course of the disorder (Scharres & Cummings, 1998). The use of antipsychotics to treat or manage the symptoms of dementia is not recommended unless psychotic symptoms cannot be managed behaviorally.

COMMUNITY RESOURCES

An increased public awareness of Alzheimer's disease and related disorders has brought about the formation of adult day care centers. These are day treatment facilities, some of which provide intensive medical, physical, or occupational therapy. Others provide primarily social activities and personal services for several hours during the day. Regionally, some units of the Area Agency on Aging (AAA) sponsor adult day care in some areas. Private day care is also available, with supervision and activities geared to the demented patient.

Support groups are sponsored by the Alzheimer's Association and community agencies. These offer family caregivers the opportunity to informally share their experiences with others. Caregiving classes are sponsored by the AAA and some local hospitals.

Respite care is available through registries of home health agencies providing homemakers, companions, and home health aides. In Southern California, the Southern Caregiver Resource Center offers grants and referrals for in-home respite. Currently, the regional resource centers in California are funded by the State Department of Mental Health and offer information and referral services, caregiver training classes, legal referrals and consultation, and counseling for the caregiver. Adult day care programs provide primary respite care in the sense that they offer caregivers time off while the patient attends a supervised, stimulating day program.

Crisis and problem-solving assistance is offered by county mental health programs. Currently in San Diego County there is a Senior Crisis Team with a 24-hr hotline. Adult protective services are available through the AAA. The AAA is an excellent resource in locating services such as home care, respite care, transportation, and telephone reassurance. Low-income persons may be eligible for Supplemental Social Security income, a federal program that makes monthly payments to the aged, disabled, and blind with incomes below federal standards. Individual states may supplement the federal benefit to cover specific groups, such as those in board-and-care facilities, and may also cover services such as home care and homemaker services.

The majority of long-term care is still delivered outside nursing homes in board-and-care homes or in the patient's home. Special Alzheimer's disease units are being promoted by some nursing homes. The bulk of informal care is delivered first by the spouse, then by children.

Research is being conducted by several centers funded by the National Institutes of Health and the National Institute for Mental Health.

Information and referral numbers include the following:

Alzheimer's Association National Clearing House
1-800-621-0379
Elder Abuse Hot Line
1-800-523-6444

Books that are helpful in educating the caregiver include the following:

- *When Your Loved One Has Alzheimer's: A Caregiver's Guide,* by David L. Carroll. New York: Harper & Row, 1989.

- *Understanding Alzheimer's Disease: What It Is, How to Cope with It, Future Directions,* edited by Miriam K. Aronson. Charles Scribner's, 1988.

- *The Loss of Self: A Family Resource for the Care of Alzheimer's Disease and Related Disorders,* by Donna Cohen, and Carl Eisdorfer. New York: NAL Penguin, 1986.

- *Care of Alzheimer's Patients: Manual for Nursing Home Staff,* by Lisa Gwyther. American Health Care Association and Alzheimer's Disease and Related Disorders Association, 1985.

- *Alzheimer's Disease: A Guide for Families,* by Lenore Powell and Katie Courtice. New York: Addison-Wesley, 1983.

- *Dementia: A Practical Guide to Alzheimer's Disease and Related Illnesses,* by Leonard L. Heston and June A. White. New York: W. H. Freeman, 1983.

- *A Guide to Alzheimer's Disease: For Families, Spouses, and Friends,* by Barry Reisberg. New York: The Free Press, 1983.

- *The Thirty-Six Hour Day: A Family Guide to Caring for Persons with Alzheimer's Disease, Related Dementing Illnesses and Memory Losses in Late Life,* by Nancy Mace and Peter Rabins (rev' ed). Baltimore: Johns Hopkins Press, 1991.

- *The Vanishing Mind: A Practical Guide to Alzheimer's Disease and Other Dementias,* by Leonard Heston & June White. New York: WH Freeman, 1991.

- *Understanding Difficult Behaviors: Some Practical Suggestions for Coping with Alzheimer's Disease and Related Illnesses,* by Anne Robinson, Beth Spencer, and Laurie White. Ypsilanti, MI: Eastern Michigan University, 1987.

- *When Bad Things Happen to Good People,* by Harold S. Kushner. New York: Schocken Books, 1981.

LEGAL ISSUES

As the disease progresses, the person with dementia will be unable, legally, to make decisions regarding medical care. Therefore, early in the course of the disease, the patient and his or her family should consider taking legal action to provide a trusted person with the authority to make any necessary decisions for the patient. Two legal devices are commonly used for this: the durable power of attorney for healthcare and conservatorship of the person. The living will previously used does not stand up in court in many states (Aronson, 1988).

Durable Power of Attorney for Healthcare

The durable power of attorney for healthcare enables one person to give another person legal authority to make medical decisions on the first person's behalf in the event of incapacity. Modern medical science can keep a patient alive long after the quality of life has deteriorated. For this reason, many persons request that extraordinary means and measures not be used to prolong their lives. The durable power of attorney for healthcare expresses the person's wishes concerning the use of life-prolonging care and treatment, such as electrical or mechanical resuscitation of the heart when it has stopped beating, the use of nasogastric or gastrostomy tubes for hydration or nutrition, a mechanical respirator for assisted breathing, and dialysis in renal failure. The durable power of attorney for healthcare allows one to specify ahead of time how one wants decisions made (Aronson, 1988).

Again, it is important that these decisions be executed while the patient is mildly impaired; he or she must be awake, alert, oriented, and legally competent to sign the document. The extent of the durable power of attorney is limited to 7 years unless the patient has become incapacitated at the end of 7 years, during which time the power of attorney continues to be valid or *durable*.

Conservatorship

Conservatorship of the person is a legal procedure that allows the conservator to assume control over a completely incapacitated individual. The conservator is responsible for making sure the conservatee is properly fed, clothed, and housed. A court hearing is required before a conservator can be appointed. Conservatorship provides an incapacitated person with as much legal protection, through court involvement, as possible. On the other hand, conservatorship can incur high and continuous legal fees, increase demands on the judicial system, and offer no guarantee that decisions always will be made in the best interests of the incompetent person or in keeping with that person's desires (Aronson, 1988).

CONSIDERING PHARMA-COLOGICAL TREATMENT

In patients with Alzheimer's disease, behavioral manifestations develop marking the degenerative changes that are occurring in the brain. It is the nurse who attempts to structure the environment to prevent problem behaviors, attempts non-pharmacological management of the behaviors when they do occur, and both assesses the patient and reports the behavior to the physician when pharmacological treatment is needed. It is vital therefore that nurses understand how to adequately assess the need for psychotropic medications.

In order to understand what pharmacological agent is appropriate for use in a cognitively impaired patient, the first step is to determine the target sign or symptom one is trying to extinguish. This not only helps prevent the inappropriate use and overuse of psychotropic medications, but also provides a standard from which to assess the effectiveness of the treatment.

The second step is to ensure that the behavior the patient is demonstrating is due to the patient's

---

TABLE 8-7

Diagnostic Criteria for Delirium Due to…(Indicate the General Medical Condition)

A. Disturbance of consciousness (i.e., reduced clarity of awareness of the environment) with reduced ability to focus, sustain, or shift attention.

B. A change in cognition (such as memory deficit, disorientation, language disturbance) or the development of a perceptual disturbance that is not better accounted for by a preexisting, established, or evolving dementia.

C. The disturbance develops over a short period of time (usually hours to days) and tends to fluctuate during the course of the day.

D. There is evidence from the history, physical examination, or laboratory findings that the disturbance is caused by the direct physiological consequences of a general medical condition.

Reprinted with permission from (DSM-IV) *Diagnostic and statistical manual of mental disorders (4th ed.).* Washington, DC: American Psychiatric Association, 1994.

---

brain disease and that any other potential causes of the behavior have been ruled out. The classic example of this is a demented patient who suddenly becomes agitated and strikes out and is later found to have an impaction or be dehydrated or suffering from some other acute medical condition. Delirium or acute confusional state is an organic psychiatric syndrome with an acute onset that causes impairment in cognition, perception, and behavior (Foreman, Fletcher & Mion, 1996). *Tables 8-7* through *8-9* list the APA's DSM-IV diagnostic criteria for delirium related to a medical condition, substance intoxication (included medications), and multiple causes (APA, 1994). Patients with a dementing illness run a higher risk for development of an overlying delirium. Therefore, any time an Alzheimer's patient shows a new behavior or change in status, one must consider the possibility that an acute delirium related to a medical condition is the cause before trying to treat the behavior with a pharmacological agent. Agitation associated with a patient's urinary tract infection requires antibiotic treatment, not a psychotropic medication. If the underlying medical condition causing the delirium is corrected early, the patient's cognitive functioning will improve.

The third step in deciding the appropriate psychotropic medication to use in a demented patient

is to understand the side-effect profile of each agent in light of the patient's other medical problems and health history. One usually picks a particular psychotropic medication by determining the side-effect profile the patient would best be able to tolerate.

The last thing to remember in the use of psychotropic medications in the patient with dementia is constantly to assess and reassess the patient's need for that particular medication at that particular dose. Alzheimer's is not a static disease. The patient shows a gradual but continually declining course. For example, early in the disease there may be a coexistent depression, because the patient is aware of his or her loss of cognitive power. As the disease progresses and the patient's self-awareness wanes, the attendant depression may clear. With the development of worsening anomia and the inability to express needs, agitation may become the major problem. Agnosia and the patient's tendency to misinterpret stimuli and situations can cause paranoia and suspiciousness. Therefore, a cognitively impaired patient on a psychotropic medication needs frequent reassessment of the need for that medication. This is even more important in light of the serious side effects that can develop with these agents. Used appropriately in judicious amounts, psychotropic medications can make a remarkable

---

TABLE 8-8
Diagnostic Criteria for Substance Intoxication Delirium

A. Disturbance of consciousness (i.e. reduced clarity of awareness of the environment) with reduced ability to focus, sustain, or shift attention.

B. A change in cognition (such as memory deficit, disorientation, language disturbance) or the development of a perceptual disturbance that is not better accounted for by a preexisting, established, or evolving dementia.

C. The disturbance develops over a short period of time (usually hours to days) and tends to fluctuate during the course of the day.

D. There is evidence from the history, physical examination, or laboratory findings of either 1 or 2:

    1. The symptoms in Criteria A and B developed during Substance Intoxication.

    2. Medication use is etiologically related to the disturbance.*

*Note: The diagnosis should be recorded as Substance-Induced Delirium if related to medication use.

Reprinted with permission from (DSM-IV) *Diagnostic and statistical manual of mental disorders (4th ed.).* Washington, DC: American Psychiatric Association, 1994.

---

difference in the quality of life for both demented patients and the patients' caregivers; however, used without a good initial assessment and frequent evaluation, these agents can cause a significant amount of morbidity in and of themselves.

THERAPEUTIC INTERACTION

Therapeutic interaction is the cornerstone of an effective, comprehensive care plan for a patient with Alzheimer's disease. A patient with dementia picks up on the stress, fatigue, and emotions the caregiver displays and cannot tolerate multiple distractions within the environment. Therefore, clear communication from a calm, unhurried caregiver within a consistent environment is vital to nursing management of a cognitively impaired patient.

Catastrophic reaction denotes when a patient's reaction to a stimulus is overblown and inappropriate for that particular situation (Hall & Buckwalter, 1987). A patient who is having a catastrophic reaction can display behaviors ranging from anger and combativeness to sadness, stubbornness, and with-

drawal. It is felt that catastrophic reactions occur in Alzheimer's disease patients when a situation overwhelms the patients' ability to handle stress (Hall & Buckwalter, 1987).

According to Hall (1991), the person with Alzheimer's disease has a diminished capacity to manage stress, and this capacity decreases even more as the disease progresses (Hall & Buckwalter, 1987). There are five causes of catastrophic reactions: (1) fatigue; (2) change of caregiver, routine, or environment; (3) multiple competing stimuli; (4) demands to achieve beyond capabilities; and (5) physiological stressors such as elimination needs or infection.

Interventions to prevent catastrophic behaviors are then targeted toward these five areas (Hall, 1991; Hall & Buckwalter, 1987; Stolley & Buckwalter, 1992; Rader, 1995). Rest periods each morning and afternoon are essential to reduce anxious behavior to more normative and relaxed behavior. Caffeine is eliminated. As much as possible, the person with dementia should have stability in routine, caregiver, and environment. The caregiver acts as a "prosthetic memory device" for the demented person who has lost his or her memory,

---

TABLE 8-9
Diagnostic criteria for Delirium Due to Multiple Etiologies

A. Disturbance of consciousness (i.e., reduced clarity of awareness of the environment) with reduced ability to focus, sustain, or shift attention.

B. A change in cognition (such as memory deficit, disorientation, language disturbance) or the development of a perceptual disturbance that is not better accounted for by a preexisting, established, or evolving dementia.

C. The disturbance develops over a short period of time (usually hours to days) and tends to fluctuate during the course of the day.

D. There is evidence from the history, physical examination, or laboratory findings that the delirium has more than one etiology (e.g., more than one etiological general medical condition, a general medical condition plus Substance Intoxication or medication side effect).

Reprinted with permission from (DSM-IV) *Diagnostic and statistical manual of mental disorders* (4th ed.). Washington, DC: American Psychiatric Association, 1994.

---

and the structure provides security to one who cannot remember. Eliminate multiple competing stimuli by monitoring or eliminating television or radio, eliminating large crowds or rooms, monitoring music, and using good communication techniques. Alternate highly stimulating with low-stimulating activities and evaluate behavior afterwards. Evaluate the patient to determine his or her capabilities and expect only what he or she is able to do at that moment. The patient may well be aware of lost abilities, and it can be overwhelming to be prodded to perform tasks he or she is no longer able to do. Finally, look for physiological causes of catastrophic reactions: stool impaction, urinary retention, pain, infections, etc. A simple intervention of taking a demented person to the bathroom at regular intervals can eliminate anxiety and dysfunctional behavior (Hall, 1991; Hall & Buckwalter, 1987; Stolley & Buckwalter, 1992; Rader, 1995).

Some specific techniques used to enhance communication and prevent problem behaviors include the following:

*   Approach the patient from the front, establishing eye contact, speaking slowly, and using short sentences and simple words.

*   Ask yes/no questions. An open-ended question is difficult to answer for a cognitively impaired patient.

*   Repeat, restate, and paraphrase as needed to help the patient understand.

*   Speak literally in concrete terms. Abstract thought is difficult for a demented patient to interpret.

*   Break down directions or tasks into simple steps, and cue the patient as needed at each step.

*   Refrain from arguing with the patient. If the patient tells you something that is untrue, use distraction and redirection instead.

Distraction and redirection are effective techniques to use in working with cognitively impaired patients. One of the benefits of a short-term memory deficit is that as a patient becomes upset or agitated over a particular situation, the caregiver can often distract the patient from that situation and redirect focus to a less upsetting subject.

It is appropriate to say a word here about *reality orientation*. This refers to a technique designed to decrease confusion and disorientation in the confused elderly. It consists of reorienting the patient to basic information on a consistent basis.

Environmental cues are used to assist in the orienting process (Hall, 1991; Hall & Buckwalter, 1987; Stolley & Buckwalter, 1992).

Although reality orientation is an appropriate process for an elderly patient temporarily confused because of an acute confusional state or a patient with Alzheimer's disease with mild cognitive impairment who is seeking information to help orient himself or herself; it is not appropriate in all cases. The goal of reality orientation is to correct the patient's misperceptions of the environment. Because of the physiological changes in the brain, Alzheimer's disease patients have lost the ability to think in the abstract, reason, and correctly interpret stimuli; therefore they have a different perception of reality. If a nurse continues to force reality on a demented patient who is too impaired to understand, a catastrophic reaction will likely ensue.

For caregivers, it is easy to forget that patients may not be able to interpret correctly the environmental cues being used to attempt orientation. For example, while walking a patient to activities, a nurse attempts to orient a demented patient, saying, "Mrs. B., you are 84 years old and live here at San Diego Nursing Facility." Mrs. B. begins to get agitated, insisting, "I'm 34 and live in New York." The nurse then walks her over to a mirror and says, "You can see you are not 34; you are 84." The patient then becomes more upset, convinced that the face she sees in the mirror is an imposter. This situation will easily escalate, with the patient interpreting incorrectly from an impaired frame of reference whatever information is presented. A catastrophic reaction then develops, with the patient becoming upset and refusing to attend activities. In this particular situation, when the patient began to get agitated and insisted she was younger and living in New York, the nurse should have changed tactics from orienting the patient to distracting and redirecting, saying something non-threatening such as, "I've heard New York is an incredible place; I'd love to visit someday. It sure gets cold in the winter, though." As the nurse is disengaging from the potential catastrophic reaction, she continues walking the patient to activities and prevents the situation from getting out of control. The nurse's comments allow the patient to respond if there are intact remote memories of New York, yet do not require the patient to answer.

Reality orientation is *not* an appropriate technique to use in working with the chronically demented elderly. The person can be oriented to reality on an informal basis through environmental cues or conversations such as, "It's really cold for October." *Validation* is more appropriate for demented persons. In validation therapy, the caregiver enters the demented person's reality, avoids confronting delusions or hallucinations, uses reminiscence, listens carefully for meaning, and provides reassurance of safety (Feil, 1984, 1994).

GENERAL SIDE EFFECTS OF PSYCHOTROPIC MEDICATIONS

There are four general areas of side effects with psychotropic medications:

1. Anticholinergic effects
2. Orthostatic hypotension
3. Level of sedation
4. Extrapyramidal symptoms

Patients with Alzheimer's disease lose a significant number of the cholinergic cells in their brain; additionally, there is diminished activity of choline acetyltransferase. These changes give the patient with Alzheimer's disease an increased sensitivity to the anticholinergic side effects of many of the psychotropic medications (Ray et al., 1993). Anticholinergic delirium, which is a frequent cause of increased confusion in elderly demented patients, can result.

The peripheral anticholinergic side effects are dry mouth, constipation, urinary retention, blurred vision, tachycardia, and dry skin and mucous membranes. Anticholinergic effects on the central nervous system can cause delirium, with symptoms including agitation, anxiety, disorientation, restlessness, assaultiveness, hallucinations, and paranoia.

A patient with Alzheimer's disease suffering from an anticholinergic delirium will appear to have worsening behavior. It is possible that the care providers may mistakenly increase the patient's dose of psychotropic medication to extinguish the behavior, when the patient actually needs a reduction in the number of medications with anticholinergic side effects. Pharmacological agents with significant anticholinergic effects therefore are used cautiously in patients with Alzheimer's disease.

Orthostatic hypotension is defined as a drop of 20mm Hg or more in the patient's blood pressure when the patient stands up. Orthostatic hypotension can be dangerous for the elderly, because it can lead to falls and associated injuries. For detection of orthostatic hypotension, the patient lies flat for 3 min. The blood pressure is then taken with the patient supine and then again immediately after the patient stands up. The elderly are at risk for orthostatic hypotension even without psychotropic treatment because of underlying atherosclerosis causing rigidity of the blood vessel walls; the body therefore takes longer to compensate for position changes. Nursing actions appropriate for patients with orthostatic hypotension include monitoring for symptoms of dizziness or falls and teaching the following safety precautions both to the patient and the patient's caregiver: Make changes in position slowly. Arise slowly from bed in several stages. From a lying position, sit at the side of the bed with the legs dangling over the side for a few moments to allow the blood pressure to stabilize before you stand up.

The degree of sedation an agent causes is also considered in choosing a psychotropic drug. If the patient needs energy and already has psychomotor retardation, then a less sedating agent would be appropriate. For highly anxious and hypervigilant patients, a more sedating agent might be a better choice.

PSYCHOSES

As Alzheimer's disease patients lose their ability to orient themselves, reason, correctly interpret their surroundings, and think logically, psychotic signs and symptoms can develop. Those usually associated with Alzheimer's disease include wandering, restlessness, agitation, paranoia, hallucinations, delusions, belligerence, and unprovoked outbursts of rage. The behavioral techniques outlined previously can help reduce the severity and frequency of these; however, the Alzheimer's disease patient *may* require a neuroleptic medication at some point to help control psychotic symptoms (Stolley & Buckwalter, 1992). These medications should be used as a last resort, however, and only after all other interventions have failed. There is little evidence that neuroleptics control behavioral symptoms of Alzheimer's disease.

Of the psychotic symptoms listed, one that is difficult for nurses to assess is agitation. In Alzheimer's disease, there is an agitation that accompanies the disorganized thought process. However, in a patient who is unable to express his or her needs, agitation can have many other possible causes. It can be a sign of fatigue; a catastrophic reaction to an overwhelming situation; a response to physical illness or pain; or the agitated restlessness of akathisia, an extrapyrimidal side effect of the neuroleptics. The symptoms the nurse observes can be the same in each of these cases; however, because of the different causes, each case would be treated in a different manner. This

TABLE 8-10
Relative Incidence of Side Effects of Neuroleptic Drugs

Generic name	Trade name	Approximate dosage range mg/day	Sedation	Hypotension	Extrapyramidal symptoms	Anticholinergic symptoms
Chlorpromazine	Thorazine Chlor PZ	10–300	Marked	Marked	Moderate	Marked
Chlorprothixene	Taractan	10–300	Marked	Marked	Moderate	Marked
Thiordazine	Mellaril	10–300	Marked	Marked	Mild-moderate	Moderate
Acetophenazine	Tindal	10–60	Moderate	Moderate	Moderate	Moderate
Perphenazine	Trilafon	4–32	Moderate	Moderate	Moderate	Moderate
Loxapine	Loxitane	5–100	Moderate	Moderate	Moderate	Moderate
Molindone	Moban	5–100	Moderate	Moderate	Moderate	Moderate
Trifluperazine	Stelazine	4–20	Moderate	Moderate	Moderate-marked	Moderate-mild
Thiothixene	Navane	4–20	Moderate	Moderate	Moderate-marked	Moderate-mild
Fluphenazine	Prolixin	0.25–6	Mild	Mild	Marked	Mild
Haloperidol	Haldol	0.25–6	Mild	Mild	Marked	Mild
Risperidone	Risperdal	1–4	Mild	Mild	Moderate	Marked
Olanzapine	Zyprexa	5–10	Mild	Mild	Mild	Mild

Adapted from: *Clinical geriatric psychopharmocology.* New York. Carl Salzman, McGraw-Hill, 1984.

requires that the nurse carefully assess agitation in any cognitively impaired patient.

In an elderly demented patient with psychotic symptoms, very low, consistent doses of the major tranquilizers are used. The antipsychotic medications are also known as major tranquilizers or neuroleptics. These medications have some significant, irreversible side effects; therefore, they should only be used to manage specific symptoms for which other interventions are not effective.

Table 8-10 lists the frequently used antipsychotics and their side-effect profiles. The side effects of concern with the neuroleptics include level of sedation, anticholinergic effects, potential for orthostatic hypotension, and extrapyramidal syndromes.

Extrapyramidal syndromes are a side effect of neuroleptic treatment. The three extrapyramidal syndromes that are most common in the elderly are parkinsonism, akathisia, and tardive dyskinesia (Ray et al., 1993).

Parkinsonism consists of bradykinesia, muscular rigidity, stooped posture, shuffling gait, masked facies, tremor, and drooling. These parkinsonian side effects occur during the first few months of treatment and then usually resolve over several months as tolerance develops (Ray et al., 1993).

Akathisia is an extrapyramidal syndrome that consists of motor restlessness and pacing. The patient has a subjective feeling of anxiety with an inability to sit still and a pressured need to move. Because akathisia can make it seem that the patient's psychotic symptoms are worsening, it can be mistakenly treated by increasing the dose of neuroleptics. This is wrong, however; when akathisia occurs, the dosage of the antipsychotic medication should be reduced.

Tardive dyskinesia is an involuntary, primarily oral- facial movement disorder. It consists of sudden movements of the tongue known as the "fly-catcher syndrome," lip smacking, lip puckering, and facial grimacing. It may be accompanied by rolling chorea movements of the arms and trunk

(Perry, Alexander, & Liskow, 1991). This frequently irreversible side effect of the neuroleptics is not only disfiguring but can also significantly interfere with the patient's ability to eat and drink. The elderly seem to be more sensitive to this effect; it develops more frequently and at smaller doses than in the young (Perry et al., 1991). Tardive dyskinesia can be reversible if detected early; therefore nurses working with patients under treatment for psychotic symptoms need to assess frequently for its early signs. These include rhythmic, wavelike movements of the tongue; mild, chorieform movements of the fingers or toes; and facial tics or frequent eye blinking (Perry et al., 1991). If any of these develops, consideration should be given to reduction of the dose or discontinuation of the neuroleptic.

DEPRESSION

The relationship between dementia and depression is a complex one. However, depression and dementia frequently coexist. It has been postulated that depression in an elderly patient is a potential early sign of an underlying dementia (Ham, 1997).

In the early stages of Alzheimer's disease, the patient is aware of cognitive losses, even while denying it to others. Additionally, once the diagnosis is made and the patient is aware of the poor prognosis, a clinical depression may develop. Because the signs and symptoms of depression in an elderly patient mimic those found in Alzheimer's disease, it can be difficult to determine if depression coexists with the patient's dementia. For this reason, any Alzheimer's disease patient who has depressive symptoms such as feelings of worthlessness, sleep or appetite disorders, or decreased energy deserves a cautious antidepressant trial (Barraclough, 1997). It must be remembered that it takes 2–4 weeks to see any therapeutic effect with antidepressant treatment, so a trial of 1

week's duration is not adequate, and neither is as needed usage.

As with other psychotropic medications, antidepressants are chosen for a particular patient according to the patient's side-effect profile. *Table 8-11* lists the frequently used antidepressants and their side-effect profiles. Each agent is evaluated in terms of its degree of anticholinergic, orthostatic hypotension, sedation, and cardiovascular effects.

The primary cardiovascular effect that the antidepressants can cause is slowing of cardiac conduction. Other than in patients with severe conduction abnormalities, however, it is now felt that most elderly patients with heart disease can be managed on antidepressants, with periodic assessment of their cardiovascular status and occasional ECGs (Fitten, 1998).

The interaction between depression and Alzheimer's disease has not been completely elucidated. Therefore, if after a full antidepressant trial the patient shows no improvement in depressive symptoms, the medication should be discontinued.

The relationship between multi-infarct dementia and depression is more clear, however, as 30–60% of stroke patients become clinically depressed following stroke. The depressive symptoms have been shown to respond to pharmacological treatment (Mosqueda & Brummel-Smith, 1997). In these patients, then, antidepressants can dramatically improve quality of life and assist in any necessary rehabilitation.

SLEEP DISTURBANCES

Cognitively impaired patients have all the potential causes for sleep disturbance that any elderly patient has, namely, anxiety, depression, pain, discomfort, and medication side effects. Additionally, as their dementia progresses, they will often acquire disrupted sleep patterns simply as a result of their brain disease. This prob-

---

TABLE 8-11
Common Side Effects Of Selected Antidepressants In Elderly Persons

Antidepressant	Anticholernigic Effects	Sedation	Blood Pressure Changes	Altered Heart Rate
Tricyclics				
Amitryptiline	Very Strong	Strong	Strong	Strong
Imipramine	Strong	Mild	Moderate	Moderate
Nortryptiline	Moderate	Mild	Mild	Mild
Desipramine	Mild	Mild	Mild	Mild
SSRI & SSNI				
(Selective Serotonin Reuptake Inhibitor & Serotonin Norepinephrine Reuptake Inhibitor)				
Fluoxetine	—	—	—	—
Sertraline	—	—	—	—
Paroxetine	—	Mild	—	—
Venlafaxine	Mild	Mild	Mild	Mild
Trazolopyridine				
Trazodone	Mild	Moderate	Moderate	Mild
Nefazodone	Mild	Mild	Mild	—

Adapted from: Fitten, L. J. Common psychiatric disorders. In *Practical Ambulatory Geriatrics*, 1998.

---

lem becomes especially difficult when the caregiver is unable to get the sleep needed to be restored and continue in the caregiving role.

Assessment of a sleep disturbance requires that the problem first be adequately determined. Is the patient having trouble falling asleep, waking up intermittently throughout the night, or having early morning awakening? Next, all potential causes of the sleep disturbance other than the patient's dementia must be ruled out. Is there anything medical that could be causing it? Arthritic pain, urinary tract infection frequency, and leg cramps are all potential causes of disrupted sleep. In these cases, a mild analgesic will be much more effective than a sedative.

Other possible causes of sleep disturbance that should be sought out before treatment with medications include excessive caffeine intake, overstimulation, staying in bed for too long at night, overfatigue, strange surroundings, change in caregiver or routine, and lack of exercise. Therefore, before medication is considered for an Alzheimer's disease patient with a sleep disturbance, the patient should be put on a structured program: arising at the same time each day, getting adequate stimulation and exercise with short rest periods throughout the day, and going to bed at the same time each night.

As caregivers, nurses need to reassure patients and the patients' families about the changes that go along with normal aging, to allow for realistic expectations. Normal aging changes in sleep pattern include lengthening of the time it takes to fall asleep and more frequent interruptions in sleep (Eliopoulis, 1995).

The next step in assessing a sleep disturbance is to do a medication review. Many medications can contribute to sleep pattern disturbance by causing nightmares, more frequent awakenings, or a lighter depth of sleep.

Finally, the environment must be assessed. Is it conducive to rest, with a comfortable temperature, soft lighting, and a reduced noise level?

If the patient continues to manifest a sleep pattern disturbance after all other potential causes have been addressed, then medications can be tried. The benzodiazepines are the most frequently used sedative-hypnotics in the elderly; however, there are some special considerations when that elderly patient is demented. *Table 8-12* lists the benzodiazepines, their rate of onset, and duration of action. The side effects of the benzodiazepines can be generalized by duration-of-action categories.

For short term use in most older individuals bensodiazepines without active metabolites are the preferred choice. These include oxazepam (Serax), lorazepam (Ativan), and temazepam (Restoril). Another short-acting non-benzodiazepine currently used for sleep is zolpidem (Ambien). The long-acting agents, diazepam (Valium), tend to accumulate in the body, leading to daytime sedation and nocturnal restlessness (Singer, 1998).

In general, hypnotics are not very effective in treating the sleep disturbances of Alzheimer's disease and can cause increased confusion, ataxia, and disinhibition. The disinhibition is particularly worrisome, because further loosening of the patient's impulse control can lead to striking out and other outburst behavior.

If the patient is displaying any other problem behavior, a sedating psychotropic medication targeting that symptom should be considered. This would prevent having to treat with two medications and compounding the potential side effects. If psychotic symptoms are present, then one of the more sedating neuroleptics would be appropriate. If there are depressive symptoms, then one of the sedating antidepressants should be used.

Finally, we must remember that sleep disturbances are often a stage the patient passes through during the course of the disease. Sleeping medications should be periodically evaluated as to their continuing need.

INCONTINENCE

Both urinary and fecal incontinence may develop in the later stages of Alzheimer's disease. Although a complete review of the various causes of incontinence is beyond the scope of discussion here, it is important to understand that a demented patient has the same potential causes of urinary incontinence as any elderly patient, and before the incontinence is attributed to dementia, the patient deserves a full workup.

Toileting is a complex task. It requires the ability to sequence activity (undress, sit on the toilet, relax the sphincter), the ability to interpret the signal that one needs to urinate, and the ability to interpret that one is in the appropriate place to urinate.

The patient with Alzheimer's disease usually loses the ability to follow complex commands, making sequencing difficult. Agnosia can make the patient unable to interpret correctly both surroundings and the urge to void.

Once a patient with Alzheimer's disease has had a thorough evaluation and the incontinence has been attributed to brain impairment, the patient is categorized as functionally incontinent. Functional incontinence is "urinary leakage associated with the inability to toilet because of impairment of cognitive and/or physical functioning, psychological unwillingness or environmental barriers." (Kane et al., 1991).

Many of the behavioral therapies used to manage functional incontinence cannot be used with demented patients because of their difficulty in

TABLE 8-12
Comparison of Benzodiazepine Anxiolytic

Drug	Rate of Onset	Half-Life (h)	Active Metabolites	Half-Life of Metabolites (h)	Doses (mg/d) Adult	Doses (mg/d) Elderly	Route of Administration
Oxazepam (Serax)	Intermediate to slow	5–15	None	—	10–60	10–30	Oral
Lorazepam (Ativan)	Intermediate	10–20	None	—	1–4	0.5–4.0	Oral, IM, IV
Diazepam (Valium)	Fastest	26–53	Yes	36–200	5–30	2–10	Oral, IM, IV†
Chloriazepoxide HCl (Librium)	Intermediate	8–28	Yes	36–200	10–100	5–30	Oral, IM, IV†
Prazepam (Centrax)	Slow	30–200	Yes	36–200	20–60	10–15	Oral
Clorazepate dipotassium (Tranxene)	Fast	30–200	Yes	36–200	15–60	7.5–15	Oral
Alprazolam (Xanax)	Intermediate	6–15	Yes	—	0.25–2.0	0.125–0.5	Oral
Halazepam (Paxipam)	Intermediate to slow	14	Yes	36–200	20–120		Oral
Triazolam (Halcion)	Fast	2–5	—	—	0.25–0.5	0.25–0.5	Oral
Temazepram (Restoril)	Intermediate to slow	12–24	—	—	15–30	15–30	Oral

*Unknown; probably about the same as the parent drug.
†IM doses unreliably absorbed.

Adapted from: *Handbook for Geriatric Psychopharmocology.* Jenicke. 1985.

learning new material and an inability to adequately perceive and report symptoms. Functional incontinence due to Alzheimer's disease is therefore managed by having the caregiver perform the techniques necessary to prevent episodes of incontinence and keep the patient dry.

Scheduled or prompted voiding is one of these caregiver-dependent techniques. For prompted voiding, the caregiver toilets the patient at regular intervals, such as every 2 hr during the day and every 4 hr at night. Timed toileting is similar to prompted voiding, but rather than keep to a regular schedule, the caregiver adjusts the schedule on the basis of the patient's pattern of incontinent episodes and continent voidings. Positive reinforcement is offered for successes, and other techniques are used as needed to trigger voiding and assist in complete bladder emptying.

Environmental manipulation is another tool in preventing incontinent episodes and keeping the patient dry. A raised toilet seat can be useful for a demented patient who becomes fearful of sitting down. A picture of a toilet on the bathroom door can help cognitively impaired patients orient themselves.

The use of protective garments and incontinence pads can make a tremendous difference in a family's ability to manage a demented patient at home. Used appropriately they can restore a sense of dignity and freedom to an incontinent patient. Nurses needs to be aware of the variety of products available on the market, as it is often necessary to individualize the products to the particular patient. For example, some patients find the adult diapers demeaning and refuse to wear them; for these patients, the products that consist of a pad worn inside normal underwear (which comes in both male and female styles) may work better.

The caregiver responsible for a patient with Alzheimer's disease also needs to remember to keep the clothing simple. A demented patient may not be able to get out of complicated garments independently, but if clothing is simplified, toileting may be continued without assistance.

WANDERING

Wandering is frequently seen in the early and middle stages of Alzheimer's disease. As with agitation, incontinence, and sleep disturbance, it is important in patients who wander to have a full assessment of why the behavior is occurring. It may be a result of the brain disease; however, a demented patient may wander as a result of physical pain, hunger, need to use the bathroom, increased confusion from medications, or an infection. Before the wandering is attributed to brain disease, a thorough evaluation must be done.

Once the patient's medical status and environment have been assessed for any potential precipitating factors, the wandering may be attributed to brain disease.

Wandering can be understood as a form of "agenda behavior" (Rader, 1995). Nurses who interpret wandering as agenda behavior view it as developing out of the fear that comes from the patient's separation from the people and environment whereby he or she previously felt connected and comfortable. The patient participates in agenda behavior to recapture past feelings of security and belonging. Wandering can be either purposeful or purposeless, but in each case, it has meaning to the patient (Algase & Struble, 1992).

An example of this is a demented woman who is living in a nursing home and keeps trying to wander away, saying "I want to go home." When her family takes her home for a visit, she continues to try to wander away, saying "I want to go home." If this is viewed as agenda behavior, this patient does not want to go home but rather to go back to a time when she felt needed, connected, and had a sense of security, feelings that Alzheimer's disease strips from its victims.

If wandering is seen as a form of agenda behavior, then rather than thinking of physical and chemical restraints as interventions, care providers will attempt to find activities for patients to make the patient feel needed and reconnected to the world. Nurses manage the wandering by distracting the patient and redirecting focus to an activity that will enhance a feeling of security and reduce the sense of isolation.

The appropriate environment for a demented patient who consistently manifests brain disease by wandering is a special care unit that is either locked or secured. In this environment, the patient can safely pace and wander and does not require sedation or restraints. Additionally, all cognitively impaired patients who have a potential for wandering should be provided an identification bracelet (e.g., Medic-Alert), with the words memory impaired inscribed on it. This makes basic medical and identifying information available to anyone finding the patient.

DRIVING

Driving is an issue that must be addressed in any patient with Alzheimer's disease. It was shown by Tune and Lucas-Blaustein at Johns Hopkins (1990) that out of 72 Alzheimer's patients studied, 40% had been involved in at least one auto accident since their illness had begun. Driving is a complex task requiring an intact short-term memory, the ability to process various competing stimuli at the same time, and the ability to orient oneself in relation to other persons and objects in space. These abilities are lost with Alzheimer's disease and can be impaired early in its course, while the patient's social skills are still intact and there is much denial of the impairment on the patient's part.

To counter this problem, many states have now passed laws requiring physicians to report the names of patients with Alzheimer's disease or other related disorders. The department of motor vehicles then decides on an individual basis, and in light of the physician's recommendation, the most appropriate action. The patient may be asked to come in for a written examination, interview, or driving test. If the patient is found to be too impaired to drive, the license will be revoked. If it is believed the patient may still drive safely, he or she will be asked to return for retesting on a regular basis, such as every year.

For families in states that do not have a reporting requirement, the car should be made inoperable in some way if the patient will not comply with the request not to drive; for example, the distributor cap could be disconnected or a kill switch installed. The easiest way, of course, may simply be to sell the car so it does not serve as a constant reminder to the patient of his or her loss. A driver can then be obtained, or the money put toward taxi fares.

MEDICAL FOLLOW-UP

Patients with a cognitive impairment require close medical follow-up after the diagnosis of Alzheimer's disease has been made. The need to establish a baseline from which any new behavior can be judged is vital. A cognitively impaired patient who is unable to express needs because of anomia, aphasia, or dysphasia, and whose brain may not be able to interpret symptoms correctly because of agnosia, requires a healthcare practitioner who is familiar with the patient's base-

line to diagnose and treat appropriately any changes in health.

ALCOHOL AND MEDICATIONS

Cognitively impaired patients require someone to monitor their medication regimen. The brain of a demented patient lacks the reserve to handle further injury, making it more sensitive to agents that exert a central nervous system effect. For this reason it is recommended that patients with Alzheimer's disease not drink alcohol and that medications, both prescription and over-the-counter, be kept to a minimum.

New healthcare providers need to be informed when a patient has a cognitive impairment so in prescribing they can, whenever possible, use an agent with minimal central nervous system effects. More important, all the medications the patient is taking should be assessed on a regular basis as to their continuing need.

NOURISHMENT AND HYDRATION

Patients with Alzheimer's disease commonly lose weight. This weight loss is felt to be multifactoral; that is, the patient forgets to eat, cannot complete the task of eating without someone cueing at each step, has become much more active with increased movement, has difficulty swallowing, or has feeding apraxia; or perhaps it is due to some as yet unexplained change in metabolism caused by the physiological changes occurring in the brain.

Whatever the cause, weight loss and inadequate protein intake put demented patients at risk for skin breakdown, particularly in combination with urinary incontinence. Therefore, adequate nutrition becomes a problem both for individual caregivers and for institutions. High-protein supplements can be bought commercially or made at home. Making sure the patient actually drinks the supplement is vital. In some patients, an occasional sweet will stimulate the appetite.

Cognitively impaired patients are also at risk for dehydration. The elderly have a diminished thirst sensation, and a demented patient, may not correctly interpret the thirst signal when it does occur. Additionally he or she may not understand environmental cues that remind a person to drink, that is, water pitchers or glasses. Dehydration can lead to delirium and puts patients at high risk for stool impaction, respiratory and urinary infections, and medication side effects. Caregivers need to offer patients with Alzheimer's disease fluids on a regular basis (See Chapter 7 for further discussion of hydration and fluid requirements). A simple reminder to drink is not adequate. A demented patient may agree that he or she should be drinking fluids but may not be able to initiate the activity or perform the necessary sequencing to actually drink the fluids. The nurse must pour the water, hand the glass to the patient, and cue the patient at each step until swallowing is completed. Because of demented patients' high risk for dehydration, fluid restriction should not be used as a technique for managing incontinence in the cognitively impaired.

The nutrition and hydration management issues for the Alzheimer's disease patient require creativity and flexibility on the caregiver's part. Early in the disease, the patient needs easy-to-eat finger foods if apraxia is affecting the ability to use utensils. Eating alone or in a small group is better than eating in the chaos of a large dining room, which may precipitate a catastrophic reaction in some patients. If a patient coughs while eating, aspiration may be developing. Aspiration begins in Alzheimer's patients as the disease progresses. A speech or occupational therapist can teach the patient's family feeding techniques to prevent aspiration, including swallowing twice, checking for

food pouching, using thickened liquids, and using different textures and temperatures of food. A feeding syringe should never be used to feed a patient at risk for aspiration. Monitoring the weight of a demented patient will allow the caregiver to detect any weight loss early. The nurse must keep a high index of suspicion regarding a developing depression when weight loss occurs early in the disease.

HOME SAFETY

Patients with Alzheimer's disease are at high risk for injury around the home. Because a patient can have significant impairment in one area of cognition while maintaining social skills, the caregiver may not be aware of the degree of the patient's impairment. Impaired judgment can prevent the patient from knowing what to do in case of emergency, the short-term memory deficit can make the patient leave pots burning on the stove, and visual agnosia can cause the patient to misinterpret a poison as something safe to drink.

Because patients with Alzheimer's disease usually have difficulty learning new material, caregivers will have more success in changing the environment to make it safe than in changing the behavior of the patient. Prevention of injury is the goal of care. Locking away toxic substances and medications can prevent accidental poisonings. A cognitively impaired patient can overdose on prescribed medications by taking double doses; therefore a caregiver needs to oversee the medication dispensing.

Patients with Alzheimer's disease are subject to hallucinations, paranoia, and outbursts of rage, so guns and other potential weapons should be locked away for both caregivers' and patients' safety.

The Alzheimer's Association has helpful brochures on how to make the home environment safe. Home health nurses can do evaluations of home safety. Many healthcare agencies, such as the

Caregiver Resource Network in California, offer caregiver training, which can be a tremendous help in assisting the caregiver in understanding the patient's deficits and making the environmental changes necessary to keep the patient safe.

EXAM QUESTIONS

CHAPTER 8
Questions 71–80

71. Normal aging is characterized by

    a. memory loss.

    b. normal response time and reflexes.

    c. increased length of time to complete mental processing.

    d. inability to learn new material.

72. Risk factors for vascular dementia include

    a. hypothyroidism.

    b. hypertension.

    c. depression.

    d. use of drugs that affect the central nervous system.

73. The onset of Alzheimer's disease is which of the following?

    a. Preceded by a stroke.

    b. Gradual and insidious.

    c. The same in each person.

    d. Characterized by delirium and confusion.

74. Agnosia is defined as difficulty in

    a. language and speaking.

    b. performing motor functions.

    c. recognizing and identifying objects.

    d. naming objects.

75. Which of the following statements about the course of Alzheimer's disease is most accurate?

    a. It fluctuates in a stepwise progression.

    b. It is predictable in all patients.

    c. It progresses through mild, moderate, and severe impairment levels and usually lasts several years.

    d. It progresses quickly in most patients.

76. Which of the following conditions could cause delirium in a demented elderly patient?

    a. Impaction, urinary tract infection

    b. Dehydration, noisy environment

    c. Hunger, change in routine

    d. Thirst, emotional upset

77. Which of the following techniques will enhance therapeutic communication with cognitively impaired patient?

    a. Speaking in abstract terms

    b. Asking open-ended questions

    c. Breaking down directions into simple steps and cueing at each step as needed

    d. Correcting repetitively spoken information from the patient

78. The early signs of tardive dyskinesia that the nurse should monitor in any elderly patient receiving neuroleptics are:

    a. Tremor, shuffling gait.

    b. Wavelike tongue movements, movements of the toes and fingers.

    c. Facial tics or eye blinking, muscle weakness.

    d. Agitated restlessness, outburst behavior.

79. A nurse monitoring the effectiveness of an antidepressant trial would expect to see improvement in the patient's signs and symptoms after

    a. 3–5 days.

    b. 1–2 weeks.

    c. 2–4 weeks.

    d. 3 months.

80. Which of the following activities is appropriate for a nurse to offer demented patients as a response to wandering when the wandering is viewed as agenda behavior?

    a. Asking them to help the more frail patients to the dining room.

    b. Letting them pace in the hallway.

    c. Having them watch television.

    d. Orienting them to reality.

CHAPTER 9

DYING AND ETHICAL DECISION MAKING

by

Susan Johnson, RN, CNA, MS

CHAPTER OBJECTIVE

After studying this chapter, the reader will be able to recognize that dying is a normal part of life and many persons will have some choice about the time and manner of their dying.

LEARNING OBJECTIVES

After studying this chapter, the reader will be able to:

1. Specify ways persons cope with death.

2. Choose nursing interventions that can help patients in the process of dying.

3. Specify ethical considerations in making treatment decisions for older persons.

4. Indicate measures that enable persons to retain autonomy in the process of dying.

5. Specify possible contributing factors in suicide in the elderly.

6. Recognize elements of bereavement.

7. Specify nursing interventions to assist grieving persons.

INTRODUCTION

A message on a bumper sticker exhorted passers-by:

AGING-CONSIDER THE ALTERNATIVE

At present, the only existing alternative to aging is, of course, dying. Eventually, everyone will die. Currently, most persons in western industrialized cultures have difficulty accepting this simple but inescapable truth. Uncounted millions have been spent on medical research in an attempt to prevent illness and postpone death. The process of dying has been removed from common experience by the practice of putting sick persons in hospitals and nursing homes. Consequently, many persons today reach the time of their own death without ever having participated in helping anyone through the dying process. This unfamiliarity with death contributes to even more fear and anxiety surrounding the idea of dying.

Another reason for difficulties in dealing with death and dying in today's culture is the development of medical technology to the point that we often have the ability to keep a person's organs functioning after normally he or she would have died. This capability creates a whole array of ethical dilemmas surrounding the care of those who can no longer care for themselves or even breathe or maintain a heartbeat without the intervention of medical machines.

This chapter first discusses the experience of death, both from the point of view of the patient and the patient's family, and from the perspective of the nurse-caregiver. A discussion of ethical considerations surrounding decisions to treat or not to treat follows, including legal considerations and the protection of patients' autonomy. Next, the issue of suicide in the elderly is addressed. Finally, bereavement and nursing interventions for persons who are grieving are described.

THE EXPERIENCE OF DYING

Filmmaker Woody Allen said, "I don't mind dying. I just don't want to be there when it happens." With this statement, he pointed out that there are really two issues to deal with concerning death. One issue is the idea of not being a living person anymore. This idea has been a central component of all religions, and different religions have come up with very different explanations and consolations for this inevitable end of life. Any person who faces terminal illness has to deal with—or avoid—this issue. In *Man's Search for Meaning* (1984), Victor Frankl, a survivor of German concentration camps, describes the method by which some persons found the strength to survive the inhumane conditions. Frankl points out that "it is a peculiarity of man that he can only survive by looking to the future" and that his fellow prisoners were able to do this by finding meaning—not in life, which had become an insane horror—but in suffering and even in death. The concept of developing ego integrity, as described by Eric Ericson, also deals with the task of finding meaning in one's own unique life. Frankl goes on to say:

> In the past, nothing is irrevocably lost, but rather, on the contrary, everything is irrevocably stored and treasured. To be sure, people tend to see only the stubble fields of transitoriness but overlook and forget the full granaries of the past into which they have brought the harvest of their lives: the deeds done, the loves loved, and last but not least, the sufferings they have gone

through with courage and dignity.

> From this one may see that there is no reason to pity old people. Instead, young people should envy them. It is true that the old have no opportunities, no possibilities in the future, but they have more than that. Instead of possibilities in the future, they have realities in the past—the potentialities they have actualized, the meanings they have fulfilled, the values they have realized—and nothing and nobody can ever remove these assets from the past.

A study of the concerns of a group of elderly men dying at home found that the threat to self-esteem and uncertainty about life after death were only part of the critical issues they faced. The men surveyed were also concerned about their immediate physical well-being. Specifically, they were worried about physical pain and suffering and risk to personal safety (Fry, 1990).

Starting in the 1960s, Elizabeth Kubler-Ross (1969) began to write about the feelings that persons experience as they face their own approaching death. Kubler-Ross notes that in her workshops, where caregivers learn from the dying, "For the patient death itself is not the problem, but dying is feared because of the accompanying sense of hopelessness, helplessness, and isolation." Those who have the opportunity to talk about their fears find they are better able to cope with those fears. Schoene-Sieffert and Childress (1986) point out that failing to inform an adult patient of a terminal illness is a violation of the patient's right to make informed decisions, and telling a family member instead of the patient is actually a violation of the patient's right of confidentiality.

One lesson Kubler-Ross learned from the terminally ill was that they are all aware of the seriousness of their illness, but that when others do not speak of it, the ill person accepts the message that the subject is too painful. Patients who were not told of their illness knew of it anyway because of the inevitable changes in the behavior of the persons around them. They welcomed being given "permission" to speak of their reactions and concerns. Some physicians adopt a paternalistic attitude and refuse to tell patients who have a terminal illness about the illness because it might reduce the patients' hope. Actually such an action on the part of a caregiver only burdens the patients with maintaining an outward denial that robs them of an opportunity to deal with what they know is true. Patients need honesty, time to arrange their affairs, and time to work through their feelings. Refusing to acknowledge their fears and concerns may be temporarily more comfortable, but it leads in the end to panic and a sense of abandonment for the patient.

A second theme that Kubler-Ross found in the coping of terminally ill patients was the tenacity of hope. People will continue to hope for the miracle cure, for the remission, for the absence of pain. Kubler-Ross states that persons who were told of a terminal diagnosis *without* allowing a sense of hope "never quite reconciled themselves to the person who presented the news to them in this cruel manner" (Kubler-Ross, 1969). She also points out that this hope can actually be a form of denial, or an attempt to find meaning in suffering. One question that nurses can ask dying patients is, "What do you hope for?" The answer to this can indicate what the patient is thinking and feeling in regard to his or her terminal illness. The hopes can range from a hope for a miracle cure, to hope for absence of pain, to hope for loved ones to become reconciled, and many other choices along the way.

A third pattern in coping with anticipated death is described by Kubler-Ross as stages in the adaptation to dying. Kubler-Ross emphasizes that these stages are not absolute; a person may move back and forth between them, more than one stage may be operating at a given time, or a stage may be skipped. By understanding the stages as a flexible framework, caregivers can gain insight into why patients may be acting in a certain way.

The initial reaction of most to the news that they are dying is one of shock and disbelief. This stage, *denial,* helps to cushion the realization of approaching death. Persons will continue to use partial denial at any point in their coping if the reality of the situation is too much to bear. It is important for nurses to realize that patients use denial as a necessary defense: it enables patients to protect themselves from information that they cannot yet cope with. It is never a nurse's job to overcome a patient's denial, because denial is the patient's needed self-protection. It is equally important not to force patients into a social kind of denial—where they use denial because it is wished on them by a caregiver who feels uncomfortable confronting the issue. Also, it is important to realize that if a patient does not want to talk, this rejection is neither personal nor permanent. The patient may want to talk tomorrow. And the nurse who has not taken the rejection personally will be available for that patient to talk with. It is through listening to the patient that nurses and other caregivers can get the clues as to what the patient knows, wants to know, and wants to avoid for now.

Anger is the primary emotion of the next stage of coping with a terminal illness. Anger can be expressed directly at the unfairness of fate, or it can be displaced and become expressed as anger at persons in the patient's life. A dying person can become enraged at his or her caregivers for not caring enough, or for not caring in the right way. A patient who feels dependent on those caregivers or who fears abandonment has further conflicted feelings added to the anger at dying. Again, it is imperative that nurses not take angry expressions personally. By understanding the source of the anger, nurses can realize that it is not really directed at them, and can continue to understand and care for the patient rather than retreat into a self-protective and non-therapeutic shell.

Anger will sometimes be expressed as "Why me?" This question is not really a request for an answer to why a particular person has been struck with a disease. Rather, it should be seen as an expression of anger at the unfairness of fate. Some persons will attempt to answer the question with explanations of their past lives. Guilt and self-blame can lead to *depression.* The idea that our behavior or feelings are the reason for our "punishment" can lead to *bargaining.* Kubler-Ross describes the stages of bargaining and depression as stepping stones toward a final acceptance of dying.

Kubler-Ross describes two types of depression for persons facing terminal illness. The first kind, which she calls a *reactive* depression, is the result of the losses that an ill person has experienced. This kind of depression is the same as for persons who are going through other types of losses: loss of roles, loss of financial security and possessions, and loss of family relationships. Nurses can know that the depression is reactive because the patient will talk of the past, and will often talk a lot. It can help patients in this type of depression to be told of resources, of options, of new ways of looking at the problem, of ways in which the problems can be solved. Reassurance can, in fact, cheer them up and increase their ability to cope.

The second type of depression Kubler-Ross calls a *preparatory* depression. This is the necessary stage of sadness that a person goes through when preparing for final separation. When we lose a relative or friend, we feel grief. When we face our own death, we face the loss of all of our friends and relations. The preparatory grief that a person undergoes in such a situation is a silent depression, and it tends to focus on the future rather than on the past. It would be a mistake to try to cheer up a person who is experiencing this type of depression. Any reassurance at this point would be a negation of the very real losses that the patient is facing. Acceptance of the patient's feelings can be expressed simply and often nonverbally just with one's presence or a simple touch. Well-meaning visitors intent on cheering up a dying patient can interfere with the progression through this phase.

The last phase of adaptation to dying, as described by Dr. Kubler-Ross, is *acceptance.* In this stage, the patient feels neither angry nor depressed. Rather he or she will be calm, quiet, and neither happy nor unhappy. Sometimes the person will seem to be withdrawn from others, or disassociated. Usually by this time a patient is very ill and tired and may sleep a lot. Family members can be helped at this time to express love and caring in an undemanding way. It is good if a loved one can sit nearby, perhaps touch gently, but without asking for the dying person to expend physical or emotional energy. It may be very hard for family members to accept the withdrawal of the dying person, especially if they are not themselves resigned to the approaching death. When family or close friends are willing to express their loving support, attending a dying person can be an intensely close and moving experience, while still a very painful one.

At the very end of the dying process, there comes a time that Kubler-Ross (1969) describes as "the silence that goes beyond words:"

> …when the pain ceases to be, when the mind slips off into a dreamless state, when the need for food becomes minimal and the awareness of the environment all but disappears into the darkness…

> Those who have the strength and the love to sit with a dying patient in the *silence that goes beyond words* will know that this moment is neither frightening nor painful, but a peaceful cessation of the functioning of the body.

If many family members are around, or if they are having difficulty offering an undemanding support, nurses may need to intervene to help the family choose one or two persons who are best able to stay with the patient during these last hours.

Whereas Kubler-Ross has studied the reactions of persons who are about to die, another physician, Raymond Moody, has studied the experiences of persons who have nearly died and of persons who were actually clinically dead and have been resuscitated. Persons who have survived these "near-death" episodes describe a remarkably similar experience. From more than 150 cases, Moody has detected several elements that appear to recur with some consistency. First there is a process of separation from the body that is sometimes peaceful and quiet, sometimes accompanied by a buzzing, ringing, or roaring noise. Then there is travel through a tunnel or valley. Persons report seeing their bodies from the outside and feeling dissociated from whatever is going on, such as resuscitation attempts. Then they are greeted by persons who have died before them and welcomed in some manner by a spirit of light that conveys a feeling of love and acceptance. At some point people become aware of a border, and for one reason or another, they turn back at this point, often with considerable reluctance to return to the living.

Throughout the experience they are filled with feelings of joy and peace. After the experience is over, they have a great deal of difficulty discussing it, especially if their descriptions are met with skepticism or denial by others. A lasting consequence of such a near-death experience for many is a change in views about life and death and a loss of the fear of dying. Because he recorded similar descriptions of the experience of near death from persons who were dying from sudden injury as well as from long-term illness, from religious persons and nonreligious persons, from persons who were taking pain medication and from persons who were not, Moody suggests that we "leave open the possibility that near-death experiences represent a novel phenomenon for which we may have to devise new modes of explanation and interpretation" (Moody, 1976). It is

also possible that understanding what others have gone through in near-death experience may comfort terminally ill patients and their families.

CAUSES OF DEATH

By understanding the major causes of death, health care planners can focus the delivery of healthcare on those conditions that are frequent and preventable or reversible. Many of the most frequent causes of death in this country are at least partially related to lifestyle. By living a healthy lifestyle including exercise, good diet, no smoking and moderate alcohol, and by being aware of early detection measures for chronic illness, persons can delay illness and death. In 1980 three of four elderly died from heart disease, cancer, or stroke. Influenza and pneumonia are also frequent causes of death after age 85. The data in *Table 9-1* indicates that heart disease, cancer and stroke remain the top three causes of death. Heart disease remains the leading cause of death among the elderly. However, among those 65 to 74, heart disease and cancer were equally prevalent as causes of death, with each accounting for about 33% of all deaths in that age group in 1990. The heart disease death rate increases in persons over age 85, accounting for 44% of deaths in that age group in 1991 (U.S. Bureau of the Census, 1996).

SPECIFIC PROBLEMS OF DYING PATIENTS AND HOSPICE CARE

Dying patients often need specific types of care to make them comfortable and to assist them in the process of dying with dignity. Nurses sometimes provide this care directly, and sometimes they teach, counsel, or assist the patients' family members in the provision of this care. The hospice movement in the United States arose to offer this kind of nursing care, and to differentiate it from the cure-oriented care provided by most healthcare institutions. Hospice care originated as a philosophy of care, based on the British model of hospice care developed by Dr. Cicely Saunders, a nurse and physician and founder of St. Christopher's Hospice in London. The U.S. government now forbids an organization from calling itself a hospice unless it is a Medicare-certified hospice. Consequently, the term in this country has come to have a fairly specific meaning. The term *palliative care* is used to describe the type of care given to provide comfort and support rather than diagnosis and cure.

Hospices in the United States are primarily home care organizations, but some inpatient hospice facilities do exist. Hospices can contract with hospitals and nursing facilities to provide inpatient services, but it can be difficult to retain the hospice philosophy of care in these settings. The long term care facility and the hospice must have an agreement spelling out the care to be given by both providers to the individual. The care of the resident must reflect the hospice philosophy which is palliative rather than curative. The care given in long term care to a hospice resident is directed at symptoms and circumstances surrounding the physical, psychosocial and spiritual needs of the individual and their family. A hospice can supply routine or continuous home care to a Medicare beneficiary who lives in a long term care facility. The Hospice has the responsibility to provide professional case management which a Registered Nurse must coordinate as well as all core services given routinely by hospice employees. Core services include medical care by a physician, nursing care such as personal care, social services and bereavement counseling. Both the long term care staff and the hospice staff are responsible for delineating and performing their respective services. Coordination and planning of care are imperative according to Medicare guidelines. Long term care facilities often become the "home" for many elderly individ-

uals. The atmosphere is often more flexible than an acute care setting. Because of these differences families and residents can disclose and carry out their wishes regarding death in a relaxed manner. Death can occur in a calm and empathic setting (Stanley & Beare, 1995).

The hospice philosophy involves a recognition that a person has a terminal illness and no longer seeks treatment aimed at providing a cure for that illness. The care is family oriented, and family members usually provide the bulk of hands-on care. Care is provided by an interdisciplinary team that includes the patient and the patient's family, primary physician and/or hospice physician, nurses, social workers, clergy, volunteers, dieticians, and physical therapists. Team members start with a common purpose: to provide care to the dying patient and the patient's family, with the understanding that death does not represent failure, but rather a natural stage of life. Through working together, team members ideally develop mutual respect, open communication, and shared decision making. The focus of hospice care is on symptom management and on coping with anticipatory grief and bereavement. Symptom management is aimed primarily at controlling symptoms before they become distressing rather than only trying to relieve them after they become a problem. It also deals with such issues as pain, hypoxia, nausea and anorexia, incontinence, constipation, and emotional reactions such as depression and anxiety.

PAIN CONTROL

One of cancer patients' greatest fears is the fear of uncontrollable pain. One of the major sources of pain in cancer is from bone cancer or from metastases to the bones. Swelling at a tumor site can also cause pain when pressure is put on nerve cells or when organs are blocked. Compassionate, terminal care involves the utmost effort to control pain while keeping the

TABLE 9-1
Top Five Causes of death for the Elderly: 1980 and 1991

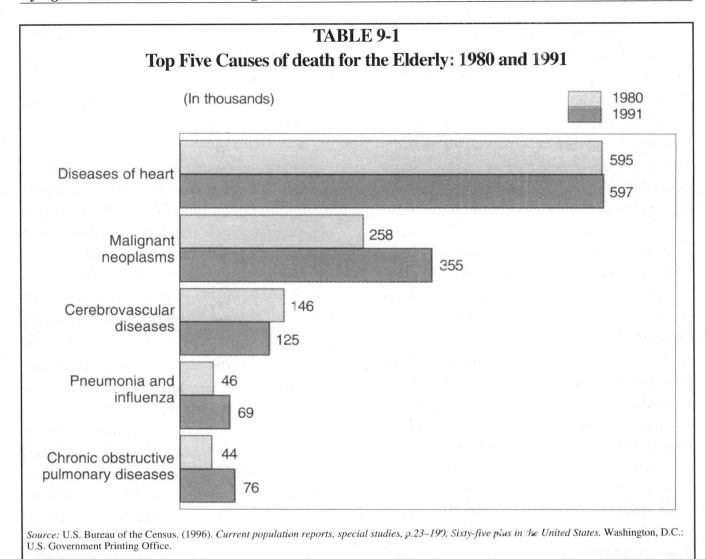

Source: U.S. Bureau of the Census. (1996). *Current population reports, special studies, p.23–190, Sixty-five plus in the United States.* Washington, D.C.: U.S. Government Printing Office.

patient as alert as possible. Controlling pain is different from alleviating pain. Control implies that the pain is never allowed to get to the point of causing distress to the patient. Nurses need to remember that a patient may have more than one source of pain. When a patient requests medication for pain, the nurse must understand which pain and how severe it is. A cancer patient whose pain is from a long-standing arthritis normally controlled with aspirin does not need Demerol (meperidine) to control that pain.

In attempting to choose the correct medication and dosage to relieve pain, nurses are usually involved in assessing the effectiveness and side effects of the medicine. Two parameters to assess are

1. Does the medicine relieve the pain?

2. Does the relief last until the time for the next dose?

If the medicine does not relieve the pain, a different medicine or a stronger dose may be needed. If the medication relieves the pain but does not last until the next dose, then the interval between doses needs to be adjusted. Many medication regimens are available to achieve the optimum effect. Some types of pain medication allow the patient to be in control of the dosing. Patient-controlled analgesia can be provided as a "pain cocktail" liquid that the patient can sip as needed or via a subcutaneous pump that allows the patient to determine the dosage needed. One type of schedule that can work well is to have a long-acting pain medication used on a schedule, with a shorter-acting drug available as needed. Frequently, additional medicines will be added to an analgesic to potentiate the pain-relieving effect.

Historically, physicians and nurses have not been comfortable allowing patients to take adequate pain medicine to control the patients' symptoms. With hospice as a model, nurses in most settings are becoming more aware of the techniques for providing adequate pain control. Nurses used to be afraid that patients might become addicted, or, of more significance in the terminally ill, that they might become tolerant and no longer get adequate relief from available medications. Obviously the problem of addiction is irrelevant for anyone who is in the process of dying. With the development of many different kinds of synthetic narcotics, tolerance is also not usually a problem. Although tolerance does develop, the reduced respiratory depression of newer drugs means that the dose can be increased when more medicine is needed without causing respiratory arrest. Eventually, high doses of pain medications may, in fact, cause impaired respirations. Many patients choose to receive adequate pain medicine even if this regimen would shorten their lives.

Table 9-2 gives examples of frequently used medications to control severe pain in terminally ill patients.

In addition to respiratory depression, another side effect of high doses of pain medication is decreased alertness. The ideal situation in pain control is to titrate the medication and the dose to the point where pain is slight, if felt at all, but the patient is alert and able to interact with others as much as he or she desires. Sometimes a person who has affairs to settle will put off requesting any more pain medicine until the need for alertness is over. Some persons have a high need for control and would rather remain more alert, even at the cost of some pain. Whenever a choice must be made between pain control and mental alertness, the patient's wishes should be followed whenever they are known.

It is important for nurses to listen when patients express the need for pain medications. Only the patient can tell when he or she is experiencing pain. Nurses may not be able to know objectively that a patient is having pain and must accept the assessment of the patient. An example of inappropriate nurse intervention is deciding that a patient who asked for pain medication does not need it because the patient is asleep. In fact, sleep can be an avoidance technique to escape pain, and a patient who falls asleep in some pain may wake in excruciating pain.

Other side effects of many pain medications include constipation and nausea. Both of these problems can be decreased by watching out for them and by taking appropriate measures to relieve them should they occur. Constipation is a common occurrence when narcotic analgesics are used, especially when factors such as decreased mobility, dehydration, and lack of roughage in the diet are added. Constipation can be helped with increased fluid and fiber if these are tolerated. Stool softeners (such as docusate sodium), mild bowel stimulants (such as bisacodyl), and suppositories can help alleviate constipation.

Nausea can sometimes be helped by using a different type of pain medication. It can also often be helped with prochlorperazine suppositories. Sometimes nausea and vomiting can be caused by the disease itself or by radiation therapy that is being given for palliative effect and is not actually a side effect of a pain medicine. When a patient is too nauseated to take an oral pain medication, other routes can be used. Transdermal patches, suppositories, and injection are all potential ways of administration pain medicine that can be easily used even in home settings. Intravenous infusion and intrathecal infusion can be used in inpatient

TABLE 9-2

Narcotics Used For The Control Of Severe Pain (with average starting doses)

MORPHINE HCL

PO: 15–30 mg, lasts 3–4 hr

IM: 10 mg, lasts 4–6 hr

SC: 10 mg, lasts 4–6 hr

LEVORPHANOL TARTRATE

PO: 3–4 mg, lasts 6–8 hr

SC: 2 mg, lasts 6–8 hr

HYDROMORPHONE HCL

PO: 1–4 mg, lasts 3–5 hr (7.5 mg PO equiv. to 10 mg morphine IM)

IM: 1.5 mg, lasts 3–5 hr

Suppository: 3 mg, lasts 4–5 hr

MEPERIDINE HCL *

PO: 50–150 mg. (PO equiv. to 1/2 IM dose), lasts 2–4 hr

IM: 80–100 mg. (eq 10 mg IM morphine), lasts 4–6 hr

OXYMORPHONE HCL

Suppository 5 mg, lasts 4–5 hr

METHADONE HCL

Has a longer duration of action, but is less effective in the elderly.

A SAMPLE COMBINATION OF ORAL MEDICATIONS FOR PAIN RELIEF:

Levorphanol, 2 mg every 6 hr

Hydroxyzine, 25 mg every 6 hr

Aspirin, 650 mg every 6 hr

Amitriptyline, 75 mg at bedtime

Docusate, 50 mg twice a day

A SAMPLE "PAIN COCKTAIL" IN 5 ML SYRUP:

Meperidine, 50 mg

Hydroxyzine, 25 mg

Acetaminophen, 325 mg

(The ingredients of a pain cocktail should be listed on the label so that the mixture can be changed or if, for instance, the meperidine needs to be increased without increasing the other ingredients.)

*Meperidine is not effective after 72 hr of administration, and is not recommended for use in the elderly.

TABLE 9-3
WHO Three-Step Analgesic Ladder

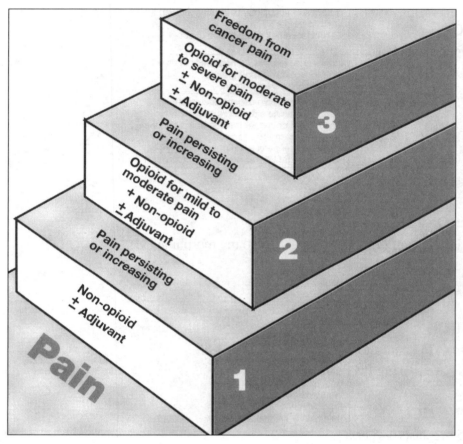

Source: World Health Organization, 1990.

settings and can control very persistent pain with minimal side effects.

Other types of medication can sometimes be added to narcotic analgesics to increase the analgesics' effectiveness. Steroids and nonsteroidal anti-inflammatory drugs (NSAIDs) can work peripherally to decrease swelling and pain. Dexamethasone is a steroid that can decrease swelling of the brain that can cause pain and delirium. Acetaminophen can sometimes potentiate a narcotic analgesic, and it is routinely added to codeine. Antianxiety drugs and antidepressants can also help patients cope with pain and with emotional states that can exacerbate the perception of pain.

Nurses need also to remember that there are many nonpharmacological approaches to alleviating pain. These include removing noxious environmental stimuli, alleviating boredom, positioning, heat, and touch. Although some have a strong sense of privacy and resist being touched, many persons benefit from it. Touch can communicate nonverbally a caring attitude by a nurse. Massage is a form of touch that can directly relax a person and provide a counterstimulus that can alleviate pain. Therapeutic touch is a developing field in which the intention and the energy of the practitioner are used to relieve pain. Guided imagery can help a person focus on more positive aspects of living and can relieve pain. Transcutaneous electrical nerve stimulation is a method of providing a counterstimulation that has worked effectively to relieve pain for some people. Medically, palliative radiotherapy, surgery, and nerve blocks are additional methods that can be used to relieve pain that does not respond to more conservative treatment.

The Agency for Health Care Policy and Research (1994) has published clinical practice guidelines for the management of cancer pain. *Figure 9-3* refers to the World Health Organization guidelines for pain management. Refer to this publication for detailed information on pain control.

LOSS OF INDEPENDENCE

One of the major problems of terminal illness is that various physical systems can fail, resulting in increased dependence on others. As energy levels, muscle strength, or coordination decrease, patients may become dependent on family members and professional caregivers to do tasks that the patients used to take for granted and do for themselves. A sensitive nurse can help patients and their families to see that "for everything there is a season," and focus on the loving exchange that such assistance can be for both the receiver and the giver. A nurse can also encourage family members to allow the patient as much control as possible, so that elements of caregiving (meals, pain control, baths, etc.) do not become power struggles as a patient attempts to retain control of his or her life.

One functional loss that causes patients and families much distress is incontinence. Bowel and bladder continence are abilities that are considered basic once a person has passed the phase of childhood toilet training. Incontinent patients are often very embarrassed, and family members are sometimes angry at facing the task of cleanup. Also, there are very real problems in providing care for incontinent patients. Urinary incontinence is sometimes managed with an indwelling catheter. Catheters are safer at home than they are in a nursing facility or a hospital where resistant organisms

can cause dangerous urinary tract infections. Even at home many indwelling catheters result in some type of bladder colonization. Whenever possible, urinary incontinence should be managed with frequent toileting or adult incontinence briefs. Sudden incontinence may be a sign of a urinary tract infection and should be assessed with a urine culture.

Bowel incontinence is even more aesthetically difficult for family members to cope with. Although trying to establish a bowel program may make management easier, such a goal needs to be balanced with the effort involved for the patient and his or her family. Again, incontinence briefs may be the best way to manage solid wastes.

For both bowel and bladder incontinence, one of the troubling consequences is skin breakdown. When added to the possibility of immobility, decreased protein intake, and increased metabolism of cancer cells, ulcers sometimes cannot be prevented. Nurses can arrange for special mattresses, frequent position changes, and prompt treatment of any skin breakdown.

Loss of control can be a major issue for patients who are facing diagnoses of a dementing illness such as Alzheimer's disease or a disease that destroys physical functioning while leaving mental function intact, such as Parkinson's. In either one of these situations, a person in the early stages of the disease faces a catastrophic loss of independence. A recent study of suicide among people more than 65 years old found that the reason given most frequently was fear of nursing home placement (Matzo, 1997). The fear of loss of independence, fear of loss of control of one's body or of decision making, are serious concerns for older persons.

One major area in which patients should be encouraged to make decisions regarding care is in deciding what kinds of treatment they want. It is hoped more and more persons will be addressing this issue before they are terminally ill. Treatment decisions are further discussed in the chapter, with the issue of advance directives.

HYPOXIA AND ANXIETY

Hypoxia can be a distressing abnormality caused by terminal illness. Hypoxia can cause anxiety and even panic, and managing it is essential to achieving a dignified death. In order to relieve patients' distress, oxygen is sometimes used. Nurses should be aware that for patients who have had long-term breathing problems, hypoxia may be the only stimulus to breathe. In such cases, giving high concentrations of oxygen can wipe out the patient's ability to breathe at all. Only low doses of oxygen, such as 2 l/min, should be used for these patients. Antihistamine sedatives such as hydroxyzine and diphenhydramine can be used to decrease anxiety, but traditional antianxiety drugs such as diazepam are rarely used. Anxiety tends not to be a problem when respirations are depressed by narcotic analgesics, but again oxygen can be administered if there is a short-term respiratory depression caused by a heavier than usual dose of narcotic. Naloxone HCl, a narcotic antagonist, can also be used in case of undesired narcotic respiratory depression, but it is very short-acting and will also have the effect of reducing the analgesic effect of the narcotic. It is also possible for a patient who is sedated more than he or she wants to be to experience anxiety as a result of loss of control. Encouraging patients to participate in care decisions whenever possible will help them to retain a feeling of control.

PHYSICAL CHANGES ASSOCIATED WITH APPROACHING DEATH

Several physical changes can signal the approach of death. Although the last stage of dying can occasionally take several days, it is usually over within a day or two unless medical intervention leads to further delays. Nurses can help patients and families by providing counseling on what to expect and how to cope with problems that develop. Recognizing these signs can also help nurses plan for a more intensive period of support for patients and the patients' families.

Persons stop eating and drinking when they have no energy or desire to force themselves to eat, or when their disease stops them from digesting food. Providing food and fluid is a basic caregiving process in our society, and persons often react to a patient's cessation of oral intake with an impulse to give food and fluids by enteral or parenteral tubes. Such feeding and hydration are actually more of a treatment for the living than for the dying. Dehydration actually seems to provide a natural anesthesia with lessening edema, less vomiting, fewer lung secretions, and even less need to void (Gallager-Alred, 1989). The Supreme Court, in the case of Nancy Cruzan, recognized that giving food and fluid to a patient who is unable to eat or drink is a medical treatment, and patients may refuse such a treatment.

Changes in breathing usually occur as death approaches, with breaths becoming shallow, noisy, and labored. Breathing patterns can become irregular, with longer and longer periods of apnea. If the decreased breathing is causing distress, the patient can be helped as described in the section on hypoxia.

Slowing circulation will occur as the heart pumps blood less strongly. Feet and hands, then arms and legs will cool and become cyanotic. Vital signs change with approaching death, but when death is expected, it is not appropriate to continually disturb a patient just to get accurate readings of temperature and blood pressure. Pulse and respirations can be measured without disturbing the patient and typically will show a tachycardia and tachypnea that become irregular in pattern.

Level of consciousness can decrease, but this is very unpredictable, and a person can regain full consciousness when least expected to do so. Nurses should always remember that hearing is the last sense to disappear. *Always speak as if the dying person can hear what you are saying.* Restlessness can occur, and effort should be made to ensure that it is not a sign of a specific physical discomfort such as pain or a need to void.

One of the most difficult occurrences for families to tolerate is bleeding. Although it is not a usual occurrence, it can be an extremely frightening one. If the bleeding is accessible, pressure on the bleeding site can reduce it. Internal bleeding can cause painful swelling that can sometimes be alleviated with ice packs. Frequent changes of towels can reduce the frightening impact of the bleeding. One hospice is reported to calmly bring out red blankets to absorb the bleeding. Families may find themselves unable to cope with significant bleeding in the home.

Finally, when a person dies, there may be an exhalation of air past collected bronchial secretions that produces a gurgle or rattle. Eyes may remain open, and family members may feel more comfortable if the eyes are gently closed. A damp gauze placed on the eyelids is usually sufficient to close them. The body should be placed in a physiologically neutral position, but tying of the hands and feet is an archaic custom that should be abandoned. When combined with the edema that occurs with the collapse of the circulatory system, this practice can result in marking the body unnecessarily. Frequently, the bowel and bladder empty, and for patients dying at home, the family may want to have a plastic sheet on the mattress to prevent soaking the mattress. Some family members want to stay with the body for a period, and this should always be accepted. For a patient dying in a hospital or nursing home, the body should not be moved until the patient's family has had a chance to see the body and sit with it if they so desire.

A nurse can help a patient and the patient's family prepare themselves for the experience of death by explaining what to expect. Knowing what may happen can help patients and their families cope without panic, especially when an emotional acceptance of the impending death has been reached. A nurse may also suggest that patients and their families make arrangements in advance for funerals, memorial services, and organ donations. When death is expected, autopsies are not generally required, and a physician's presence is not required to complete a death certificate. In some locations, calls to an emergency medical system will result in compulsory cardiopulmonary resuscitation (CPR) and transport to a hospital. When this is not the desired outcome, families need to be warned not to call an emergency number. One of the advantages of hospice involvement is that many of these arrangements are made more easily in a system where the providers have had much experience in coping with death.

SUDDEN DEATH

Unexpected death presents a different array of problems and responses than those that occur when a death is anticipated. When death is immediate, family members will not have had time to adapt. When a patient is being maintained on medical machinery and the patient's family members are asked whether to turn off the machines, they will usually need time to get used to the idea of the loved one dying. Families that are initially resistant to the termination of life support may change their minds as they become more reconciled to the idea, and as it becomes more probable that recovery is impossible. Families can be helped in making these decisions if the patient has previously made his or her wishes about life support known. After a general discussion of ethical and legal principles surrounding the provision of health care, the chapter discusses advance directives, which can be a valuable tool to inform others of one's wishes.

ETHICAL AND LEGAL PRINCIPLES IN CARING FOR OLDER ADULTS

General ethical principles apply to all human relationships. "It is by following ethical rules that a person develops desirable qualities and attitudes. Good people tend to do good acts; and people become good in part by repeated performance of morally appropriate acts, such as personally providing supportive care to a terminally ill or severely demented patient" (Reese & Faryna, 1990). Although our society attempts to translate ethical principles into law, the legal system cannot address all such issues. General principles of good behavior include respect for others, regardless of physical or mental impairment, *honesty* in communicating with others, and *compassion* in working with persons who are having trouble. These general principles of behavior carry through into four ethical principles that are central to the provision of health care: *justice, autonomy, beneficence,* and *fidelity* (Fitting, 1990).

Respect for the worth of each person leads to the principles of autonomy and justice. Autonomy is the right of each person to make decisions that affect his or her life. Autonomy does not give a person the right to impose unlimited burdens on others, such as family members or healthcare providers. Autonomy is becoming an evermore recognized right in the United States. The 1990 Supreme Court decision in the case of Nancy Cruzan recognized autonomy in agreeing that a person has the right to make decisions about accepting or rejecting medical treatment. In healthcare, the principle of autonomy has led to the legal principle of *informed consent,* which assures a person the right to be informed of the benefits and risks of proposed treatment options and the right to

consent or to refuse consent for medical care. Specifically informed consent requires that a patient receive an explanation of the proposed procedure to the extent of his or her ability to understand, including

- knowledge of possible hazards or possible complications of the procedure

- expected results (benefits) of treatment and reasonable alternatives (Feutz, 1990).

Healthcare providers need to have some idea about a patients' abilities to understand the consequences of his or her decisions. In situations in which a patient is thought to be unable to understand the consequences of his or her decisions, a physician will usually consult the patient's family members to make a decision. This practice is usually workable when all family members agree. However, when someone in the family disagrees, or even when a healthcare provider, state regulator, or district attorney disagrees, then a consensus decision by family members becomes unworkable. In the Cruzan case, for instance, the state acted to prevent withdrawal of tube feedings because the state of Missouri has "an unqualified interest in the preservation of life."

A major finding in the Cruzan case was that the court does not recognize "substituted judgment." Although the court recognizes the right of a person to make decisions about life-sustaining treatment, and the court also accepts that tube feeding constitutes a medical treatment; none of Nancy Cruzan's family or friends could say that she had ever expressly stated her preference for life-support continuation or termination. In other words, if someone could say, "Nancy told me that she would never want to be kept alive in these circumstances," the court would have accepted her wishes. But the court was not willing to accept someone else's judgment in substitution for the individual patient. The formal mechanism for persons to inform others of wishes concerning life support is some kind of *advance directive* (AD).

When a person is no longer able to understand the consequences of his or her actions, nurses and other health providers need to be aware that a consent that cannot be truly informed is not valid. Great care must be taken not to evaluate a person as unable to understand the consequences of his or her actions just because the person's decision does not agree with the doctor's or nurse's beliefs about what the decision should be. The determination of whether a person is competent or not is actually made by the courts. Caregivers may be asked questions such as the following:

- Can the person make choices regarding life?

- Are the outcomes of choices reasonable?

- Are the choices based on rational reasons?

- Is the person able to understand the implications of the choices made? (Feutz, 1990)

If a person is judged to be incompetent, the court will appoint a conservator. If no family member or close friend is available to act as a conservator, public conservators are available.

The ethical principle of justice creates a duty to distribute resources fairly, to treat others without discrimination on the basis of irrelevant characteristics. There is some controversy in this country over whether healthcare is a right or something persons may purchase. So far, however, healthcare is not a right of everyone, and health providers may discriminate on the basis of the ability to pay. In other words, doctors, nurses, and others are not required to provide care if the person receiving the care is unable to pay for that care. Ethically, many healthcare providers have trouble with discrimination based on the ability to pay. The President's Commission on Securing Access to Health Care proposed that health care is different from other goods and services because health is beyond a person's control. Illness is distributed unevenly, and an individual cannot always know the best actions to

take to maximize health (Feutz, 1990). But so far our society has not chosen to ensure that everyone has equal access to healthcare. Even if our society were to recognize basic healthcare as a right, and if we developed universal healthcare coverage, there would still be questions about what constitutes basic healthcare, and how much each person is entitled to. Although universal healthcare coverage may solve some problems about access to healthcare, it will not necessarily guarantee justice for all.

Another limit to access to healthcare is that physicians have no duty to offer futile treatment. For instance, a person who has multiple metastases may not be offered surgery to remove a tumor if physicians judge that such an operation will not significantly prolong life or improve its quality. In deciding that a treatment is futile, a physician should be sure that the principle of justice is being followed: would this treatment be futile for anyone with the same clinical picture? A treatment cannot be futile for an uninsured patient but reasonable for an insured patient.

Beneficence is another central ethical principle. It is the duty to help others. Closely related, *nonmalfeasance* is the duty to do no harm. The Hippocratic oath, still sworn to by some physicians, promises to "first, do no harm." In today's complex medical and social systems, it is often not easy to decide how to help others, how to do no harm. When a caregiver makes a decision that is different from a patient's decision, the intention to help others may lead the caregiver to impose the decision on the patient. This is called *paternalism* and is in conflict with the patient's right to autonomy. Paternalism used to be the rule in health care, but with the increasing value of autonomy, paternalism is less and less acceptable. Some older persons will still take the attitude that the doctor knows best and will defer to their physician's opinion.

One more ethical principle that applies to healthcare is fidelity. This is the duty to keep promises, and is central to contractual relationships. A nurse who is providing professional care has a duty to follow through on promises made to a patient, including the implied promise to provide competent care. Any nurse who makes a commitment to follow the ethical principles of justice, autonomy, beneficence, and fidelity can be fairly confident of doing his or her best for others.

ADVANCE DIRECTIVES

An AD is a document that a competent adult may complete and share with health care providers that tells what that person would want to happen in case he or she becomes unable to make his or her wishes known. Different states have approved different types of ADs, but the principle remains the same: that a person has a right to make an autonomous decision that should be respected and followed even if that person becomes unable to communicate the decision in the future.

To learn about advance directives in your state, contact

Concern For Dying/Society for the Right To Die

250 W. 57th St., New York, NY 10107

Tel: (212) 246-6962

or your local medical society or medical association.

Within a year of the Supreme Court decision in the case of Nancy Cruzan, Congress passed the Patient Self-Determination Act (PSDA). This law requires hospitals, nursing homes, home care agencies, hospices, and Medicare HMOs to inform each adult patient, on admission, of the patient's rights in that state to make an AD. Patients will also be asked if they have an AD. The institutions must document their action and the patient's answer in the medical record and are strongly urged to place a copy of any AD in the record. It is important to note that the patient is not required to make deci-

sions about an AD at this point, but is only asked if he or she has already made such decisions. The institution may also give additional information to those patients who are interested in finding out how to make an AD.

Advance directives are sometimes called Living Wills, but this term can be confusing because in some states this term means a document that meets specific guidelines, such as the requirement that a person must be terminally ill before completing the directive. Most states have some mechanism by which a person can do two things: inform health care providers of the person's wishes and designate a surrogate decision-maker to speak for the person if necessary. Because the durable power of attorney for healthcare (DPAHC) allows a person to do both of these, this form of AD is discussed here. This power of attorney is called *durable* because it endures even when a person is no longer competent, which is not the case for a regular power of attorney. It is a power of attorney for healthcare because it limits the decision-making authority to healthcare decisions and does not empower the surrogate to make decisions about the patient's estate. As long as the patient is able to make and communicate decisions, questions about treatment decisions should be referred to the patient. Only when the person becomes unable to make or communicate decisions does the DPAHC go into effect. Forms for DPAHC are available that include instructions on how to *execute* it. A lawyer is not required, but states have different regulations about who can witness the patient's signature. It is possible that admission to a hospital is not the best time to bring up the subject of ADs, but it is hoped that having such a requirement will encourage patients to discuss the issue more with their families and physicians and make their wishes known. In a recent study of 9,015 patients treated in five teaching hospitals (Haynor, 1998), only 688 patients, or less than 10%, had written advanced directives, with two-thirds of those in the form of durable power of attorney. Three out of every four physicians were unaware of these patients' advanced directives (even though they were included in the clinical record), and only 3% of the advanced directives were specific enough to affect care decisions.

In discussing ADs with patients, nurses need to avoid imposing their own values on the patient. However, it may be helpful to give information about the treatment options. For example, CPR is one form of medical treatment. A study of CPR done on 503 patients more than 69 years old found that only 8% survived to be discharged from the hospital, and that half of these went to a nursing home. Of the the 116 patients in this study who had an unwitnessed cardiopulmonary arrest, only 1 survived to be discharged from the hospital (Murphy et al., 1989). Sensible reasons for refusing medical treatment include low chance of success, poor quality of life or terminal illness, and ethical or religious beliefs.

It is essential that all caregivers understand that having an AD does *not* mean that a patient refuses CPR. Each AD is an individual expression of that person's wishes, and it can vary from wanting all possible treatment to refusing hospitalization or even refusing antibiotics or tube feedings. Some persons may want all possible treatment unless it is determined that they are in a coma from which it is unlikely that they would recover. Having stated one's treatment decisions on an AD does not guarantee that all eventualities will be planned for, and this is the reason that designating a surrogate decision-maker is a good idea. It should also be noted that a person can change his or her mind at any time about treatment decisions, and a verbal statement will legally supercede a previously written ADs.

One last point about treatment decisions is that there is no difference, ethically or legally, between withholding a treatment and withdrawing it after it

has started. Many persons have an emotional reaction that withdrawing a treatment is much closer to actively participating in the termination of life, but there is no ethical or legal background to this belief. If a caregiver feels more comfortable not starting a new tube feeding rather than removing an existing one, the short delay it might cause is usually not a problem, but the caregiver should realize that the delay is on behalf of the caregiver and not the patient.

SUICIDE

I will not escape by death from disease so long as it may be healed and leaves my mind unimpaired... But if I know I must suffer without hope of relief, I will depart.

—Seneca

Closely related to the issue of accepting or refusing medical treatment is the right of a person to choose to terminate his or her own life. Many believe that when a person has a terminal illness and faces a lengthy period of physical pain and distress, loss of awareness, or loss of independence, he or she should have the ability to end his or her own life. Some believe that physicians should be able to prescribe a lethal dose of medicine so that a person can end her or his own life peacefully and with dignity, with loved ones present. Others believe that approving assisted suicide is the first step toward the slippery slope of condoning legalized murder and that the absolute prohibition against actively helping someone to die is the best protection humans have against abuses that could result in murder.

In today's society, with so much emotional, legal, and moral conflict about the issue of suicide, it is impossible to evaluate the true incidence of suicide for geriatric patients, but documented suicide is the ninth leading cause of death for people over 65 and the eighth leading cause for people over 85 (U.S. Bureau of the Census, 1996). Older people have fewer failed suicide attempts than younger people. This can be attributed to greater seriousness of intent and to poorer physical health and reduced ability to recover. Suicide among seniors frequently has more than one cause, and reasons can range from grief and loss to belief that one is worthless or a burden to others, loss of independence or self-esteem, or even being faced with the prospect of placement in a nursing home (Matzo, 1997).

One alternative to suicide is to make sure that the physical comfort of the dying person is maximized. Liberal use of medication for pain control as offered by hospices has helped many people face dying with more assurance. However, some persons pain cannot be controlled, and some patients' have other reasons for believing their quality of life is insufficient to warrant further struggle. A major example is the person with dementing illness who faces a long period of dependence and loss of control. Sometimes people who become paralyzed or who suffer deforming surgery have a persistent belief that the quality of their lives is insufficient to justify the pain and suffering they endure. In many cases, the fear of waiting "too long" to be able to end one's own life could be reduced if people were able to get help from loved ones or from caring and involved physicians. Derek Humphry (1991) has written a book, *Final Exit,* that supports physician-assisted suicide, and describes specific methods of "self-deliverance."

In June of 1997, the Supreme Court, in a 9–0 decision, refused to recognize a constitutional right to die. This was done by upholding New York and Washington state statutes criminalizing physician-assisted suicide. The Supreme Court then invited state legislatures to examine the issue and pass legislation allowing physician-assisted suicide if the state could articulate a legitimate state interest for doing so (Beder, 1998). This decision has successfully moved the focus for decision-making about physician-assisted suicide from the federal to the state locale. Several states including Florida and Oregon have attempted to pass laws legalizing physician-assisted suicide. Public opinion strongly supports physician-assisted-suicide. A Gallop Poll in 1997 showed 57% of Americans believe such assistance should be legally available to the terminally ill.

One study of gerontological nurses (Beder, 1998) revealed that, although physician-assisted suicide is still illegal, more than 40% of nurses surveyed had received requests for assistance in dying. The patient and family realize that this is illegal, but still make the requests of nursing staff. Awareness of the frequency of these requests and the burden this places on staff nurses could lead to a more proactive stance in preparing nurses for these discussions, according to the author. The nurse can adopt the role of advocate, nurturer and teacher.

For nurses as caregivers and as family members, assisting someone to commit suicide is still against the law. There are two situations in which nurses should actively intervene if they know a person is contemplating suicide: if the person is suffering from a depression that is potentially reversible, and if the person is being pressured by someone else to consider suicide as a solution. Nurses can help patients and physicians detect signs and symptoms of depression, and can also help patients understand that depression will often end, allowing a resumption of a satisfying life. Anyone dealing with a person who is contemplating suicide should avoid talking the person into it. Humphry suggests that others should always try, up to a point, to dissuade a person from suicide, as this encourages the person to examine other possible solutions.

BEREAVEMENT

When a person is terminally ill, he or she goes through a preparatory grief process. At the same time, the person's family and friends go through a period of anticipatory grief. This grief can parallel the reaction of the dying person, although not necessarily at the same time. After the loved one dies, the family continues to feel grief during the period of bereavement. Although time frames are different for everyone, it is a commonly held belief that persons who have accomplished a lot of "grief work" during the anticipatory period will be better able to cope with bereavement. Families of persons who die suddenly do seem to stay in the initial phase of shock and denial for a much longer time than those of persons who have had time to prepare (Browning, 1995). Several other factors can affect the survivors' ability to cope with bereavement. Persons who feel that they had a good relationship with the dead person, and who believe that they did everything they could to help, will feel less guilt and will move through bereavement more easily. Widows or widowers who have someone to confide in are known to cope more effectively than those who do not. Similarly, the surviving spouse who has strong religious beliefs recovers sooner than those without such faith.

Initially, when a person dies, loved ones go through a period of shock and numbness, even when the death was expected. As the numbness wears off, it is usually followed by a period of yearning, holding on to memories of the deceased. This period may also be characterized by protest, with feelings of guilt, loneliness, anxiety, fear, and irritability. The bereaved can also have ambivalent feelings about the deceased, having anger at being left behind. Another form of ambivalence can occur when the family had a poor relationship with the deceased. For some women, for instance, widowhood can be a release from the stressors of a difficult marriage and a chance to explore and meet their own needs. Such ambivalent feelings can increase feelings of guilt. Nurses can support the bereaved by accepting all of the bereaved person's feelings and allowing him or her to explain what those feelings are without advance expectations by the nurse (Perrin, 1997; Ebersole & Hess, 1998).

Persons report dreams and visualizations, even hallucinations, of the loved one and preoccupation with possessions of the dead person, with places and experiences shared. Physically, survivors often experience many symptoms such as nausea, restlessness, sleep disturbances, and appetite changes. Socially, the bereaved may withdraw or may enter into a frenzied period of activity.

Usually, there is a gradual decline in mourning and a return of interest in life, a resumption of previous patterns of living. Sometimes bereavement is prolonged. Major indicators of this include the following (Browning, 1995)

- Severe identification phenomenon, incorporating traits of the deceased.

- Multiple physical signs and symptoms without apparent illness.

- Prolonged social isolation.

- Self-destructive behavior.

- Severe insomnia and/or anorexia.

- Prolonged feelings of depression, despair, worthlessness, or guilt.

- Denial of grief feelings.

The nurse's role in the case of prolonged grief is to encourage the grieving person to get help, both in terms of professional therapeutic help and from the person's informal support system. Hospice nurses often remain actively involved with families during the period of bereavement. If nurses are aware of the losses their patients have suffered and understand the emotional, social and physical effects of bereavement, they can adapt their plans of care to focus on the needs of the grieving patient and family. One caution is that a bereaved person may say he or she is fine because that is the socially expected response when, in fact, the person is still deep in the process of grieving. Nurses can help in such instances by accepting the bereaved person's sad and angry thoughts, by giving the person social permission to grieve. It is never helpful to tell a grieving person that he or she has grieved too long; it's better to focus on the potential of a positive outcome.

SUMMARY

Dying is a very complex issue. Nurses can help patients and patients' family members cope with the physical and emotional problems of anticipating death and coping with bereavement. Although it is a general goal of healthcare to increase duration of life, the quality of that life is often more important to the patient than the quantity of time. Maintaining a balanced view about the value of life, the inevitability of death, and the right of a person to make autonomous decisions, nurses can provide care to patients in many different circumstances. Many people alive today will participate to some extent in decisions about the end of their lives, and as medical science continues to blur the line between life and death, personal decisions will become an ever larger part of the dying process.

EXAM QUESTIONS

CHAPTER 9
Questions 81–90

81. The major cause of death in the elderly is

    a. accidents.

    b. suicide.

    c. flu/pneumonia.

    d. heart disease.

82. Pain control for terminal cancer patients may be complicated by the problems of

    a. dehydration.

    b. diarrhea.

    c. tachycardia.

    d. nausea.

83. The preparatory depression that precedes the acceptance of death does which of the following?

    a. Focuses on the past.

    b. Can be relieved by reassurance.

    c. Will be expressed with much talking.

    d. Is related to the anticipation of multiple losses.

84. Which of the following is a key factor in determining the dosage of pain medications for a cancer patient?

    a. Risk of addiction.

    b. The patient's weight.

    c. Whether the medication relieves the pain.

    d. The needs of the family or caregiver needs.

85. Hospice nursing philosophy includes which of the following?

    a. Curing the disease

    b. Physical care only

    c. Using high technology

    d. Symptom control

86. What is the most important thing for a nurse to do for a dying patient?

    a. Provide pain relief.

    b. Explain how to cope with physical signs and symptoms.

    c. Check vital signs regularly.

    d. Listen to the needs expressed by the dying person.

87. Which of the following characterizes an advance directive?

    a. It means the patient does not want CPR.

    b. It means the caregivers should talk to the family and not to the patient.

    c. It tells the caregivers what treatment options a patient chooses.

    d. It needs to be drawn up by a lawyer.

88. Which of the following statements about ethics is true?

    a. Ethical decisions are legally correct.

    b. Withdrawing a treatment is more serious than withholding it.

    c. Ethical principles will enable caregivers to make a single correct decision.

    d. Ethics apply to everyone equally.

89. Advance directives are a way to carry out the ethical principle of

    a. justice.

    b. beneficence.

    c. autonomy.

    d. nonmalfeasance.

90. Which of the following is illegal?

    a. Withholding medical treatment at the patient's request

    b. Self-deliverance

    c. Nurse-assisted suicide

    d. Giving pain medication that may depress respirations

CHAPTER 10

CONTINUUM OF CARE

by

Barbara Santamaria, MPH, RN, C &

Deborah Lubow, MS, RN, C

CHAPTER OBJECTIVES

After studying this chapter, the reader will be able to recognize the needs of the elderly in a variety of settings and specify strategies to promote healthy aging.

LEARNING OBJECTIVES

After studying this chapter, the reader will be able to:

1. Specify strategies to promote healthy aging.

2. Specify areas to be considered in evaluating elderly clients in the community and other settings.

3. Recognize situations in which home health or hospice care would be available under current Medicare and Medicaid guidelines.

4. Recognize resources available to aging clients in the community to support independent living.

5. Indicate common problems of the elderly in the acute care setting and appropriate interventions.

6. Specify situations in which rehabilitation would be appropriate.

7. Specify issues involved in selecting a nursing home.

INTRODUCTION

Today people are talking about and planning for growing old. During the past decade, the over-65 population has grown twice as fast as the general population and now accounts for 30 million people. In the course of this century, average life expectancy has increased 60%, from 47 years in 1900 to 75 years in 1987. This progress has largely been due to the advances of science and public health in conquering life-threatening communicable diseases (U.S. Public Health Service, 1990). People who reach the age of 65 now can expect to live into their eighties. In fact, the most rapid population growth over the next decade will be among those 85 years of age and older. Although many think of health problems in old age as inevitable, most of these problems are either preventable or can be controlled (U.S. Public Health Service, 1990). As health professionals, our challenge in the years ahead will be to maximize the active and independent years of our elderly population—to prevent the ill from becoming disabled and to help people with disabilities preserve function and prevent further disability. This chapter reviews a strategy including guidelines for promoting healthy aging, community resources available to support the patient, and various institutional options. Nurses need to be familiar with the entire continuum of care *(Figure 10-1)* in order to provide comprehensive, coordinated care to elderly patients in any setting (Burton, 1990).

PREPARING FOR HEALTHY AGING

Some changes associated with aging are inevitable, but others can be modified by changes in lifestyle. We now recognize that changes in health behaviors can increase life expectancy and reduce disability from chronic disease. It is thought that good preventive care can extend the period of independent functioning until shortly before death. In the following section, we look at four areas that influence health: preventive services, exercise, nutrition, and smoking/alcohol.

Appropriate Use of Preventive Services

A periodic health examination every 1–3 years is recommended for those in the 40–64 age group and yearly after age 65 (U.S. Preventive Services Task Force, 1989). The examination should include at least a check of weight and blood pressure and selected screening examinations. Common screening examinations include breast examinations, mammograms, pap smears, fecal occult blood testing and digital rectal exams. The recommendations are summarized on the following pages.

The American Cancer Society recommends annual PSA (Prostate-Specific Antigen) and DRE (digital rectal examination) for prostate cancer detection for all men over age 50 whether symptomatic or not (American Cancer Society, 1998). Additionally, younger men at high risk such as African-American men with a strong familial history should be screened. There is some controversy among national organizations about the use of the routine PSA test. This test is a prostate-specific enzyme test not a prostate-cancer-specific enzyme (Carson, 1998). PSA can be elevated in a number of benign conditions including urinary retention, instrumentation, prostatitis, prostatic infarction and BPH (Benign Prostatic Hypertrophy). If the PSA is above the normal range of 4.0 ng/mL further urologic investigation is done.

Adults need to keep their immunizations current. Tetanus, influenza, and pneumococcal vaccines are recommended. Although uncommon, tetanus continues to be reported in the United States. A number of years ago during 1985-1986, 147 cases of tetanus were reported to the Centers for Disease Control. More than 70% of these cases occurred among persons more than 50 years old, and in 30%, there was no evidence of an acute injury as a cause for their disease. Twenty-nine cases were associated with chronic wounds (e.g., skin ulcers, abscesses, and gangrene), particularly in nursing home patients (Korn & Poland, 1989). Tetanus vaccine is usually given in combination with diphtheria vaccine. Adults of all ages should receive the vaccine every 10 years after they receive the primary series. Longer periods between booster immunizations may be acceptable in individual instances (Reed, 1998).

Influenza vaccine is given yearly in the fall to allow time for immunity to develop, because influenza is most prevalent in the winter. The vaccine is recommended for the well elderly (over age 65) as well as for the chronically ill, because both groups are at risk for complications from influenza infection—the well elderly at moderate risk, the chronically ill at high risk. The vaccine is also recommended for residents of nursing and other long-term care facilities.

Pneumonia is the sixth leading cause of death. There is controversy regarding the efficacy of the vaccine, particularly in older patients with multiple health problems. The vaccine is recommended for persons over age 65 and the chronically ill. It is probably most effective in younger, healthier adults. New guidelines recommend vaccination of persons 65 or over who have not been previously vaccinated or those whose vaccination status is

FIGURE 10-1
Continuum of Geriatric Care

Outreach	Monitoring services	
	Homemaker	In home
	Home healthcare	
Information/referral	Nutritional programs	
	Legal/protective services	Community
	Senior centers	
Assessment	Community medical services	
	Dental services	
Case management	Community mental health	
	Dental services	
Linkages	Respite care	
	Hospice care	
Evaluation/quality assurance	Retirement villages	
	Life care	
	Services	
	Domiciliary care	
	Foster home	
Special housing	Personal care home	Institutional
	Group home	
	Congregate care	
	Meals	
	Social services	
	Medical services	
	Housekeeping	
	Nursing facilities	
	Mental hospitals	
	Acute care hospitals	

Adapted from Brody, S. J. & Masciocchi, C. "Data for long-term care planning by health systems agencies. *American Journal of Public Health,* 70, pp. 1194–1198, 1980.

unknown. Revaccination is recommended for those who were both previously vaccinated when they were less than 65 years of age and have had five or more years elapse since the last vaccination if they did not have a significant reaction to their first pneumococcal vaccine (Centers for Disease Control & Prevention, 1997).

Exercise

Exercise is one of the most active areas of clinical research in aging. It is felt that much of the decline in physical performance seen in later years is the result of inactivity. Regular exercise can improve physical capacity and functioning. Regular physical exercise and activity aid in reducing obesity, improving hyperglycemia, lowering blood levels of lipids, and reducing blood pressure. It protects against the development and progression of coronary artery disease, hypertension and non-insulin-dependent diabetes mellitus (NIDDM). Physically inactive persons are almost twice as likely to develop coronary heart disease as those who engage in regular physical activity. Exercise helps to extend normal walking patterns into old age, thus reducing risk of falls, and increases bone mineral content, thus reducing risk for osteoporotic fractures. It may also lead to increased feelings of well-being and better sleep by reducing depression and anxiety. In general, patients who are healthy can begin a moderate exercise program, (i.e., walking) without medical clearance; however, persons with known cardiovascular, pulmonary, or metabolic diseases (diabetes, thyroid disorders, renal or liver disease) should have a thorough medical evaluation before beginning. In addition, persons who respond yes to any of the following seven questions (Harris, Casperson, DeFriese, & Estes, 1989) should consult a health care provider before beginning an exercise program.

1. Has your doctor ever said that you have heart trouble?

2. Do you frequently have pains in your heart or chest?

3. Do you often feel faint or have spells of severe dizziness?

4. Has a doctor ever said that your blood pressure was too high?

5. Has your doctor ever told you that you have a bone or joint problem such as arthritis that has been aggravated by exercise or might be made worse by exercise?

6. Is there a good physical reason not mentioned here why you should not follow an activity program even if you wanted to?

7. Are you over age 65 and not accustomed to vigorous exercise?

Although the precise amount of exercise required to prevent premature disability or death is unknown, it appears that many sedentary persons would be healthier if they simply walked 30–60 min every other day (Pate et al., 1991) *Healthy People 2000* is a report of the U.S. Public Health Service (1990) that outlines a national strategy for improving the health of the nation. It sets as a goal 30 min daily of light-to-moderate exercise (walking, swimming, cycling, dancing, and gardening) performed at less than 60% of maximum heart rate or 30 min three times per week of vigorous exercise at greater than 60% of maximum heart rate. Maximum heart rate or MHR roughly equals 220 beats per minute minus age. Brisk walking is an activity that many find easily adaptable to their lifestyle. Many large shopping malls have early openings allowing older persons to walk in a climate-controlled environment before the commercial stores open for business. It is important for healthcare professionals to encourage physical activity suited to clients' physical condition at all ages.

Nutrition

Another area to be considered is nutrition, as dietary factors contribute substantially to preventable illness and premature death. The Dietary Guidelines for Americans recommend that to stay healthy, a person should eat a variety of foods; maintain a healthy weight; choose a diet low in fat, saturated fat, and cholesterol; choose a diet with plenty of vegetables, fruits, and grain products; use sugar only in moderation; and if alcoholic beverages are consumed, do so in moderation. Intake of dietary fat needs to be assessed and kept at approximately 30% of total calories consumed. Saturated fat intake should be kept at less than 10% of total daily calories. Excessive consumption of fat is linked to a higher risk of heart disease, breast and colon cancer, and gallbladder disease.

Obesity is a common nutritional problem of public health concern in the United States. Approximately 26% of white American males aged 65 to 76 years are overweight, 37% of white American women are overweight (Morley, 1998). Obesity is more common among African Americans. Older persons tend to have abdominal fat and less peripheral weight, with an increase in waist-to-hip ratio. Although the mortality associated with obesity tends to decrease with aging, obesity with increased age is correlated with hypertension, sleep apnea, pulmonary embolism, gallbladder disease, diagnostic problems and increased surgical risk (Morley, 1998).

Obesity is, also, closely linked to impaired glucose metabolism and the development of NIDDM. It increases the work of the heart and can lead to cardiac enlargement and can lead to osteoarthritis of the weight-bearing joints. Excess weight tends to "creep up on" persons. Most Americans gain 15–25 lb between the ages of 25 and 50 because of decreased activity and a reduced metabolic rate. Because obesity (defined as 30% or more over desirable weight) can cause new health problems or worsen existing ones, weight reduction should be recommended to those who are 30% or more over their desirable weight. Traditionally, a formula such as the following has been used as a guide (Davidson, 1976):

Men (medium frame): 106 lb for the first 5 ft plus 6 lb for each additional inch.*

Women (medium frame): 100 lb for the first 5 ft plus 5 lb for each additional inch.*

There are other methods of determining desirable weight. *Table 10-1* compares Metropolitan weight recommendations with the age-specific recommendations developed by Andres et al. (1985). The age-specific weight standards are felt to be more accurate for young adults and for those in their 50s and 60s. Diet combined with exercise has proved to be effective for weight reduction.

Calcium intake is particularly important for women, because osteoporosis is a major cause of fractures, immobility, and death in the elderly. Risk of osteoporosis can be decreased by adequate calcium intake in middle life and continued adequate calcium intake with exercise older women. Postmenopausal women should have a daily calcium intake of 1200 to 1500mg (Lyles, 1998). Post-menopausal women can increase bone mass in the spine and hip and reduce the rate of vertebral compression fractures by 50% through the use of estrogen. Estrogen replacement therapy can be given either orally or by transdermal patch. Evidence indicates a greatly reduced risk of heart disease in women taking estrogens after menopause and appears to tip the scales in favor of estrogen supplementation for women.

Smoking/Alcohol

According to *Healthy People 2000*, tobacco use is the most important single preventable cause of death in the United States, accounting for 1 of every 6 deaths or 390,000 deaths annually. It is a major risk factor for diseases of the heart and blood vessels; chronic bronchitis and emphysema; cancer

TABLE 10-1
Comparison of the Weight-for-Height Tables from Actuarial Data (Build Study): Non-Age-Corrected Metropolitan Life Insurance Company and Age-Specific Gerontology Research Center Recommendations[a]

Ht. (ft.-in.)	Metropolitan 1983 Weights pounds) for Ages 25-59[b]		Gerontology Research Center Weight Range for Men and Women (pounds)[c]				
	Men	Women	Age 25	Age 35	Age 45	Age 55	Age 65
4-10	–	100-131	84-111	92-119	99-127	107-135	115-142
4-11	–	101-134	87-115	95-123	103-131	111-139	119-147
5-0	–	103-137	90-119	98-127	106-135	114-143	123-152
5-1	123-145	105-140	93-123	101-131	110-140	118-148	127-157
5-2	125-148	108-144	96-127	105-136	113-144	122-153	131-163
5-3	127-151	111-148	99-131	108-140	117-149	126-158	135-168
5-4	129-155	114-152	102-135	112-145	121-154	130-163	140-173
5-5	131-159	117-156	106-140	115-149	125-159	134-168	144-179
5-6	133-163	120-160	109-144	119-154	129-164	138-174	148-184
5-7	135-167	123-164	112-148	122-159	133-169	143-179	153-190
5-8	137-171	126-167	116-153	126-163	137-174	147-184	158-196
5-9	139-175	129-170	119-157	130-168	141-179	151-190	162-201
5-10	141-179	132-173	122-162	134-173	145-184	156-195	167-207
5-11	144-183	135-176	126-167	137-178	149-190	160-201	172-211
6-0	147-187	–	129-171	141-183	153-195	165-207	177-219
6-1	150-192	–	133-176	145-188	157-200	169-213	182-225
6-2	153-197	–	137-181	149-194	162-206	174-219	187-232
6-3	157-202	–	141-186	153-199	168-212	179-225	192-238
6-4	–	–	144-191	157-205	171-218	184-231	197-244

[a] Values in this table are for height without shoes and weight without clothes. To convert inches to centimeters, multiply by 2.54; to convert pounds to kilograms, multiply by 0.455.

[b] The weight range is the lower weight for small frame and the upper weight for large frame.

[c] Data from Andres R: Mortality and obesity: The rationale for age specific height-weight tables. In Andres R, Bierman EL, Hazzard WR (eds) *Principals of Geriatric Medicine.* New York, McGraw-Hill, 1985, 311–318.

Source: US Public Health Service (1990). *Healthy People 2000: National Health Promotion and Disease Prevention Objectives* (CDHHS Publication. No. PHS 91-502127). Washington DC: US Government Printing Office.

of the lung, larynx, pharynx, oral cavity, esophagus, pancreas, and bladder; and other problems such as respiratory infections and stomach ulcers. Smoking is responsible for 85% of all lung cancer deaths. There is some evidence showing that long-term smokers can benefit from stopping smoking by reducing their risk of heart disease, increasing their life expectancy, and improving respiratory

function and circulation. There is also epidemiological evidence showing that even in the elderly, cessation of smoking is accompanied by decreased risk of death due to heart disease. Efforts to promote smoking cessation should occur at all ages.

Excessive drinking is a significant risk factor for many serious health problems, including cirrhosis of the liver, injuries, and suicidal behavior. It has been estimated by the National Institute on Alcohol Abuse and Alcoholism that as many as 40% of hospital beds are filled at any one time with patients whose illness is caused (at least in part) by alcohol.

It is estimated that 12% of men and 1% to 3% of women over 60 have severe problems related to alcohol abuse. Some speculate that heavy drinking gradually subsides until age 70, when an increase occurs (Ebersole & Hess, 1998). It may be that the stresses of aging activate alcohol abuse and this may in turn increase the stresses of aging. Older women tend to credit increased drinking to stress while older men blame boredom.

Since about one third of the population is abstinent, the consumption of alcohol is concentrated in the approximately 94 million drinking Americans. About one third of that number (30 million) consume approximately 70% of all the alcohol produced. It is this group that uses the healthcare system more frequently, is most at risk of trauma, and has the recurring problems that constitute the disease alcoholism. In spite of these data, alcoholism is frequently overlooked and remains largely untreated.

The multiple dangers of alcohol abuse are well documented and publicized, and although the danger must not be negated, there are some established benefits to moderate alcohol intake. Numerous studies have shown a decreased incidence and prevalence of the major cause of death in all industrialized societies—coronary heart disease—among those who consume moderate amounts of alcohol compared with those who abstain. A recent study of Japanese men undergoing coronary angiography for suspected coronary artery disease showed that those who consumed a moderate amount of alcohol (1–1.5 oz daily) had significantly less coronary stenosis than those who drank less or more. Although the serious consequences of excessive acute or chronic alcohol intake should

not be underestimated, the benefit of moderate alcohol use should not be dismissed (Kaplan & Saddock,1994).

COMMUNITY SETTING

Although nursing facilities are often thought of as the place for aging members of society, the truth is that only 5% of the elderly population are in nursing facilities at any point in time. Most older persons live outside of institutions. There are a growing number of resources available to assist elders to maintain their independence. Many grew out of the increasing political activism of elderly people. The Gray Panther movement of the seventies and the Pepper Commission of the eighties focused the attention of Congress and the public on the dramatic increase occurring in the old and older populations. Senior centers and other community-based agencies expanded their services to meet the growing need of health provision and screening for the elderly. Most states, either through the health department or Office on Aging, have created many sources of information for elderly persons and those who are caregivers for the elderly. As these vary from state to state, it is helpful to contact these resources and become aware of the services provided.

ASSESSMENT

Because of the variety of needs of older patients, a comprehensive approach to assessment has been advocated (Fretwell, 1992; Ebersole & Hess, 1998). This assessment looks beyond medical diagnoses and considers a wide range of areas that affect a person's capability for independent function. This is an approach that can be used in the community setting, as well as others. The following areas should be considered:

1. Activities of daily living (ADL) and Instrumental activities of daily living (IADL)

FIGURE 10-2 *(1 of 2)*
Ages 40 - 64, Schedule: Every 1–3 Years*

Leading Causes of Death:
Heart disease • Lung cancer
Cerebrovascular disease
Breast cancer • Colorectal cancer
Obstructive lung disease

SCREENING

History
Dietary intake
Physical activity
Tobacco/alcohol/drug use
Sexual practices

Physical Exam
Height and weight
Blood pressure
Clinical breast exam[1]
High-Risk Groups
    Complete skin exam (HR1)
    Complete oral cavity exam
      (HR2)
    Palpation for thyroid nodules
      (HR3)
    Auscultation for carotid bruits
      (HR4)

Laboratory/Diagnostic
  Procedures
Nonfasting total blood cholesterol
Papanicolaou smear[2]
Mammogram[3]
High-Risk Groups
    Fasting plasma glucose (HR5)
    VDRL/RPR (HR6)
    Urinalysis for bacteriuria
      (HR7)
    Chlamydial testing (HR8)
    Gonorrhea culture (HR9)
    Counseling and testing for
      HIV (HR10)
    Tuberculin skin test (PPD)
      (HR11)
    Hearing (HR 12)
    Electrocardiogram (HR13)
    Fecal occult blood/sigmoi-
      doscopy (HR14)
    Fecal occult
      blood/colonoscopy (HR15)
    Bone mineral content (HR16)

COUNSELING

Diet and Exercise
Fat (especially saturated fat), cholesterol, com-
    plex carbohydrates, fiber, sodium, calcium[4]
Caloric balance
Selection of exercise program

Substance Use
Tobacco cessation
Alcohol and other drugs:
Limiting alcohol consumption
Driving/other dangerous activities while under
    the influence
Treatment for abuse
High-Risk Groups
    Sharing/using unsterilized needles and
      syringes (HR19)

Sexual Practices
Sexually transmitted diseases: partner selection,
    condoms, anal intercourse
Unintended pregnancy and contraceptive
    options

Injury Prevention
Safety belts
Safety helmets
Smoke detector
Smoking near bedding or upholstery
High-Risk Groups
    Back-conditioning exercises (HR20)
    Prevention of childhood injuries (HR21)
    Falls in the elderly (HR22)

Dental Health
Regular tooth brushing, flossing, and dental
    visits

Other Primary Preventive Measures
High-Risk Groups
    Skin protection from ultraviolet light
      (HR23)
    Discussion of aspirin therapy (HR24)
    Discussion of estrogen replacement therapy
      (HR25)

IMMUNIZATIONS
Tetanus-diphtheria (Td)
  booster[5]
High-Risk Groups
    Hepatitis B vaccine
      (HR26)
    Pneumococcal vaccine
      (HR27)
    Influenza vaccine (HR28)[6]

This list of preventive services
is not exhaustive. It reflects
only those topics reviewed by
the U.S. Preventive Services
Task Force. Clinicians may
wish to add other preventive
services on a routine basis and
alter considering the patient's
medical history and other individual circumstances.
Examples of target conditions
not specifically examined by
the Task Force include:
    Chronic obstructive pul-
      monary disease
    Hepatobiliary disease
    Bladder cancer
    Endometrial disease
    Travel-related illness
    Prescription drug abuse
    Occupational illness and
      injuries

Remain Alert For:
Depressive symptoms
Suicide risk factors (HR17)
Abnormal bereavement
Signs of physical abuse or
  neglect
Malignant skin lesions
Peripheral arterial disease
  (HR18)
Tooth decay, gingivitis, loose
  teeth

*The recommended schedule applies only to the periodic visit itself. The frequency of the individual preventive services
  listed in this table is left to clinical discretion, except as indicated in other footnotes.

1. Annually. 2. Every 1–2 years for women until age 75, unless pathology detected. 3. For women. 4. Every 1–3 years.
    5. Every 10 years.

Source: US Public Health Service (1990). *Healthy people 2000: National Health Promotion and Disease Prevention Objectives* (CDHHS Publication.
No. PHS 91-502127). Washington DC: US Government Printing Office.

FIGURE 10-2 *(2 of 2)*
Ages 40 - 64, High-Risk Categories

HR1 Persons with a family or personal history of skin cancer, increased occupational or recreational exposure to sunlight, or clinical evidence of precursor lesions (e.g., dysplastic nevi, certain congenital nevi).

HR2 Persons with exposure to tobacco or excessive amounts of alcohol, or those with suspicious symptoms or lesions detected through self-examination.

HR3 Persons with a history of upper-body irradiation.

HR4 Persons with risk factors for cerebrovascular or cardiovascular disease (e.g., hypertension, smoking, CAD, atrial fibrillation, diabetes) or those with neurologic symptoms (e.g., transient ischemic attacks) or a history of cerebrovascular disease.

HR5 The markedly obese, persons with a family history of diabetes, or women with a history of gestational diabetes.

HR6 Prostitutes, persons who engage in sex with multiple partners in areas in which syphilis is prevalent, or contacts of persons with active syphilis.

HR7 Persons with diabetes.

HR8 Persons who attend clinics for sexually transmitted diseases. attend other high-risk health care facilities (e.g.. adolescent and family planning clinics), or have other risk factors for chlamydial infection (e.g., multiple sexual partners or a sexual partner with multiple sexual contacts).

HR9 Prostitutes, persons with multiple sexual partners or a sexual partner with multiple contacts, sexual contacts of persons with culture-proven gonorrhea, or persons with a history of repeated episodes of gonorrhea.

HR10 Persons seeking treatment for sexually transmitted diseases; homosexual and bisexual men; past or present intravenous (IV) drug users; persons with a history of prostitution or multiple sexual partners; women whose past or present sexual partners were HIV-infected, bisexual, or IV drug users; persons with long-term residence or birth in an area with high prevalence of HIV infection; or persons with a history of transfusion between 1978 and 1985.

HR11 Household members of persons with tuberculosis or others at risk for close contact with the disease (e.g., staff of tuberculosis clinics, shelters for the homeless, nursing homes, substance abuse treatment facilities, dialysis units, correctional institutions); recent immigrants or refugees from countries in which tuberculosis is common (e.g., Asia, Africa, Central and South America, Pacific Islands); migrant workers: residents of nursing homes, correctional institutions, or homeless shelters; or persons with certain underlying medical disorders (e.g. HIV infection).

HR12 Persons exposed regularly to excessive noise.

HR13 Men with two or more cardiac risk factors (high blood cholesterol, hypertension, cigarette smoking, diabetes mellitus, family history of CAD); men who would endanger public safety were they to experience sudden cardiac events (e.g., commercial airline pilots); or sedentary or high-risk males planning to begin a vigorous exercise program.

HR14 Persons aged 50 and older who have first-degree relatives with colorectal cancer: a personal history of endometrial, ovarian, or breast cancer; or a previous diagnosis of inflammatory bowel disease. adenomatous polyps, or colorectal cancer.

HR15 Persons with a family history of familial polyposis coli or cancer family syndrome.

HR16 Perimenopausal women at increased risk for osteoporosis (e.g., Caucasian race, bilateral oopherectomy before menopause, slender build) and for whom estrogen replacement therapy would otherwise not be recommended.

HR17 Recent divorce, separation, unemployment, depression, alcohol, other drug abuse. serious medical illnesses, living alone, or recent bereavement.

HR18 Persons over age 50, smokers, or persons with diabetes mellitus.

HR19 Intravenous drug users.

HR20 Persons at increased risk for low back injury because of past history, body configuration, or type of activities.

HR21 Persons with children in the home or automobile.

HR22 Persons with older adults in the home.

HR23 Persons with increased exposure to sunlight.

HR24 Men who have risk factors for myocardial infarction (e.g., high blood cholesterol, smoking, diabetes mellitus, family history of early-onset CAD) and who lack a history of gastrointestinal or other bleeding problems, and other risk factors for bleeding or cerebral hemorrhage.

HR25 Perimenopausal women at increased risk for osteoporosis (e g., Caucasian, low bone mineral content, bilateral oopherectomy before menopause or early menopause. slender build) and who are without known contraindications (e. g., history of undiagnosed vaginal bleeding, active liver disease, thromboembolic disorders, hormone-dependent cancer).

HR26 Homosexually active men, intravenous drug users, recipients of some blood products, or persons in health-related jobs with frequent exposure to blood or blood products.

HR27 Persons with medical conditions that increase the risk of pneumococcal infection (e.g., chronic cardiac or pulmonary disease, sickle cell disease, nephrotic syndrome, Hodgkin's disease, asplenia, diabetes mellitus, alcoholism, cirrhosis, multiple myeloma, renal disease or conditions associated with immunosuppression).

HR28 Residents of chronic care facilities and persons suffering from chronic cardiopulmonary disorders, metabolic diseases (including diabetes mellitus), hemoglobinopathies, immunosuppression, or renal dysfunction.

Source: US Public Health Service (1990). *Healthy people 2000: National Health Promotion and Disease Prevention Objectives* (CDHHS Publication. No. PHS 91-502127). Washington DC: US Government Printing Office.

FIGURE 10-3 *(1 of 2)*
Ages 65 and Over, Schedule: Every Years*

Leading Causes of Death:
Heart disease • Cerebrovascular disease
Obstructive lung disease
Pneumonia/influenza
Lung cancer • Colorectal cancer

SCREENING

History
Prior symptoms of transient
    ischemic attack
Dietary intake
Physical activity
Tobacco/alcohol/drug use
Functional status at home

Physical Exam
Height and weight
Blood pressure
Visual acuity
Hearing and hearing aids
Clinical breast exam[1]
High-Risk Groups
    Auscultation for carotid bruits
        (HR1)
    Complete skin exam (HR2)
    Complete oral cavity exam
        (HR3)
    Palpation of thyroid nodules
        (HR4)

Laboratory/Diagnostic
    Procedures
Nonfasting total blood cholesterol
Dipstick urinalysis
Mammogram[2]
Thyroid function tests[3]
High-Risk Groups
    Fasting plasma glucose (HR5)
    Tuberculin skin test (PPD)
        (HR6)
    Electrocardiogram (HR7)
    Papanicolaou smear[4] (HR8)
    Fecal occult
        blood/Sigmoidoscopy
        (HR9)
    Fecal occult
        blood/Colonoscopy
        (HR10)

COUNSELING

Diet and Exercise
Fat (especially saturated fat), cholesterol, com-
    plex carbohydrates, fiber, sodium, calcium[3]
Caloric balance
Selection of exercise program

Substance Use
Tobacco cessation
Alcohol and other drugs:
    Limiting alcohol consumption
    Driving/other dangerous activities while
        under the influence
    Treatment for abuse

Injury Prevention
Prevention of falls
Safety belts
Smoke detector
Smoking near bedding or upholstery
Hot water heater temperature
Safely helmets
High-Risk Groups
    Prevention of childhood injuries (HR12)

Dental Health
Regular dental visits, tooth brushing, flossing

Other Primary Preventive Measures
Glaucoma testing by eye specialist
High-Risk Groups
    Discussion of estrogen replacement therapy
        (HR13)
    Discussion of aspirin therapy (HR14)
    Skin protection form ultraviolet light
        (HR15)

IMMUNIZATIONS
Tetanus-diphtheria (Td)
    booster[5]
Influenza vaccine[6]
Pneumococcal vaccine
High-Risk Groups
    Hepatitis B vaccine
        (HR16)

**This list of preventIve ser-
vices is not exhaustive.** It
reflects only those topics
reviewed by the U.S.
Preventive Services Task
Force. Clinicians may wish to
add other preventive services
on a routine basis and alter
considering the patient's medical history and other individual circumstances. Examples
of target conditions not specifically examined by the Task
Force include:
    Chronic obstructive pul-
        monary disease
    Hepatobiliary disease
    Bladder cancer
    Endometrial disease
    Travel-related illness
    Prescription drug abuse
    Occupational illness and
        injuries

Remain Alert For:
Depression symptoms
Suicide risk factors (HR11)
Abnormal bereavement
Changes in cognitive function
Medications that increase risk
    of falls
Signs of physical abuse or
    neglect
Malignant skin lesions
Peripheral arterial disease
Tooth decay, gingivitis, loose
    teeth

*The recommended schedule applies only to the periodic visit itself. The frequency of the individual preventive services
    listed in this table is left to clinical discretion, except as indicated in other footnotes.

1. Annually for women. 2. Every 1–3 years for women. 3. Every 1–2 years for women beginning at age 50 (age 35 for
    those at increased risk). 4. For women. 5. Every 10 years. 6. Annually.

Source: US Public Health Service (1990). *Healthy people 2000: National Health Promotion and Disease Prevention Objectives* (CDHHS Publication.
No. PHS 91-502127). Washington DC: US Government Printing Office.

FIGURE 10-3 *(2 of 2)*
Ages 65 and Over, High-Risk Categories

HR1 Persons with risk factors for cerebrovascular or cardio-vascular disease (e.g., hypertension, smoking, CAD, atrial fibrillation, diabetes) or those with neurologic symptoms (e.g., transient ischemic attacks) or a history of cerebrovascular disease.

HR2 Persons with a family or personal history of skin cancer, or clinical evidence of precursor lesions (e.g., dysplastic nevi, certain congenital nevi), or those with increased occupational or recreational exposure to sunlight.

HR3 Persons with exposure to tobacco or excessive amounts of alcohol, or those with suspicious symptoms or lesions detected through self-examination.

HR4 Persons with a history of upper-body irradiation.

HR5 The markedly obese, persons with a family history of diabetes, or women with a history of gestational diabetes.

HR6 Household members of persons with tuberculosis or others at risk for close contact with the disease (e.g., staff of tuberculosis clinics, shelters for the homeless, nursing homes, substance abuse treatment facilities, dialysis units, correctional institutions); recent immigrants or refugees from countries in which tuberculosis is common (e.g., Asia, Africa, Central and South America, Pacific Islands); migrant workers: residents of nursing homes, correctional institutions, or homeless shelters; or persons with certain underlying medical disorders (e.g., HIV infection).

HR7 Men with two or more cardiac risk factors (high blood cholesterol, hypertension,. cigarette smoking, diabetes mellitus, family history of CAD); men who would endanger public safety were they to experience sudden cardiac events (e.g., commercial airline pilots); or sedentary or high-risk males planning to begin a vigorous exercise program.

HR8 Women who have not had previous documented screening in which smears have been consistently negative.

HR9 Persons who have first-degree relatives with colorectal cancer: a personal history of endometrial, ovarian, or breast cancer: or a previous diagnosis of inflammatory bowel disease, adenomalous polyps, or colorectal cancer.

HR10 Persons with a family history of familial polyposis coli or cancer family syndrome.

HR11 Recent divorce, separation, unemployment, depression, alcohol or other drug abuse, serious medical illnesses, living alone, or recent bereavement.

HR12 Persons with children in the home or automobile.

HR13 Women at increased risk for osteoporosis (e.g., Caucasian, low bone mineral content, bilateral oopherectomy before menopause or early menopause, slender build) and who are without known contraindications (e.g., history of undiagnosed vaginal bleeding, active liver disease, thromboembolic disorders, hormone-dependent cancer).

HR14 Men who have risk factors for myocardial infarction (e.g., high blood cholesterol, smoking, diabetes mellitus, family history of early-onset CAD) and who lack a history of gastrointestinal or other bleeding problems, or other risk factors for bleeding or cerebral hemorrhage.

HR15 Persons with increased exposure to sunlight.

HR16 Homosexually active men, intravenous drug users, recipients of some blood products, or persons in health-related jobs with frequent exposure to blood or blood products.

Source: US Public Health Service (1990). *Healthy people 2000: National Health Promotion and Disease Prevention Objectives* (CDHHS Publication. No. PHS 91-502127). Washington DC: US Government Printing Office.

---

2. Cognitive function

3. Fall risk

4. Medication

5. Hearing and vision

6. Socialization and family resources

The central focus of the assessment is on function, because a person's functional abilities will greatly influence the amount of care and support services needed. Physical function can be evaluated easily by using a scale such as that developed by Katz et al., which looks at ADLs such as bathing, dressing, toileting, transferring, feeding, and continence *(Figure 10-4)*. Ability to perform IADLs, including use of the telephone, shopping, preparing food, and housekeeping, should also be assessed *(Figure 10-5)*. The latter activities are especially important for elderly people living independently.

Cognitive function is evaluated quickly and easily by using a scale such as Folstein's mini-mental status examination *(Figure 10-6)*. This is a 30-point scale that can be given in about 10 min and is reliable. Scores of less than 24 suggest impairment, and scores of less than 20 may be indicative of dementia (Reuben, 1998). It often happens that acute illness in the elderly will be manifested as a change in mental status.

FIGURE 10-4
Activities of Daily Living (ADL) Scale

EVALUATION FORM

Name_____Day of Evaluation_____

For each area of functioning listed below, check description that applies. (The word "assistance" means supervision, direction, or personal assistance.)

BATHING: either sponge bath, tub bath or shower.

☐ Receives no assistance *(gets in and out of tub by self, if tub is usual means of bathing).*

☐ Receives assistance in bathing only one part of the body (such as back or a leg).

☐ Receives assistance in bathing more than one part of the body (or not bathed).

DRESSING: gets clothes from closets and drawers, including underclothes, outer garments, and using fasteners *(including braces, if worn).*

☐ Gets clothes and gets completely dressed without assistance.

☐ Gets clothes and gets dressed without assistance, except for assistance in tying shoes.

☐ Receives assistance in getting clothes or in getting dressed, or stays partly or completely undressed.

TOILETING: going to the "toilet room" for bowel and urine elimination; cleaning self after elimination and arranging clothes.

☐ Goes to "toilet room," cleans self, and arranges clothes without assistance *(may use object for support such as cane, walker, or wheelchair and may manage night bedpan or commode, emptying same in morning).*

☐ Receives assistance in going to "toilet room" or in cleansing self or in arranging clothes after elimination or in use of night bedpan or commode.

☐ Doesn't go to room termed "toilet" for the elimination process.

TRANSFER

☐ Moves in and out of bed as well as in and out of chair without assistance *(may be using object for support, such as cane or walker).*

☐ Moves in and out of bed or chair with assistance.

☐ Doesn't get out of bed.

CONTINENCE

☐ Controls urination and bowel movements completely by self.

☐ Has occasional "accidents".

☐ Supervision helps keep urine or bowel control; catheter is used or person is incontinent.

FEEDING

☐ Feeds self without assistance.

☐ Feeds self except for getting assistance in cutting meat or buttering bread.

☐ Receives assistance in feeding or is fed partly or completely by using tubes or intravenous fluids.

Adapted from: Katz, S., Ford, A. B., Moskowitz, R. W., et al. (1963). Studies of illness in the aged. The index of ADL: A standard measure of biological and psychosocial function. *Journal of the American Medical Association,* 185, 914.

FIGURE 10-5

Instrumental Activities or Daily Living (IADL) Scale

Self-Rated Version Extracted from the Multilevel Assessment Instrument (MAL)

1. Can you use the telephone:
   without help, — 3
   with some help, or — 2
   are you completely unable to use the telephone? — 1

2. Can you get to places out of walking distance:
   without help, — 3
   with some help, or — 2
   are you completely unable to travel unless special arrangements are made? — 1

3. Can you go shopping for groceries:
   without help, — 3
   with some help, or — 2
   are you completely unable to do any shopping? — 1

4. Can you prepare your own meals:
   without help, — 3
   with some help, or — 2
   are you completely unable to prepare any meals? — 1

5. Can you do your own housework:
   without help, — 3
   with some help, or — 2
   are you completely unable to do any housework? — 1

6. Can you do your own handyman work:
   without help, — 3
   with some help, or — 2
   are you completely unable to do any handyman work? — 1

7. Can you do your own laundry:
   without help, — 3
   with some help, or — 2
   are you completely unable to do any laundry at all? — 1

8a. Do you take medicines or use any medications?
   (If yes, answer Question 8b) Yes — 1
   (If no, answer Question 8c) No — 2

8b. Do you take your own medicine:
   without help (in the right doses at the right time), — 3
   with some help (take medicine if someone prepares it for you and/or reminds you to take it), or — 2
   (are you/would you be) completely unable to take your own medicine? — 1

8c. If you had to take medicine, can you do it:
   without help (in the right doses at the right time), — 3
   with some help (take medicine if someone prepares it for you and/or reminds you to take it), or — 2
   (are you/would you be) completely unable to take your own medicine? — 1

9. Can you manage your own money:
   without help, — 3
   with some help, or — 2
   you completely unable to handle money? — 1

FIGURE 10-6
Mini-Mental Health State Exam

Patient_____Date_____Examiner_____

Maximum Score	Score	ORIENTATION

5   [   ]   What is the (year) (season) (date) (day) (month)?

5   [   ]   Where are we: (state) (county) (town) (hospital) (floor)

REGISTRATION

[   ]   Name 3 objects: 1 second to say each. Then ask the patient all 3 after you have said them.

3

Give 1 point for each correct answer. Then repeat them until he learns all 3. Count trials and record.

Trials_____

ATTENTION AND CALCULATION

[   ]   Serial 7's. 1 point for each correct. Stop after 5 answers. Alternatively spell "world" backwards.

RECALL

5

[   ]   Ask for 3 objects repeated above. Give 1 point for each correct.

LANGUAGE

[   ]   Name a pencil, and watch (2 points)

3   Repeat the follow "No ifs, ands or buts." (1 point)

Follow a 3-stage command: "Take a paper in your right hand, fold it in half, and put it on the floor." (3 points)

9   Read and obey the following: "Close your eyes" (1 point)

Write a sentence. (1 point)

Copy design. (1 point)

_____

TOTAL SCORE

ASSESS level of consciousness along a continuum

_____

Alert   Drowsy   Stupor   Comatose

In validation studies using a cut-off score of 23 or below, the MMSE has a sensitivity of 87%, a specificity of 82%, a false positive ratio of 39.4%, and a false negative ratio of 4.7%. These ratios refer to the MMSE's capacity to accurately distinguish patients with clinically diagnosed dementia or delirium from patients without these syndromes.

Adapted from: Folstein, M. F. & Spenser, M. P. The Mini-Mental State Examination, in Keller, P. A.: *Innovations in Clinical Practice: A Source Book.* (1985).

Fall-risk assessment is also important because fall incidence and severity of fall-related complications rise steadily after middle age (Rubenstein, 1998). Accidents are the fifth leading cause of death in older persons, and falls cause two thirds of these accidental deaths. About three fourths of the deaths caused by falls in this country occur in the over 65 population which is only 13% of the total population.

In addition, one third to one half of people more than 65 years of age suffer at least one avoidable fall a year. Many lead to hip fractures. Older disabled persons should have appropriate assistive devices (i.e., cane or walker if needed for balance or support). Lighting in the home should be adequate both inside and outside. Torn or loose rugs should be replaced. There should be appropriate bathroom safety equipment, if needed (Rubenstein, 1998).

Medications need to be evaluated. Many elders use a variety of medications both prescribed and over-the-counter. There may be interactions among drugs, as well as adverse effects from particular medications. Because of reduced liver and renal function in the elderly, many drugs need to be prescribed in dosages that are lower than those required by the general adult population in order to avoid toxic effects.

Hearing and vision assessments may uncover problems that can correct and thus may improve the patient's quality of life.

An evaluation of social supports is critical. Isolated elderly patients will be more prone to depression and need more community support in the event of functional decline than those with a strong social network. In addition, the needs of caregivers must be considered and balanced along with the needs of the patient. Caregivers, often spouse or family members, need support to avoid "burn-out."

HOME HEALTH AND HOSPICE CARE

Not infrequently, an elderly person will have an acute illness or accident that may lead to the need for continued health services in the home. For those patients more than 65 years of age, Medicare is the principal public health insurance. Medicare consists of Part A, or hospital insurance, and Part B, or supplementary medical insurance.

Part A covers four kinds of care:

1. Inpatient hospital care
2. Medically necessary inpatient care in a skilled facility
3. Home health care
4. Hospice care

Home health care may be provided if these criteria are met:

1. Patient is homebound.
2. Physician develops and certifies a plan of care.
3. Skilled care, (e. g. nursing, physical therapy) is required.

Home health care provides in-home part-time or intermittent skilled nursing care and physical and/or speech therapy. Home health aides may also be provided as long as skilled needs are necessary.

Part B of Medicare, a voluntary program paid for by the elderly person, pays a portion of the cost of a physician, outpatient care, outpatient physical or speech therapy services, some home health care services, and supplies not covered by Part A.

Home health care includes many services, not all of which may be covered by Medicare. Most communities have home health agencies that can provide a wide range of services, such as skilled nursing; physical; speech; occupational therapy; medical and social services; nutritional services; meals; homemaker services; home health aides;

respiratory and IV therapy; and medical supplies and appliances.

Hospice services may be provided by a Medicare-certified hospice program if a physician certifies that a patient is terminally ill (less than 6 months to live) and the patient chooses hospice care instead of regular home care.

Medicaid (Medical Assistance) is available to a person in need of home care if he or she meets the state's income and asset requirements. These will vary from state to state. Medicaid, Title XIX of the Social Security Act, will provide medically necessary care on an intermittent basis under a treatment plan by a physician. Provided is nursing care, home health aides, and medical supplies and equipment, if the patient meets the eligibility requirements. Other sources for reimbursement are the Older American Act Title III and VII for persons over 60 with low income, which provides coverage for senior center day care, Meals-on-Wheels, transportation, home repair, information, and referral. The Social Services Act, Title XX of the Social Security Act, will provide homemaker chore service workers on the basis of need.

RESOURCES

The following is a listing of other resources available to older persons and their families. These can help provide needed support and avoid institutionalization. Currently, many of these resources are not covered by Medicare.

1. **Legal and protective services:** Legal services are sometimes available to elderly persons at minimal cost. Protective services are designed for elders who are judged incapable of caring for themselves or who are at risk for abuse or neglect by others.

2. **Monitoring services:** Services intended to supervise or keep in touch with frail, elderly persons living alone. These include telephone networks and friendly visitors, as well as alarm systems (e.g. Lifeline).

3. **Special housing:** These vary from continuing care retirement communities that provide a range of types of housing and health care services to congregate care in which elders have their own apartment but can receive selected services to personal care homes.

4. **Senior centers:** These were developed in the 1940s with the initial purpose of providing social and recreational activities (Kern, 1990). Health fairs may be held where screening tests for vision, hearing, blood pressure, cervical cancer, and rectal cancer are done.

5. **Homemaker or chore services:** Housekeeping services that allow elderly persons to remain at home include house cleaning, shopping, meal preparation, and errands.

6. **Adult day care:** Centers provide places where disabled elders can go during the day; they are often used to relieve caregivers' burdens. Eligibility varies from center to center.

7. **Transportation or mobility:** Elderly persons are often eligible for reduced fares on public transportation as well as for special modes of transportation if handicapped.

8. **Support groups:** These are groups that bring together persons with similar concerns, (e.g., Parkinson's disease, stroke clubs, caregiver groups). They provide education and peer interaction.

9. **Nutrition programs:** Senior centers and other community-based agencies often provide "eating together" programs that meet nutritional needs and provide opportunity for social contact, educational programs, and outreach efforts. For those who are unable to shop or prepare meals, there are Meals-on-Wheels programs that deliver a hot meal and snack daily to the patient's home.

ACUTE CARE

People over age 65 constitute the greatest consumers of acute hospital services in the United States. (Eliopoulous, 1990). More than 5 million persons over age 65 are hospitalized yearly. Admission to the hospital often results in complications and adjustment problems not seen in younger persons as hospitalized individuals with functional disabilities often regress to a state of helplessness rapidly (Ebersole & Hess, 1998). In addition, many elderly patients tend to have chronic problems that hospitals are poorly equipped to handle. Hospitalization is often followed by an irreversible decline in functional status and quality of life. Many studies support this contention (Creditor, 1993). Elderly patients often experience problems that lengthen their hospital stay and make illnesses more difficult to treat. At its worst, hospitalization can result in permanent institutionalization or death—the so-called cascade of disasters. For example, an elderly woman experiences hypotension and falls as a result of too vigorous treatment for hypertension. Having broken a hip, she is admitted to the hospital for surgical repair. Following surgery, she initially does well for a day or two. Fever then develops, and it is determined she has pneumonia. She becomes disoriented and, as a result, cannot participate in rehabilitation. Her hospital discharge is delayed, and she eventually needs to go to a nursing facility until she is able to independently care for herself.

A systematic assessment of elderly patients soon after admission is critical to promote timely interventions for minimizing disability and maximizing independence. The assessment should include the following:

- Social functioning, including family systems and significant relationships

- Morale

- Sensory impairments

- Prosthetic aids used

- Economic resources

- Home environment and management

- Availability of community resources that could provide assistance after discharge

- Patient's goals

Care should be taken not to put elderly patients into a passive role while they are hospitalized. Though it can be more time-consuming for staff, elderly patients should be allowed to do as much of their ADLs as possible. This is of particular importance for patients who were independent before their hospitalization.

The following sections briefly discuss common problems of the elderly in the acute care setting: immobility, cognitive impairment, incontinence, skin breakdown, and falls

Immobility

Other than hypotension, an acute neurological or cardiovascular event, recent surgery, and unstable fractures, there are very few reasons for immobilizing hospitalized older patients. Factors that cause immobilization in the hospital without legitimate reasons include environmental barriers such as bedrails, restraints, high beds, lack of staff to help with mobility, cognitive impairment, pain with movement, affective disorders, sensory changes, terminal illness, overuse of sedative and psychoactive drugs, and acute episodes of illness. Immobility or bedrest can result in severe deconditioning because, the rate of recovery for lost strength is much slower than the speed of the loss. A person at bedrest can lose 1–3% of his or her muscle strength per day. It may take 6 weeks to recover from 3 weeks of immobilization (Rubenstein, 1998). In addition, the immobilized patients are at risk for the development of other complications, including stiffness or contractures of joints, pressure sores pneumonia, constipation, fecal impaction, and deep-vein thromboses.

Prevention involves mobilizing patients as soon as possible and doing daily range of motion exercises.

Cognitive Impairment

Delirium or acute confusional state occurs in one third to one half of elderly patients at some point in their hospitalization and puts them at risk for complications. Delirium is a disturbance of cerebral function with global cognitive impairment that has an abrupt onset; is brief in duration; and is characterized by evident concurrent disturbances in attention, sleep-wake cycle, and psychomotor behavior. Delirium can be caused by environmental dislocation, adverse drug reactions, including postanesthesia effects; urinary tract infection, malnutrition, hypoglycemia or hyperglycemia, and fluid and electrolyte disturbances. Treatment of delirium should include addressing all reversible problems and providing for patient's safety in the interim. One effective intervention is the continuous presence of a reliable family member or friend who can reassure the individual that the terrifying experience is temporary (Ebersole & Hess, 1998). Delirium or confusion may be manifested as the following (Fretwell, 1992).

- Verbal or behavioral manifestations of disorientation to place.

- Inappropriate behaviors such as pulling dressings or tubes, physical combativeness.

- Inappropriate communication such as incoherent speech, verbal combativeness.

- Visual or auditory hallucinations.

Whenever possible, one should try to prevent the occurrence of delirium. Nursing measures that may be helpful in preventing delirium include the following:

- Visit the patient frequently, especially in the beginning of the hospitalization. Provide a supportive environment.

- Orient the patient to hospital routines.

- Explain diagnostic tests and treatments. Explain rationale for various steps.

- Use drugs appropriately and judiciously for the treatment of anxiety, agitation, and insomnia.

- Anticipate common problems, such as nocturnal falls, incontinence, missed meals, and lack of sleep. Take appropriate prophylactic measures (Fretwell, 1992).

- Place the patient in a quiet, well-lighted room in which a clock, a calendar, and a few familiar objects are clearly visible (Lipowski, 1989).

Incontinence

Because it is a leading cause of social isolation and institutionalization of the elderly, incontinence should not be ignored or viewed as an inevitable consequence of aging. The major causes of incontinence in the acute care setting are medications, mental status changes, fecal impaction, immobility, restraints, and psychological regression. Often indwelling catheters are inserted, putting the patient at risk for urinary tract infections, instead of addressing the underlying causes. Incontinence has been cited as a major reason for institutionalization in the United States and other countries. Besides displacement from one's home and the sequelae of the relocation, incontinence often causes psychological distress, lowered self-esteem, and withdrawal from society and social activities. Untoward physical effects of incontinence have also been reported, including skin breakdown and urinary tract infection, especially with fecal incontinence (Joffrion & Leuszler, 1995).

Once incontinence begins, it tends to persist and becomes more severe with advanced age and other infirmities, such as immobility. Nurses must target appropriate groups for health education, clinical assessment, and interventions necessary to alleviate or at least modify incontinence. Incontinence can be treated. There are behavioral therapies such as habit training, contingency management, bladder retraining, pelvic-floor exercises, and biofeedback that can be used to modify or eliminate incontinence (McDowell, Burgio, & Candid, 1990).

The Agency for Health Care Policy and Research (AHCPR) has published clinical practice guidelines regarding urinary incontinence in adults (AHCPR, 1992). This publication provides valuable information regarding diagnosis and treatment of incontinence.

Skin Breakdown

Pressure sores are predictable, preventable problems in most hospitalized older patients. The best intervention is prevention. Elderly patients who are at risk for skin problems should be placed on appropriate pressure-relieving devices early in their hospitalization and a regular turning schedule implemented. Various scales have been developed to detect at-risk patients.

The Norton Scale shown here *(Figure 10-7)* addresses general physical condition, mental condition, activity, mobility, and incontinence. Each area is graded on a scale of 1 to 4. If the sum of all five categories together is less than 14 or 15, there is significant risk of pressure sore development, and appropriate interventions should be instituted. The AHCPR (1992), has published clinical practice guidelines for the prevention of pressure sores. Guidelines for treatment of pressure ulcers were published in December, 1994, and remain the standard for clinicians.

Falls

Falls are a common problem among hospitalized elderly patients. Patients are considered as being at risk for falls if one or more of the following conditions are present:

- A known fall before or after admission
- Confusion, disorientation, uncontrolled restlessness, sedation
- Unsteady gait because of pain, fatigue, arthritis or osteoporosis
- Muscle weakness or interference with sense of balance
- Unwillingness or inability to call for help when walking
- An interruption of cerebral oxygenation with dizziness, syncope or vertigo
- A history of crawling out of bed
- Incontinence of bowel and/or bladder

Interventions such as providing bedside commodes, nonskid footwear, night lights, low bed positions, and frequent checks can result in a greatly reduced prevalence of falls.

Rather than make patients safer from falls in the hospital or acute care setting, physical restraints have been found to increase risks for patients. Typically, nursing staff initiate the use of physical restraints to manage patients' problem behaviors and to protect patients from hurting themselves. In the hospital milieu alone, the rate of restraint use in older patients is estimated to be between 13% and 20% (Matthiesen et al., 1996). Nurse in acute care setting have reported increased use of physical restraints when they felt that they were working short-staffed. OBRA and the Joint Commission for the Accreditation of Hospitals have taken stands recognizing the potential negative outcomes associated with the use of physical restraints. Alternatives to the use of physical restraints include: assessing for the underlying cause of the restlessness or other behavior, such as pain, itching, need to be toileted; reality orientation, active listening, therapeutic touch, beds closer to the floor, electronic alarms for beds and wheelchairs, accessible call lights, and— most important—adequate supervision by staff. The study by Matthiesen et al. showed that staff need role models who can help them problem solve and examine alternatives to the use of restraints. Reducing the use of restraints in the acute care setting is a priority for gerontological nurses.

FIGURE 10-7
The Norton Scale
Patient Assessment Form

Name	Date	Physical Condition		Mental Condition		Activity		Mobility		Incontinent		Total Score
		Good	4	Alert	4	Ambulant	4	Full	4	Not	4	
		Fair	3	Apathetic	3	Walk/help	3	Sl. limited	3	Occasional	3	
		Poor	2	Confused	2	Chairbound	2	V. limited	2	Usually/Urine	2	
		V. Bad	1	Stupor	1	Bed	1	Immobile	1	Doubly	1	

Adapted from: Norton, D., McLaren, R. & Exton-Smith, A. N. (1962). *An investigation of geriatric nursing problems in hospitals.* Edinburgh: Churchill Livingstone.

DISCHARGE PLANNING

Shortened hospital stays due to the implementation of the Medicare prospective payment plan based on diagnosis-related groups (DRGs) has resulted in the earlier discharge of patients, many of whom still have significant health problems. Discharge planning is essential and should begin when the patient is hospitalized. Older patients, the patients' families, and all members of the health care team should be involved. Discharge planning involves assessing the needs and limitations of patients and their caregivers during hospitalization, planning for continuity of health care on discharge, and coordinating needed individual, family, hospital, and community resources to implement the discharge plan. Some patients are likely to resume their lives as before, but others will require community supports or institutionalization. Comprehensive discharge planning is especially important for patients being discharged to the community. Discharge planning sessions with the family and patient are invaluable in giving information, clarifying understanding of the illness, and answering questions. Information can be shared regarding community agencies and other available resources.

In assessing the amount of support a patient will need in the community, the following guide (Cooney, 1990) is helpful:

1. **24-hr supervision**
   a. Patient cannot independently get from bed to chair or chair to toilet.
   b. Patient unsafe with transfers and walking.
   c. Patient incontinent.

2. **8 hr a day supervision**
   a. Patient cannot eat independently.

3. **2–4 hr a day supervision**
   a. Patient cannot dress independently.
   b. Patient cannot prepare own meals, but can manage with Meals-on-Wheels.

4. **Daily supervision**
   a. Patient needs help with medications.
   b. Patient needs help administering insulin, etc.

5. Three times a week

  a. Patient cannot bathe independently.

Other important factors to consider are environmental factors such as stairs; distance from bedroom to bathroom; needed medical equipment, and safety hazards, particularly with respect to risk of falling. The weeks following hospitalization are crucial. The patient and the patient's family will need as much support as possible. Nurses, who are most likely to view patients holistically, can pull together the resources needed to plan and coordinate to meet the physical, psychosocial and functional needs of the patient (Ebersole & Hess, 1998).

Inpatient and outpatient geriatric evaluation units are becoming more available. These are units where a geriatric patient can be evaluated more comprehensively and appropriate management plans made.

Patients without a primary caregiver who are not capable of caring for themselves or those who are in need of special rehabilitation services may need to be discharged to a nursing facility or rehabilitation facility.

REHABILITATION

Rehabilitation is defined as the restoration of physical and psychological health necessary for independent living and functional independence. Principles of rehabilitation are of major importance in working with elderly patients in all settings. The primary health problems of older adults are chronic: heart disease, high blood pressure, hearing loss, glaucoma or cataracts, arthritis, diabetes. Eighty percent of older adults have at least one chronic illness, and most have several. For many, chronic illness will mean a complete change in lifestyle. Patients will need support in adjusting to their limitations. Personal fulfillment in old age comes not only from reacting successfully to the challenges of loss, illness and change, but from continuing to direct one's own life and maintain dignity and self-worth (Stromberg, 1998). Listening to concerns and clarifying any confusion about the illness is important. Education needs to focus on the how and why of restructuring patients' lives and must extend to their family members and friends. Rehabilitation efforts for older adults should do the following (Matteson & McConnell, 1988):

1. Promote the patient's functional independence.

2. Prevent secondary disabilities.

3. Control underlying disease or impairment.

4. Preserve dignity of the individual.

Effective rehabilitation can enable elderly patients to improve their level of independence and live in a preferred and less costly community setting.

Rehabilitation can occur in many settings. Often the determining factor is the patient's medical insurance and what it will cover. Medicare will allow rehabilitative therapies in the acute care setting if there is an appropriate diagnosis and significant deficit. Often patients are discharged before they regain function and must seek further rehabilitation in other settings such as rehabilitation units or hospitals, or nursing facilities or through home health care. Medicare will pay for acute needs, but not for maintenance or chronic needs. There must be documentation of daily progress. Patients who are poorly motivated are quickly dropped from rehabilitation programs.

Successful rehabilitation is dependent on the positive outlook and the mutually agreeable goals of both staff and patient. Three frequently encountered attitudinal stumbling blocks in geriatric rehabilitation are ageism or negative attitudes toward the elderly, feelings that dependency is a right that elders have earned by virtue of their longevity, and apathy towards therapy that results from fatigue.

Negative attitudes toward aging and the elderly lead to a defeatist attitude with respect to rehabilitation. Elderly patients, their families and sometimes even health care staff may feel that being old is synonymous with functional decline, and thus little effort will be made to promote independence. A patient who has undergone an above-the-knee amputation may not be motivated to transfer or ambulate independently because he or she feels that increasing disability goes along with increasing age. There may be little faith in what rehabilitation can accomplish. Other elderly persons may feel they have earned the right to be dependent because of their age and may expect their family members to care for them. This attitude also interferes with rehabilitation efforts. Finally, some patients may not have the energy, both physical and emotional, to cooperate with a strenuous program. For these patients, setting small, limited goals may be helpful.

Common problems that will require rehabilitation in elderly patients include deconditioning, stroke, amputation, and hip fracture. Other conditions that may benefit from rehabilitative therapies include Parkinson's disease and arthritis.

NURSING FACILITIES

At any point in time, only about 5% of the elderly population are residing in nursing facilities, but an estimated 20% of the elderly population will spend some time in a nursing facility over the course of a year. Generally, there are several ways to pay for nursing facility care: private pay, nursing facility insurance, Medicare, and Medicaid. Patients paying privately should know that nursing facility care currently costs approximately $30,000 per year. Nursing facility insurance is expensive and has in the past had severe limitations and restrictions. Patients considering buying insurance should look closely at benefits. Medicare is the federal program that helps pay for doctor and hospital bills after age 65. Almost everyone who receives Social Security is covered by Medicare. Medicare rarely pays for nursing facility stays (see following). The majority of nursing facility care is paid for by Medicaid, a state program that receives federal aid for meeting health care expenses of persons in certain categories of need. Medicaid pays for nursing facility care if the patient does not have enough money to do so.

Occasionally following hospitalization for an acute illness, especially because of early discharge related to use of DRGs, patients will need a stay in a nursing facility before returning to their own home. Patients who have need of continued skilled nursing may be admitted to a skilled nursing facility, which Medicare will pay for up to 150 days subject to a copayment for the first 8 days. These services must be certified as needed by a physician. The critical point is in the definition of skilled care. Skilled care is care that can be performed only by or under the supervision of licensed nurses or professional therapists pursuant to a doctor's orders. Medicare will not cover custodial care.

Medicaid programs vary from state to state; each state determines the payment, duration, and scope of covered services. The Medicare Catastrophic Act of 1988 provided for protection from spousal impoverishment in order to be eligible for Medical Assistance (Medicaid). For example, when a husband or wife is Medicaid eligible and in a nursing facility, the spouse in the community may keep a minimum of about $810/month income as a maintenance allowance. The spouse may keep at least $12,000 in assets (in addition to care and home) or one half of the couple's assets, whichever is greater but not more than $60,000. This is unique to each state so the individual needs to examine the requirements for the state in which he resides. This is a complicated issue, and persons with substantial assets should get legal advice.

Patients should be encouraged to visit nursing facilities they are considering before they make a decision. If the patient is too ill, family members or friends should be encouraged to do so. The following checklist *(Figure 10-8)* can serve as a guide. (Maryland Attorney General's Office, 1990).

The nursing facility industry has suffered from a poor public image. The reality is that nursing facilities, as a whole, try to provide good services to a very frail and ill population with limited resources. When patients enter a nursing facility, they must adapt to a totally different environment from their own home. Privacy is diminished, and personal effects are minimal and may be lost or stolen. There is a need to conform to the schedules for bathing, eating, sleeping, and activities as determined by the nursing facility staff. A patient may be forced to spend time in the company of persons with whom he or she has little in common. It is important that family members maintain close contact with a patient in a nursing facilities, to help alleviate feelings of depression and loss of self-esteem. Patients and their families should be made aware of the Patient's Bill of Rights for Nursing Facility and the complaint procedure of the nursing facility. Although placement in a nursing facility can be difficult, with proper and adequate preparation, patients and their families may find the quality of family relationships really improved, to the benefit of all.

FIGURE 10-8 *(1 of 2)*
What to Look for Checklist

	Yes	No
Look at the Residents:		
Do they seem well cared for?	☐	☐
Are they dressed and involved in activities?	☐	☐
Are their clothes clean? Shoes on? Nails clipped? Is their hair combed? Are they clean shaven?	☐	☐
Are they up and moving? Are those in wheelchairs frequently moved from place to place?	☐	☐
Do they do more than just sit and stare at the walls or TV?	☐	☐
Are they talking among themselves?	☐	☐
The Residents' Rooms:		
Are they bright and cheerful?	☐	☐
Is the home definitely clean?	☐	☐
Is the temperature comfortable? Are the rooms well-ventilated? Air-conditioned? Individual thermostats?	☐	☐
Is there counter space for personal items?	☐	☐
Are residents allowed to decorate their own rooms? Hang pictures?	☐	☐
Are bathing and toilet areas private?	☐	☐
Are there grab bars on toilets and bathtubs?	☐	☐
Is fresh drinking water within easy reach of the bed? Is the pitcher clean?	☐	☐
Does each bed have a curtain or screen for privacy?	☐	☐
Is there adequate closet space? Can possessions be kept reasonably secure?	☐	☐
Does each resident have a sink and mirror? An adjoining bathroom?	☐	☐
Does each room have private phones?	☐	☐
Look at the Staff:		
Do employees show respect to the residents?	☐	☐
Do employees only discuss residents' medical problems privately?	☐	☐
Are residents treated like adults?	☐	☐
Are enough nurses and aides on duty?	☐	☐
Is the staff friendly toward you?	☐	☐
Is the administrator open to your questions?	☐	☐
Are employees dressed neatly?	☐	☐
Do residents seem at ease with the staff?	☐	☐
Are the activity rooms filled with residents?	☐	☐
Are the staff members in sight?	☐	☐
The Residents' Safety:		
Are emergency exit doors well-marked, unobstructed, and unlocked?	☐	☐
Are there wheelchair ramps?	☐	☐

FIGURE 10-8 *(2 of 2)*
What to Look for Checklist

Are there sufficient smoke detectors and sprinklers?   ☐ ☐
Are lobby and floors clean?   ☐ ☐
Are patient areas well-lighted?   ☐ ☐
Do halls have handrails?   ☐ ☐
Are fire, evacuation and disaster plans posted?   ☐ ☐
Do tubs have non-slip surfaces? Grab bars?   ☐ ☐
Does each resident's bed have a call button within easy reach?   ☐ ☐
Are there no-smoking areas? If so, is this enforced?   ☐ ☐
Are hallways wide enough for 2 wheelchairs to pass?   ☐ ☐
Are there press-down door handles rather than doorknobs?   ☐ ☐

Food:
Are the dining room and kitchen clean?   ☐ ☐
Are they reasonably odor-free, without the smell of heavy insecticides?   ☐ ☐
Do residents appear to like the food?   ☐ ☐
Does the staff feed the residents who can't feed themselves?   ☐ ☐
Will the home provide special diets such as low cholesterol or low salt?   ☐ ☐
Are the tables easily accessible to wheelchairs?   ☐ ☐
Can residents eat in their rooms if they prefer?   ☐ ☐
Can snacks be brought into the home?   ☐ ☐

Services and Programs:
Does the facility have arrangements with a nearby hospital to transfer residents in an emergency? ☐ ☐
Does the facility have arrangements with a nearby pharmacy to deliver medications for residents?   ☐ ☐
Can you continue to use your current pharmacy?   ☐ ☐
Is there an adequate physical therapy program?   ☐ ☐
Is the unit dose method of dispensing drugs used?   ☐ ☐
Is a social worker on staff?   ☐ ☐
Does the home have a resident council?   ☐ ☐
Is it possible to attend religious services?   ☐ ☐
Is personal laundry done regularly?   ☐ ☐
Are special events or holiday parties held for the residents?   ☐ ☐

Source: Maryland Attorney General's Office. (1990). *Nursing homes: What you need to know*, pp. 17–19.

EXAM QUESTIONS

CHAPTER 10
Questions 91–95

91. What age population is predicted to grow most rapidly in the next decade?

    a. 19–39

    b. 40–65

    c. 85 and over

    d. Over 65

92. Regular physical exercise and activity aid in which of the following?

    a. Preparing one for marathon running

    b. Reducing obesity, blood pressure, and blood lipids

    c. Preventing accidents

    d. Increasing osteoporosis

93. People with which of the following disease(s) will need medical clearance to begin a moderate walking exercise program?

    a. Cardiovascular, pulmonary, or metabolic disease

    b. Poliomyelitis

    c. Crohn's disease

    d. Benign prostatic hypertrophy

94. Reduction of weight is recommended to persons who are what percentage over their desirable weight?

    a. 10

    b. 20

    c. 30

    d. 5

95. On an average, most Americans tend to gain how many pounds between the ages of 25 and 50?

    a. 100

    b. 10

    c. 15–25

    d. 50

CHAPTER 11

ELDER ABUSE/MISTREATMENT
by
Joan Cagley-Knight, MSN, ARNP

CHAPTER OBJECTIVE

After studying this chapter, the reader will be able to discuss types of elder abuse or mistreatment, characteristics of abusers and victims, and legal obligations for nurses.

LEARNING OBJECTIVES

After studying this chapter, the learner will be able to:

1. Differentiate and describe signs of four (4) types of elder abuse or mistreatment.

2. Discuss legal and moral obligations of nurses as mandatory reporters.

3. Describe characteristics of victims and abusers.

4. Identify at least four (4) risk factors for elder abuse.

5. Identify the relationship between spousal abuse and elder abuse.

6. Explain crisis nursing interventions for elder abuse.

INTRODUCTION

For two decades elder abuse has become an increasingly visible problem and is recognized as a legitimate concern of nurses as healthcare providers. Elder abuse, a social atrocity that can lead to death, remains deeply shrouded in the secrecy that surrounds family violence. Estimates range from 1.5 to 2 million cases per year, but it is also believed that less than one case in 14 is reported to a public agency (AHCA Health Policy Issue Brief, 1998). Most states spend less than $3 per elder for protective services despite the extent of the problem.

One way to look at abuse or mistreatment is to look for *unmet needs* of the elderly. Unmet needs can include inadequacy of nutrition, personal care, medical attention, and psychosocial needs. This way of looking at abuse and neglect enables the healthcare practitioner to remain non-judgmental while helping the elderly individual to meet those needs. Nurses also have a legal commitment as well as helping responsibilities for persons who experience elder abuse. The commonly recognized types of abuse and mistreatment will be discussed in this chapter, followed by a brief discussion of legal obligations of nurses. Next, is a look at who are the abusers as well as who are the victims. A description of interventions and potential barriers to intervention conclude the chapter.

DEFINITIONS

The National Center for Elder Abuse has identified two important characteristics that occur in several types of elder abuse which can be seen in any practice setting. These are:

An elder's frequent and unexplained crying; and

an elder's unexplained suspicion or fear of a particular person in the care setting.

Generally four categories of elder abuse and mistreatment are recognized:

• Physical abuse

• Neglect by caregiver or self

• Psychological abuse or

• Financial abuse or exploitation (Lynch, 1997).

Keep in mind that it is not rare for elderly individuals to experience several types of abuse at the same time.

PHYSICAL ABUSE

Physical abuse is defined as the use of physical force resulting in bodily harm, physical pain or impairment, including sexual abuse or misconduct. Physical abuse or mistreatment typically, includes hitting, slapping, beating, pushing, punching, shoving, shaking, kicking, pinching and burning. The inappropriate use of drugs or physical restraints, force-feeding and any other type of physical punishment are examples of physical abuse.

Suspicious Signs and Symptoms

Quinn and Tomita (1997) identify four possible signs to watch for that indicate abuse:

1. *The individual is brought to the hospital emergency room by someone other than the caregiver, or the person is found alone.* Mrs. Abbot is brought to the hospital emergency room (ER) by a neighbor who stopped by for a visit and noted her lethargic and lying in bed.

2. *There is a prolonged period between injury or illness and presentation for medical care.* Mrs. Abbot experienced a serious eye injury and laceration of the head, but was not brought for medical attention for a week. This raises serious questions about her nephew who lives with her.

3. *There is a suspicious history. Doctor or facility "hopping" as well as explanations of injuries that are not consistent with the injury are suspect.* Mrs. Abbot's nephew, when located, states that his aunt "fell off a stool" injuring her eye and head and just needed some rest.

4. *There is noncompliance with prescribed medications or suggested treatments.* The nephew refuses to allow medical treatment or antibiotic or pain medications, stating that his aunt does not want any type of surgical intervention and doesn't believe in taking medication.

In this instance, or in any incident, it is important to assess and interview the individual privately and immediately. Competence or capacity to make decisions may be an issue which will need to be addressed as well.

Sexual abuse is considered another form of physical abuse. It is defined as nonconsensual sexual contact with an elderly individual. Sexual contact with any person incapable of giving consent is also considered sexual abuse (National Center on Elder Abuse). Sexual abuse includes unwanted touching, rape, sodomy, coerced nudity and sexually explicit photographing. Some signs to watch for include: torn, bloody underclothes, bruises on the breasts or genitals, unexplained venereal disease or unexplained vaginal or anal bleeding.

NEGLECT (ACTS OF OMISSION)

Frequently emergency rooms are the primary point of entry to the health care system for the elderly abused or neglected person. Mr. Tyson was an 83-year-old man brought to the emergency room in a large city. He was suffering from dehydration and exposure. He had been found by the police after being without food or water for at least two days while he lay curled in the trunk of his car. When he was found, he reported that he saw the light of day only when his niece lifted the trunk lid to check the authenticity of her forgery of his check and signature. After he was brought to the emergency room, he was confused about why his niece who "loved him" had turned on him. His concern was that his family not be treated too harshly and that she "get a break." "After all," he said, "she didn't kill me." Mr. Tyson endured a harrowing experience of neglect and continued to protect his caregiver.

Neglect refers to "omissions" either by self or others. It describes situations in which the basic needs of an elder are not being met (Lynch, 1997; Quinn & Tomita, 1997). The lack of attention can be to the person or his environment. Neglectful actions can include lack of adequate nutrition, personal care, medications, medical attention or a safe well-maintained home or place to live. Neglect may be either intentional or unintentional. The neglect may be intentional if withholding the necessities of life and physical care is done willfully. Unintentional neglect is usually done due to lack of experience or information of the caregiver.

In cases of self-neglect, the decision to intervene, following recognition of the problem, may be more difficult than in cases of caregiver neglect or physical abuse. The need to respect the person's right to self-determination may supercede your need as a healthcare provider to ensure patient safety. Assessing the functional and educational needs of any elder experiencing self-neglect is vital.

PSYCHOLOGICAL ABUSE

Psychological abuse inflicts emotional pain and distress on the elderly individual. It may be difficult to detect unless witnessed. Psychological abuse includes name-calling, saying unkind things about the elder within their hearing, and mocking them (Quinn & Tomita, 1997). Threats, insults or humiliation are psychological abuse. Ignoring or isolating an elderly person and excluding them from day-to-day activities is psychological neglect. Manifestations of this abuse in the individual may be confusion, disorientation, fearfulness, trembling, and fidgeting when certain subjects are discussed, changing the subject frequently, and cowering when the caregiver is present. Lack of eye contact, withdrawal and clinging are signs as well.

After knee surgery, Mrs. McNulty age 85 went to stay with her son and his wife. Her daughter-in-law began to refer to the fact that she needed so much help to get to the bathroom, could no longer fix her own meals and "had to be waited on all the time." The daughter-in-law referred to herself as the "unpaid maid" for Mrs. McNulty. She reminded her of how she used to care for her own home and yard and now couldn't even make it to the bathroom without help from the daughter-in-law. After several weeks, Mrs. McNulty began to withdraw from the family and spent the day in her room watching "soaps" or talk shows. On the revisit to the clinic, the nurse noticed the depression and suggested a talk with a local counselor. Mrs. McNulty agreed and, as a result, during several sessions which included the family, the daughter-in-law recognized the part she played in the depression of Mrs. McNulty. The discussion of how overwhelmed she felt about caring for her mother-in-law helped the counselor and family to develop new strategies for improving the relationships during the convalescence.

FINANCIAL ABUSE OR EXPLOITATION

Financial abuse occurs when family members, caregivers, or "friends" take control of the assets of an elder either through coercion, misrepresentation or outright stealing (Lynch, 1997). The victims often have cognitive or physical impairments. Financial abuse occurs in about one third of the cases of elder abuse.

Indicators of financial abuse include:

- Sudden and unusual activity in bank accounts.

- Withdrawals of large sums of money indicating radical changes by an elder including sudden use of ATM and credit cards.

- Abrupt changes in wills or other financial transactions.

- Sudden transfer of assets to distant relatives or caregivers.

- Large bills for care either not given or poorly given.

- Forged signatures and documents to be signed by the elder which they do not understand.

- Disappearance of personal items such as art work, jewelry, silverware, etc.

Any allegation by an elder of financial exploitation should be taken seriously. Typically, someone who the elderly person trusts is handling their finances with or without authorization. The financial abusers have strong personalities and offer the elder someone to rely on and become dependent on. The data on the extent of financial exploitation is difficult to come by since banks, lawyers and judges, who typically see financial abuse and report to the police, are not mandated to report, in most states, to the agencies who keep the statistics about abuse and neglect.

LEGAL OBLIGATIONS

Strategies for dealing with elder abuse and neglect must balance the elderly individual's needs for safety against their need for autonomy and self decision-making. Regardless of this dilemma, most states have mandatory reporting laws which require the full disclosure of *suspected* elder mistreatment. State legislation addresses specific elder abuse statutes for both community and institutionalized elderly. The laws of each state indicate the age limits to be considered elderly, but it is not less than 60 years of age in any state (Capezuti, Brush & Lawson, 1997). 42 states have Adult Protective Service (APS) laws that outline which practitioners are mandatory reporters. In most states, nurses, physicians, psychologists, social workers and pharmacists are required by law to report possible cases of elder abuse or mistreatment. APS or the responsible state agency is mandated to investigate all reports often within specific time frames.

Nurses are specifically identified as mandatory reporters in 23 states and are referenced as "health care professionals" in 16 other states (Tatara, 1995) *(Table 11-1)*. Civil and criminal penalties for failure to report range from fines of $100 to $1,000 and/or 3 months to 6 years in jail. Only five states—Florida, Montana, California, Utah and West Virginia—actually prosecuted mandatory reporters for failing to report. Several states do not identify any penalties for failing to report. Eight states have voluntary reporting laws—Colorado, Illinois, New Jersey, New York, North Dakota, Pennsylvania, South Dakota and Wisconsin. Mandatory and voluntary reporting is based on *suspected* abuse or neglect identified by the reporter. APS or another agency is responsible for investigation and validation of the mistreatment. APS laws provide immunity for reporting suspected abuse or neglect in "good faith." You, as the nurse, must be able to show that you acted without malice and with good intentions. Additionally, some states assure confidentiality to reporters and the reports.

The Joint Commission for Accreditation of Health Care Organizations (JCAHO) has set standards which require emergency room nurses to make reports of elder mistreatment or domestic violence. Recent studies have suggested that a significant portion of elder abuse may be accounted for as spousal abuse which could have been occurring for years. Health care providers need to recog-

TABLE 11-1
Elder Mistreatment Statutes*

State	APS Law	Minimum Year of Age	Reporting Requirement[1]	Penalty[2]	Reporter Protection[3]	Self-Neglect[4]	Services[5]
Alabama	1977	18	M-O	$500/6 months	L,C		E,T,H
Alaska	1988	18	M-O	M-PNS	L,C,E		T,CM
Arkansas	1977	18	M-N	M-PNS	L,C		E,T,CR,M,L
Arizona	1980	18	M	$1,000/6 months	L,C	No	CM,S,P,B,M
California	1986	18	M-N	NA	L,C,E	No	CM
Colorado	1991	18	V	NA	L,C,E		CM
Connecticut	1977	60	M-N	$500	L,C		T,CM,CR,S,H,P,B,M
Delaware	1982	18	M-O	None	L,C		E,T,CM,S,H,B,M,L
District of Columbia	1985	18	M-O	$300	L,C,E	No	E,T,CM,S,P,B,M,L
Florida	1974	18	M-N	FNS/2 months	L,C,E		E,T,CR,CM,S,H,M,L
Georgia	1981	18	M-N	$1,000/1 year	L,C	No	P,B,M,L
Hawaii	1989	Adult	M-N	M-PNS	L,C		E,CR,CM,M
Idaho	1991	18	M-N	$300/6 months	L,C	No	CM,M
Illinois	1988	60	V	NA	L,C		T,CM
Indiana	1985	18	M-O	None	L,C,E		E,T,M
Iowa	1983	18	M-O	Civil damages	E		T,CM,CR,P
Kansas	1985	18	M-N	$1,000/6 months	L,C,E		T,CM,CR,H,B,M,L
Kentucky	1976	18	M-N	$250/1 year	L,C		E,T,M
Louisiana	1982	18	M-O	$500/6 months	L,C		T,CM
Maine	1981	18	M-N	$500*	L,C		E,T,CM,H,M
Maryland	1977	65	M-O	None	L,C		E,T,CM,P,L
Massachusetts	1983	60	M-N	$1,000	L,C,E	No	E,T,CM,S,P,M,L
Michigan	1982	18	M-O	$500 plus damages	L,C		CM,M,L
Minnesota	1980	18	M-O	Civil damages	L,C		
Mississippi	1986	18	M-N	$1,000/1 year	L,C,E		E,T,CR,S,P,B,M,L
Missouri	1980	18	M-N	M-PNS	L,C		T,CM,CR,H,M
Montana	1975, 1983	60, 18	M-N	FNS	L,C,E		E,T,H
Nebraska	1988	18	M-N	M-PNS	L,C		T,CM,CR,S,H,P,B,M,L
Nevada	1981	60	M-N	1-6 years	L,C		CM,CR
New Hampshire	1978	18	M-O	M-PNS	L,C		T,CM,CR,M
New Jersey	1993	18	V	NA	L,C,E		CR,M,L
New Mexico	1989	18	M	None	L,C		E,CM,H,P,M,L
New York	1975	18	V	None	L,C		E,CM,H,M
North Carolina	1973	18	M-O	None	L		CM,S,P,B,M,L
North Dakota	1989	18	V	NA	L,C		E,CM,S,H,P,B,M,L
Ohio	1981	60	M-N	None	L,E		E,T,CM,S,P,B,M
Oklahoma	1977	18	M-N	M-PNS	L,C	No	T,CR
Oregon	1975, 1981	18, 65	V	NA	L,C,E	No	E,S,P,B,L
Pennsylvania	1987	60	M-O	$1,000/1 year	L,C	No	T,CM,M,L
Rhode Island	1981	60	M-N	$2,500/1 year	L,C		E,M,L
South Carolina	1974	18	M-N	NA	L,C,E	No	
South Dakota	1976	18	V	NA	L		
Tennessee	1978	18	M-N	$500/3 months	L,C,E		E,CM,S,H,P,B,M,L
Texas	1981	18	M-O	M-PNS	L,C		E,T,CM,H,P,M,L
Utah	1985	18	M-N	$500	L,C,E		E,CR
Vermont	1985	18	M-N	$1,000	L,C,E		T,CM,CR
Virginia	1974	18	M-N	None	L,C	No	E
Washington	1984	60	M-N	None	L,C	No	CM
West Virginia	1981	18	M-N	$100/10 days	L,C		T,CM,P,M
Wisconsin	1983	60	V	NA	L,C,E		
Wyoming	1981	18	M-O	None	L,C		E,T,CM,P,M

*The information in this table is based on a study conducted in 1993 (Tatara, 1995) and a review of each state's statute and amendments current as of 1/1/96 (Westlaw computer-assisted legal research service).

[1] M=mandatory reporting; V=voluntary reporting; N=law specifically names nurses as mandated reporters; O=law does not name nurses specifically but names health care professionals or anyone with the knowledge or case to believe.

[2] Penalty=fine and/or jail term; M-PNS=misdemeanor, penalty not specified; FNS=fine but not specified; NA=not applicable for states with voluntary reporting laws.

[3] L=law guarantees protection from civil and criminal liability; C=law stipulates that reporting records, including the reporter's name, are confidential; E=law specifically prohibits retaliation by an employer against any employee who reports mistreatment.

[4] Each APS law includes self-neglect as a category with the exception of those listed as "no."

[5] Key to services: E=emergency intervention; T=24-hour, statewide and/or toll-free telephone service; CR=central registry; CM=case management, including counseling and information and referral services; S=shelter; H=housing, relocation service, or respite; P=personal care, homemaker and/or chore services; B=basics such as food, clothing, home energy assistance; M=medical and mental health services; L=legal services.

Used with permission of the National Center for Elder Abuse.

nize this possibility and screen all women and persons over age 60 for possible abuse, utilizing your facility policies and procedures.

Many policies and procedures exist to promote the documentation and reporting of elder mistreatment or abuse. These procedures include:

- Call the abuse Hot Line listed in your telephone directory.

- Notify the individual delegated the responsibility in your agency or facility, usually a social worker or administrator.

- If you identify immediate danger to the elderly person, call the police.

- Contact your state agency such as APS for assistance.

- Document all circumstances, including the name, sex, race, and address of the abused as well as the current location of the abused and the type of abuse that occurred or is *suspected.*

Make sure your documentation is accurate, detailed and objective. As much as possible, write down the exact words of the elder and their caregiver. All nurses should know the community resources available to the abused person and to the abuser. Know the limits on your states APS laws in regard to emergency shelter, help with basics like food or clothing, medical and psychiatric care, case management services, and legal assistance.

VICTIMS AND ABUSERS

Who are the abusers and who are the victims? Throughout the years studies have identified the characteristics of the victim or the victim's situation (Hwalek, et al., 1996) while some have looked at the abuser. Usually abusers are described as middle-aged adult children or other relatives of the victim. Often, the abuser is also the caregiver to the victim. A 1988 study by Pillemer and Finkelhor found that men were as likely to be abused as women, but the surprising finding was that 58% of elder abuse is spousal abuse whether by men or women. Elder abuse may be spousal abuse grown old (Ebersole & Hess, 1998). It should be noted that more elderly men than elderly women are likely to be living with an elderly spouse since there are many more elderly widows than widowers. The 1996 study by Hwalek, et al. identified two characteristics of abusers that strengthened their dependence on the victim. The most common barrier to the abuser being independent from the victim was substance abuse followed closely by the abuser's financial dependence on the victim. Other risk factors for being an abuser are a history of mental illness, a family history of violence, stressful events and increasing dependency.

Cultural differences exist in identifying what actions are abusive to the victim. Korean-American women tend not to perceive certain situations as abusive that other American woman might (Moon & Williams, 1993). Differences exist in perception of abusive behavior between African-American women, Hispanic women and Caucasian American women. No universal agreement about what constitutes abuse exists.

Frail elders with dementia and Alzheimer's Disease are often at risk for abusive behavior. The dependence of the individual and their unrelenting needs for personal care and supervision lead to frustration and abusive behavior. One telephone study of in-home caregivers who had called a help line showed that almost 18% had pinched, kicked, struck, hit or shoved the demented individual in their care (Coyne et al., 1993).

The significance of spousal abuse in relation to elder abuse needs to be recognized by all nurses. Although abuse in institutional settings has been recognized for many years, it is only recently that domestic violence and spousal abuse towards the elderly have become evident. Caregiver burden and stress are significant in abusive relationships in the community, but spousal abuse which has occurred for years can be much more dangerous and deadly. Nurses must screen all dependent elderly and be alert to potential abuse situations.

LOCATION OF ELDER MISTREATMENT

Where does abuse occur? Abuse of the elderly in long term care has been discussed and written about for many years. One study conducted by telephone in 1988 by Pillemer and Moore (and still considered up-to-date) examined the scope and nature of physical and psychological abuse in nursing homes. Staff were interviewed randomly and asked to comment on what they had seen others do and what actions they had personally taken. The results were disturbing. 36% of those questioned had seen at least one incident of physical abuse in the previous year and 10% reported that they themselves had committed one or more physically abusing acts. Excessive restraining was the most common type of physical abuse observed and action taken by the staff person. Pushing, grabbing, shoving or pinching residents were the next most commonly observed and done by staff. Others reporting seeing staff throw things at residents, kick or hit residents with a fist or try to hit them with an object.

Even more distressing was that 81% of those questioned reported seeing incidents of psychological abuse during the preceding year, and 40% reported they had committed at least one act of psychological abuse themselves within the past year. Over two thirds saw a staff member yelling at a resident in anger and one-half had seen another staff member insult or swear at a resident. 33% of staff reported that they had yelled at a resident while one in 10 described insulting or swearing at a resident themselves within the past year.

Other studies have identified nursing assistants as making up the largest group of abusers and male employees as responsible for the majority of abuse incidents (Payne & Cikovic, 1996). The abusers justified their actions as responses to stressful situations in which they had been provoked. Administrators and owners of nursing homes must provide better working conditions, stress management techniques, and humane treatment of staff in order to provide more humane treatment to residents in long term care. Modification of the attitudes of staff toward residents—and staff towards any one who abuses residents is imperative. Recognition of the harmful and debilitating effects of physically restraining residents in long term care settings has improved the quality of life and lessened injuries from this form of physical abuse.

The fact is that most abuse of the elderly occurs in their homes by their own family. However, with astonishing frequency, abuse occurs in the home by paid caregivers. Theft of personal effects is the most common problem in the home (Ebersole & Hess, 1998). Many times elderly are accused of being "paranoid" or "confused" about where they have put their belongings Abusers have even escalated to murder in home care settings. More care must be taken in investigating the background of home care workers and in training and supervision.

"The home is the place where, when you go there, they have to take you in."

—Robert Frost

Most elderly live at home and receive care at home as they age. Most of this care is given by the family who may or may not be willing and able to assume this care. While many steps have been taken to combat elder abuse and neglect, much remains hidden and secret. Violence and neglect in the home are volatile issues. The home, especially in this country, has been seen as safe from government interference, a haven. Because behavior inside the home has traditionally been private and beyond the reach of public policy, secrecy and isolation are common in a victim/abuser relationship. Nurses may be the initial visitor in the home to recognize the problem of elder abuse. Becoming a patient advocate for individual rights and autonomy as well as protection requires skill and dedication.

Interventions

The first phase of intervention is identification of the elder abuse. The risk factors for abuse that need to be considered are:

The family history:

- Is there a history of violence or mental illness?

The living arrangements:

- Who lives in the home?
- Is either person isolated?

The lifestyle of the potential victim or abuser:

- What recent stressful events have occurred and what happened as a result?
- What do family interactions reveal about how stressors are handled?
- What are the emotional stressors in the current situation?
- What is the health status of each?
- What is the cognitive status of the potential victim?

The resources available:

- What is the financial status of the potential victim/abuser?
- How dependent are they on one another?
- What social support system is available to either victim or abuser?

Since elder abuse tends to be episodic and reoccurring, review of past emergency room visits and accidents must be undertaken (Quinn & Tomita, 1997).

As nurses we need to overcome the barriers to recognition and intervention of abuse and violence.

The barriers according to Shea et al. (1997) are personal, social and sociocultural. Knowing a lot about something like elder abuse or domestic violence does not necessarily reduce the incidence of these occurrences. If you have had a personal experience with domestic violence, which many nurses have, you may be acutely sensitive to caring for victims. Your powerful emotions such as anger, shame and helplessness, may prevent you from caring and advocating for an abuse victim. Social norms about the use of physical punishment and the family's right to privacy may prevent the recognition or reinforce the conspiracy of silence fostered by the abuser. Some nurses may blame the victim for not seeking help sooner. In some institutions there may be medical, economic, political, legal and ethical barriers to identifying abuse. There may be sanctions for your attempt to go beyond the medical aspects of care because they take time and resources that are limited. As mentioned before, JCAHO and major professional organizations such as the American Nurses Association and the American Medical Association have policy statements supporting the need for advocacy. Living in an abusive situation can destroy a victim's quality of life no matter when or where it occurs. As a nurse you have the power and privilege to restore damaged self-esteem and promote health.

Interventions for elder abuse focus on stopping the exploitation of the individual while protecting their safety and autonomy. Crisis intervention strategies to handle medical and legal emergencies are available. Most procedures are outlined by the court following civil and criminal statutes. Since many victims of abuse will remain with the abuser, it is necessary to intervene with both the victim and abuser. Counselors utilize environmental changes, reality orientation, and education to prevent further abusive incidents.

Legal interventions, specifically in a home situation, may include a guardianship or conservator-

---

TABLE 11-2
National and Community Resources

LOCAL COMMUNITY
Local police
Adult Protective Services
State elder abuse HOTLINES
(see local directory)

NATIONAL
National Center on Elder Abuse
American Public Welfare Association
810 First ST, NE, Suite 500
Washington D.C. 20002-4267
(202)682-2470

American Association of Retired Persons
Criminal Justice Services
601 E ST NW
Washington D.C. 200049
(202)434-2222

National Association of State Units on Aging
National Eldercare Institute on Elder Abuse
& State Long Term Care Ombudsman
  Services
1225 I Street, NW, Suite 725
Washington DC 200005
(202)898-2578

National Coalition Against Violence
(202)638-6388
(303)839-1852

National Organization for Victim Assistance
1-800-TRY-NOVA
(202)232-6682

Adapted from Lynch, S. (1997).

---

ship. The focus is on using the least restrictive options with the least amount of court intrusion. While one goal is to hold the abuser accountable for his or her actions, another goal is to allow the victim the autonomy to return to the situation she chooses. Emergency shelters have been established in some communities to provide care during crisis situations.

SUMMARY

Elder abuse is an escalating problem and recognizing risk factors for abuse and knowing interventions that are available in your community may help *(Table 11-2)*. Your willingness to interrupt an abusive situation by listening and asking questions may encourage elderly abused individuals to seek and accept help. Since many elderly abuse victims are unable to ask for help due to cognitive impairment or dependence, there is an additional burden to be a proactive advocate for elderly, report all suspected abuse of any type, recognize the impact of spousal abuse on elder abuse and train non-professional staff to develop skills with geriatric patients.

EXAM QUESTIONS

CHAPTER 11
Questions 96–100

96. How much do states typically spend for adult protective services for the elderly?

    a. More than $10 per individual.

    b. Less than $3 per individual.

    c. Less than $20 per individual.

    d. More than $5 per individual.

97. Which of the following statements is true about sexual abuse?

    a. It is not very common.

    b. Bilateral bruising on the upper arms is often a sign.

    c. This often results in non-compliance with medication or treatments.

    d. Sexual contact with any elderly person unable to give consent is considered sexual abuse.

98. The primary point of entry into the health care system for an elderly person who has been abused is:

    a. Home health care.

    b. Public housing units.

    c. Community health clinics.

    d. Emergency rooms.

99. Which of the following is a risk factor for elder abuse?

    a. Educational status of the victim.

    b. Number of persons living in the home.

    c. Large amounts of money inherited by the victim.

    d. Mutual dependence by victim and abuser.

100. Which states have prosecuted mandatory reporters for failing to report suspected abuse?

    a. New York, Colorado, Illinois, New Mexico, Arizona.

    b. California, Florida, Montana, Utah, West Virginia.

    c. Wisconsin, Minnesota, North Dakota, Iowa, Montana.

    d. Colorado, Illinois, Pennsylvania, South Dakota, Wisconsin.

GLOSSARY

Activities of daily living (ADL) - the basic activities of daily living, including bathing, dressing, toileting, transferring, feeding, and continence.

Advance directive - a document that a competent adult can complete and share with a health care provider that tells what the person would want to happen in case he or she become unable to make his or her wishes known.

Agnosia - Failure to recognize a stimulus (visual, auditory, tactile) although primary sensory receptors are intact.

Akathisia - an agitated motor restlessness that is one of the extrapyramidal side effects of the neuroleptics.

Alzheimer's disease - a type of senile dementia occurring in older persons; progressive loss of mental abilities occurs.

Anemia - a hemoglobin level of less than 12 g/dl.

Anomia - the inability to remember names of objects.

Anosmia - a decrease in the sense of smell.

Anticholinergic effects - result from a drug blocking the parasympathetic nerve impulses; include urinary retention, blurred vision, constipation, tachycardia, and delirium.

Antidepressants - a form of drug therapy used to treat depression.

Aphasia - absence or impairment of the ability to communicate through speech, writing, or signs because of dysfunction of brain centers; expressive aphasia is secondary to affected motor areas; receptive aphasia is due to affected sensory areas.

Apraxia - the inability to perform previously learned motor activities in the presence of intact motor and sensory systems, (e.g. inability to use a fork to eat).

Brain enzyme - a protein that accelerates a specific chemical reaction in the brain.

Cataracts - a clouding or opacity occurring in the normally crystalline lens that leads to vision changes.

Catastrophic reaction - an overblown or exaggerated response to the precipitating situation; results when a cognitively impaired patient is overwhelmed by a situation; reactions include agitation, sadness, refusal to comply, or outburst behavior.

Cerebrovascular accident - more commonly referred to as a stroke results from the disruption of the cerebral blood supply.

Cerumen - ear wax.

Choline acetyltransferase - an enzyme that stimulates the production of acetylcholine, a chemical active in the transmission of nerve impulses.

Congestive heart failure - a decrease in the pumping ability of the heart; usually results from underlying conditions such as coronary artery disease or myocardial infarction.

Conservatorship - a legal procedure that allows the conservator to assume control over a completely incapacitated person.

Coronary artery disease - narrowing of the coronary arteries resulting in diminished blood flow to the myocardium; usually the result of atherosclerosis.

Delirium - a state of clouded consciousness with inattention, sensory misperception, disordered stream of thought, and disturbances of psychomotor activity.

Dementia - a loss of previously existing intellectual abilities severe enough to interfere with occupational or social functioning.

Depression - a serious mental disorder that may be characterized by deep depression or melancholia; it is a common psychiatric problem in older adults.

Discharge planning - an ongoing process consisting of the assessment of patients' needs before and during hospitalization, planning for the continuity of care on discharge, and the coordination of resources needed on discharge.

Durable power of attorney for health care - a legal procedure that enables one person to give another person the legal authority to make health care decisions on behalf of the first person.

Dyskinesia - abnormal involuntary movements.

Electroencephalography (EEG) - recording of the electrical activities of the brain by means of wires placed painlessly on the scalp; useful in detecting tumors, epilepsy, and brain damage.

Extrapyramidal syndrome - side effects of the neuroleptics; includes akathisia, parkinsonism, and tardive dyskinesia.

Functional incontinence - urinary leakage due to the inability to toilet because of a cognitive impairment, physical functioning, psychological unwillingness, or environmental barriers.

Geriatric - describes the field of applied gerontology; includes medical care.

Gerontic nursing - describes the field of nursing care of older patients.

Gerontology - the study of older adults.

Gout - a common inflammatory disease in men over 40 resulting from hyperuricemia and development of crystals in the joints.

Habit training - a technique to manage functional incontinence in which the caregiver adjusts the patient's toileting schedule on the basis of the patient's pattern of incontinent episodes and continent voidings.

Hayflick phenomenon - a theory of aging that proposes that cells loose the ability to reproduce themselves after 50 divisions.

Hospice - an alternative type of healthcare setting where the focus of care is to assist the patient, who is terminally ill, to die in comfort and with dignity.

Hypertension - the persistent elevation of the arterial blood pressure to levels greater than or equal to 95mm Hg diastolic and 160mm Hg and greater systolic.

Hypoalbuminemia - a decrease in the level of serum albumin level; results in a decrease of the immune response.

Infarct - an area of tissue in an organ or part that undergoes necrosis following cessation of blood supply. It may result from occlusion or stenosis of a supplying artery.

Lacunar syndromes - clinical manifestations of infarcts up to 20mm (mostly 10mm) size located in the subcortical cerebrum and in the brainstem resulting from occlusion of small arteries; frequently associated with hypertension.

Marasmus - the result of an inadequate supply of calories resulting in weight loss and decreased weight for height values.

Myoclonus - brief contractions of muscles, usually irregular in rhythm and amplitude.

Neurofibrillary tangle - an accumulation of abnormal fibers in the nerve cells in the cerebral cortex.

Neuroleptics - also known as the antipsychotic or major tranquilizer medications; used to treat the psychotic symptoms that can occur in Alzheimer's disease.

Orthostatic hypotension - a drop of 20mm Hg or more in blood pressure when a person rises.

Osteoarthritis - a noninflammatory, progressive, degenerative disorder of the movable, weight-bearing joints.

Osteoporosis - a metabolic bone disorder characterized by loss of bone mass resulting in fractures.

Pharmacokinetics - study of the metabolism and action of drugs, including absorption, distribution, metabolism, and elimination.

Presbycusis - hearing loss caused by changes in the neural, sensory, metabolic, and mechanical structures of the inner ear; characterized by a decreased ability to hear consonants.

Primary prevention - interventions aimed at detecting and reducing risk factors that predispose persons to disease.

Proband - a subject who is being studied and whose family history is being constructed to determine if other members of the family have had the same disease discovered in the subject.

Prompted voiding - a technique to manage functional incontinence in which the caregiver toilets the patient at regular intervals.

Proprioception - sensation pertaining to stimuli originating from within the body regarding spatial position and muscular activity or to the sensory receptors that they activate.

Psychoses - mental disturbances of such magnitude that there is personality disintegration and loss of contact with reality.

Psychotropic drugs - medications that exert an influence on the mind.

Restorative feeding - a philosophy of feeding that attempts to increase elderly patients' level of independence and to improve or maintain nutritional and health status.

Secondary prevention - the early detection of a disease before it becomes dangerous or disabling.

Tardive dyskinesia - an often irreversible, involuntary movement disorder (either generalized or in single muscle groups), that may occur as a side effect of the neuroleptics.

Tertiary prevention - detecting a disease that is symptomatic and taking action to maximize recovery.

Tinnitus - a ringing or buzzing in the ear.

Xerostomia - dry mouth; in the elderly may result from decreased salivary production.

Definitions based on *Taber's Cyclopedic Medical Dictionary,* 15th ed., Philadelphia: F. A. Davis, 1985; and *The Little Black Book of Neurology.* Thurston, S., Chicago: Year Book Medical, 1987.

BIBLIOGRAPHY

Abrass, I. B. (1987). A study of training in clinical pharmacology of the elderly. *Clinical Pharmacology and Therapeutics, 42,* 693–695.

ADA Reports. (1998). Position of The American Dietetic Association: Liberalized diets for older adults in long-term care. *Journal of the American Dietetic Association, 98*(2), 201–204.

Agency for Health Care Policy and Research. (1992). *Pressure ulcers in adults: Prediction and prevention.* (Publication no. 92-0047). U.S. Government Printing Office.

Agency for Health Care Policy & Research (AHCPR). (1993). *Clinical Practice Guideline. Number 5, Depression in primary care.* (AHCPR Publication No. 93-0551).

Agency for Health Care Policy and Research. (1994). *Clinical practice guideline #9, management of cancer pain.* (AHCPR Publication No. 94-0592) Rockville, MD: U.S. Government Printing Office.

Agency for Health Care Administration (1998). *AHCA health policy issue brief: Violence as a health epidemic.* Tallahassee: Florida AHCA, Office of Health Policy.

Aging America Trends and Projections, (1985-86 edition). (1985). U.S. Senate Special Committee on Aging: AOA USDHHS PF 3377.

Algase, D. L. & Struble, L. M. (1992). Wandering behavior: What, why, and how? In K. C. Buckwalter (ed.), *Geriatric mental health nursing: Current and future challenges.* Thorofare, NJ: Slack.

Allman, R. M. (1989). Pressure ulcers among the elderly. *New England Journal of Medicine, 320,* 850–853.

American Cancer Society. (1998). *Cancer Facts & Figures - 1998.* Atlanta: Author.

American Diabetes Association. (1997). Translation of the diabetes nutrition recommendations for health care institutions: Position statement. *Journal of the American Dietetic Association, 97*(1), 52–53.

American Psychiatric Association. (1994). *Diagnostic and statistical manual of mental disorders: DSM-IV* (4th ed.). Washington, DC: American Psychiatric Association.

Anderson, F. & Williams, B. (1989). *Practical management of the elderly.* (5th ed, pp.78–99). Oxford, England: Blackwell Scientific.

Andres, R., Elahi, D., Tobin, J., Muller, B. & Brant, L. (1985). Impact of age on weight goals. *Annals of Internal Medicine, 103*(6), 1030–1033.

Angelucci, D. & Lawrence, M. (1995). Death and dying. In Stanley, M. & Beare, P. (eds). *Gerontological Nursing.* Philadelphia: FA Davis.

Aronson, M. K. (1988). *Understanding Alzheimer's disease,* New York: Charles Scribner's Sons.

Avolio, A. P., Deng, F. Q. & Li, W. Q. (1985). Effects of aging on arterial distensibility in populations with high and low prevalence of hypertension: Comparison between urban and rural communities in China. *Circulation,* 71, 202–10.

Avorn, J., Dryer, P., Connelly, K. & Soumerai, S. B. (1989). Use of psychoactive medication and the quality of care in rest homes. *New England Journal of Medicine,* 320, 227–232.

Baillie, S. P., Bateman, D. N. & Coates, P. E. (1989). Age and the pharmacokinetics of morphine. *Age and Aging,* 18, 258–262.

Baran, D., Sorensen, A. & Grimes, J. (1990). Dietary modification with dairy products for preventing vertebral bone loss in premenopausal women: A three-year prospective study. *Journal of Clinical Endocrinology and Metabolism,* 70, 246–270.

Barash, R. A. (1991). How aging affects sexual functioning. *California Nursing,* May-June, 25–28.

Barraclough, J. (1997). ABC of palliative care: Depression, anxiety, and confusion. *British Medical Journal, 315*(7119), 1365–1368.

Bauer, D. (1993). Factors associated with appendicular bone mass in older women. *Annals of Internal Medicine,* 118:157.

Baum, H. M. & Manton, K. G. (1987). National trend in stroke related mortality: Comparison of multiple cause mortality data with survey and other health data. *Gerontologist,* 27, 293–300.

Baylis, E. M., Hall, M. S. & Lewis, G. (1972). Effects of renal function on plasma digoxin levels in elderly ambulant patients in domiciliary practice. *British Medical Journal,* 1, 338–341.

Beck, C. & Chumbler, N. (1997). Planning for the future of long term care: Consumers, providers, and purchasers. *Journal of Geronontological Nursing, 23*(8) 6–13.

Beder, J. (1998). Legalization of assisted suicide. *Journal of Gerontological Nursing, 23*(4) 14–20.

Benet, S. (1971). Why they live to be 100, or even older, in Abkhasia. In Kart, C. S. & Manard, B. B. (Eds), *Aging in America: Readings in social gerontology.* Alfred Publishing Co.

Berkey, D. & Valdez, I. (1997). The mouth and teeth. In Ham, R. & Sloane, P. (eds). *Primary Care Geriatrics,* (3rd ed). St. Louis: Mosby.

Berkow, R., Butler, R. & Sunderland, J. (1995). Cognitive failure, delirium, and dementia. In Abrams, W., Beers, M. & Berkow, R. (eds). *Merck Manual of Geriatrics,* (2nd ed). Whitehouse Station, NJ: Merck Research Laboratories.

Bettis, S. (1979). Depression: The "common cold" of the elderly. *Generations,* III (4), Spring.

Bienenfeld, D. (Ed). (1990). V*erwoerdt's clinical geropsychiatry.* Baltimore: Williams and Wilkins.

Birren, J. E. (1964). *The psychology of aging.* Englewood Cliffs, NJ: Prentice-Hall.

Bistrian, B. R. (1977). Nutritional assessment and therapy of protein-calorie malnutrition in the hospital. *Journal of the American Dietetic Association,* 71, 393–397.

Black, J. S. & Kapoor, W. (1990). Health promotion and disease prevention in older people. *Journal of the American Geriatrics Society,* 38, 168–172.

Blazer, D. (1995). Depression. In Abrams, W., Beers, M. & Berkow, R. (eds). *The Merck Manual of Geriatrics* (2nd ed). Whitehouse Station, NY: Merck Research Laboratories.

Blum, H. L. (1980). Social perspective on risk reduction, family and community health. *The Journal of Health Promotion and Maintenance, 3* (1), 41–61.

Bock, J. C. (1991). *Geriatric review syllabus.* New York: American Geriatrics Society.

Demaagd, C. (1995). High-risk drugs in the elderly population. *Geriatric Nursing, 16*(5), 198–207.

Bombardier, C. H., D'Amico, C. & Jordan, J. S. (1990). The relationship of appraisal and coping to chronic illness adjustment. *Behavior Research and Therapy, 28*(4), 297–304.

Bowles, S. (1991). In Rogers-Seide, F. F., *Geriatric Nursing Care Plans.* St. Louis: Mosby-YearBook.

Bowman, B. B. & Rosenberg, I. H. (1982). Assessment of the nutritional status of the elderly. *American Journal of Clinical Nutrition, 35*, 1142–1151.

Braun, B. I. (1991). The effect of nursing home quality on patient outcome. *Journal of the American Geriatrics Society, 39*, 329–338.

Breschneider, J. & McCoy, N. (1988). Sexual interest and behavior in healthy 80 to 102 year olds. *Archives of Sexual Behavior, 17*, 109–29.

Bronstein, K. S., Popovich, J. M. & Amider, C. S. (1991). *Promoting stroke recovery.* St. Louis: Mosby-YearBook.

Browning, M. A. (1995). Depression. In Hogstel, M. O. (Ed). *Geropsychiatric nursing* (2nd ed). St. Louis: Mosby.

Brummel-Smith, K. (1998). Rehabilitation. In Yoshikawa, T., Cobb, E. & Brummel-Smith, K. (eds). *Practical Ambulatory Geriatrics* (2nd ed). St. Louis: Mosby.

Buckwalter, K. (1995). Depression and suicide in Stanley, M. & Beare, P. (Eds). *Gerontological nursing.* Philadelphia: FA Davis & Co.

Buffum, M. & Buffum, I. (1997). The pharmacologic treatment of depresson in elders. *Geriatric Nursing, 18*:144–149.

Bullock, B. L. & Rosendahl, P. P. (1984). *Pathophysiology adaptations and alterations in function.* Boston: Little, Brown.

Bulpitt, C. J. & Fletcher, A. E. (1990). Drug treatment and quality of life in the elderly. *Clinical Geriatric Medicine, 6*(2), 309–317.

Burns, A., Howard, R. & Pettit, W. (1995). *Alzheimer's disease: A medical companion.* Cambridge, MA: Blackwell Science.

Burton, J. (1990). Long-term care. In Beack, J. C., Abrass, I. B., Burton, J. R., Cummings, J. L., Makinodan R. & Small, R. W. (Eds). *Yearbook of geriatrics and gerontology* (p. 71). Chicago: YearBook Medical.

Butler, R. N. & Lewis, M. I. (1977). *Aging & mental health.* St. Louis: Mosby.

California Association of Health Facilities. (1989, February 10). *Guidelines Bulletin No. 89-05: The withdrawal or withholding of life-sustaining procedures in long term care facilities.*

Campbell, J. (1997). Alcoholism. In Ham, R. & Sloane, P. (eds). *Primary Care Geriatrics* (3rd ed). St. Louis: Mosby.

Capezuti, E., Brush, B. & Lawson, W. (1997). Reporting elder mistreatment. *Journal of Gerontological Nursing, 23*(7) 24–32.

Carid, F. I., Dall, J. L. C. & Williams, B. O. (1985). The cardiovascular system. *Textbook of geriatric medicine and gerontology* (3rd ed.). New York: Churchill Livingstone.

Carotenuto, R. & Bullock, J. (1980). *Physical assessment of the gerontologic client.* Philadelphia: F. A. Davis.

Carson, C. (1998). Update on benign prostatic hyperplasia. *The Clinical Advisor, 8*(1):57–65.

Caspersen, C. J., Christenson, G. M. & Pollard, R. A. (1986). Status of the 1990 physical fitness and exercise objectives: Evidence from the N.H.I.S. 1985. *Public Health Reports* 101, 587.

Cello, M. B., Johnson, J. L. & Finch, W. R. (1991). Evaluating arthritis complaints. *Nurse Practitioner, 16*(2), 9–20.

Centers for Disease Control. (1988). Recommendations of the Immunization Practices Advisory Committee, Centers for Disease Control: Prevention and control of influenza. *Journal of the American Geriatrics Society,* 36, 963–968.

Centers for Disease Control and Prevention. (1994). *HIV/AIDS Surveillance Report.* Atlanta: Author.

Centers for Disease Control & Prevention. (1997). Prevention of pneumococcal disease: recommendations of the Advisory Committee on Immunization Practices (ACIP). *MMWR 46* (No. RR-8):1.

Chenitz, W. C., Stone, J. T. & Salisbury, S. A. (1991). *Clinical gerontological nursing.* Philadelphia: Saunders.

Chestnut, C. H., Cumming, S. R. & Drinkwater, B. L. (1988). New options in osteoporosis. *Patient Care,* 22, 160–187.

Chopra, D. (1993). *Ageless body timeless mind: The quantum alternative to growing old.* NY, NY: Random House Audiobooks.

Chaisson-Stewart, G. M. (1985). An integrated theory of depression. In Chaisson-Stewart, G. M. (Ed). *Depression in the elderly: An interdisciplinary approach.* New York: John Wiley and Sons.

Chernoff, R. (1991). *Geriatric Nutrition, The Health Professional's Handbook.* Aspen Publishers, Inc.

Chidester, J. C. & Spangler, A. A. (1997). Fluid intake in the institutionalized elderly. *Journal of the American Dietetic Association, 97*(1), 23–38.

Christian, E., Dluby, N. & O'Neill, R. (1989). Sounds of silence. *Journal of Nursing,* 15, 11.

Cobbs, E. & Brummel-Smith, K. (eds). *Practical Ambulatory Geriatrics* (2nd ed). St. Louis: Mosby.

Cohen, G. (1998). Health modifiability and human potential with aging. In Yoshikawa, T., Congress of the United States, Office of Technology. (1987). *Losing a million minds: Confronting the tragedy of Alzheimer's disease and other dementias.* Washington, DC: U.S. Government Printing Office.

Cockcroft, D. W. & Gault, M. H. (1976). Prediction of creatinine clearance from serum creatinine. *Nephron,* 16, 31–41.

Col, N., Fanale, J. E. & Kronholm, P. (1990). The role of medication noncompliance and adverse drug reactions in hospitalization of the elderly. *Archives of Internal Medicine,* 150, 841–846.

Collman, G. W., Shore, D. L., Shef, C. M., Checkoway, H. & Luria, A. S. (1988). Sunlight and other risk factors for cataracts: An epidemiologic study. *American Journal of Public Health, 78* (11), 1459–1462.

Cooney, L. M. (1990). Transitional rehabilitation: An approach to the patient with a new disability. In Hazzard, W., Andres, R., Brierman, E. & Blass, J. (Eds). *Principles of geriatric medicine and gerontology* (2nd ed). New York: McGraw-Hill.

Costa, P. T. & McCrae, R. R. (1988). Personality in adulthood: A six-year longitudinal study of self-reports and spouse ratings on the NEO personality inventory. *Journal of Personality and Social Psychology, 54*(5), 853–863.

Costa, P. T., Jr., McCrae, R. R., Zonderman, A. B., Barbano, H. E., Lebowitz, B. & Larson, D. M. (1986). Cross-sectional studies of personality in a national sample: 2. Stability in neuroticism, extraversion, and openness. *Psychology and Aging, 1*(2), 144–149.

Coyne, A., Reichman, W. & Berbig, L. (1993). The relationship between dementia and elder abuse. *American Journal of Psychiatry, 150*(4): 643.

Creditor, M. C. (1993). Hazards of hospitalization of the elderly. *Annals of Internal Medicine, 118*(3), 219–223.

Cunningham, W. R. & Bookbank, J. W. (1988). *Gerontology: The psychology, biology, and sociology of aging.* New York: Harper & Row.

Cutrona, C., Russell, D. & Rose, J. (1986). Social support and adaptation to stress by the elderly. *Psychology and Aging, 1*(1), 47–54.

Dalton, C. (1995). Complementary therapies in arthritis treatment. *Advance for Nurse Practitioners, 3*(11), 33.

Davidson, J. K. (1976). Controlling diabetes with diet therapy. *Postgraduate Medicine, 59*(1), 114–119.

Davies, P. (1979). Neurotransmitter-related symptoms in SDAT. *Brain Research, 171,* 319–327.

DeMaagd, G. (1995). High risk drugs in the elderly population. *Geriatric Nursing,* 16:178–207.

Dolan, M. B. (1980). Being old is not the same as being ill. *Nursing, 80,* 41–42.

Doll, R. (1997). One for the heart. *British Medical Journal,* Dec 20–27, 315 (7123), 1664–1668.

Ebersole, P. & Hess, P. (1998). *Toward healthy aging: Human needs and nursing response,* (5th ed). St. Louis: Mosby.

Eliopoulos, C. (Ed). (1990). *Caring for the elderly in diverse care settings* (pp. 257–265). Philadelphia: Lippincott.

Eliopoulis, C. (1995). *Manual of Gerontologic Nursing.* St. Louis: Mosby.

Erikson, E. (1963) *Childhood and society,* (2nd ed). New York: W.W. Norton.

Esberger, K. K. & Hughes, S. T., Jr. (1989). *Nursing care of the aged.* Norwalk, CT: Appleton & Lange.

Ettinger, B. (1987). Overview of the efficacy of hormonal replacement therapy. *American Journal of Obstetrics and Gynecology, 156*(5), 1296–1303.

Ettinger, W. H. (1988). Approach to the diagnosis and management of musculoskeletal disease. *Clinics in Geriatric Medicine, 4*(2), 269–277.

Evans, J. G. (1984). *Aging and disease.* Ciba Foundation Symposium 134.

Fal, T., Herrmann, F. & Rapin, C. H. (1991). Prognostic role of serum albumin and prealbumin levels in elderly patients at admission to a geriatric hospital. *Archives of Gerontology and Geriatrics,* 12, 31–39.

Farmer, M. E., Kittner, S. J., Abbott, R. D., Wolz, M. M., Wolf, P. A. & White, L. R. (1990). Longitudinally measured blood pressure, antihypertensive medication use, and cognitive performance: The Framingham Study. *Journal of Clinical Epidemiology,* 43, 475–480.

Farrell, J. (1990). *Nursing care of the older person.* Philadelphia: Lippincott.

Featherman, D. L. & Peterson, T. (1986). Markers of aging. *Research on Aging, 8*(3), 339–365.

Feil, N. (1984). Communicating with the confused elderly patient. *Geriatrics,* 39, 131–132.

Feil, N. (1994). *The validation breakthrough.* Baltimore: Health Professions Press.

Ferri, F. F. (1997). Selected organ system abnormalities. In Ferri, F. F. & Fretwell, M. D., *Practical guide to the care of the geriatric patient,* (2nd ed). St. Louis: Mosby.

Ferri, F. F. (1992). Geriatric rehabilitation. In Ferri, F. F. & Fretwell, M. D., *Practical guide to the care of the geriatric patient.* St. Louis: Mosby.

Ferri, F. F. & Fretwell, M. D. (1997). *Practical guide to the care of the geriatric patient,* (2nd ed). St Louis: Mosby.

Feutz, S. A. (1990). Legal aspects of gerontological nursing. In Eliopoulos. (pp. 157–177). *Caring for the elderly in diverse care settings.* Philadelphia: Lippincott.

Field, D. & Minkler, M. (1988). Continuity and change in social support between young-old and old-old or very-old age. *Journal of Gerontology, 43*(4), 100–106.

Fifth Report of the Joint National Committee on Detection, Evaluation, and Treatment of High Blood Pressure. (1993). *Archives of Internal Medicine, 153*(2), 154.

Fitten, L. J. (1998). Common psychiatric disorders. In Yoshikawa, T., Cobbs, E. & Brummel-Smith, K. (eds). *Practical Ambulatory Geriatrics,* (2nd ed). St.Louis: Mosby.

Fitting, M. D. (1990). Ethical issues. In Eliopoulos, C. *Caring for the elderly in diverse care settings.* (pp. 178–188). Philadelphia: Lippincott.

Flowers, C. & Baker, R. (1998). Eye disorders. In Yoshikawa, T., Cobb, E. & Brummel-Smith, K. (eds). *Practical ambulatory geriatrics.* St. Louis: Mosby.

Folstein, M. F., et al. (1975). *Journal of Psychiatric Research, 12*(3), 189–190.

Forbes, E. J. & Fitzsimmons, V. M. (1981). *The older adult: A process for wellness.* St. Louis: Mosby.

Foreman, M., Fletcher, K., Mion, L. & Simon, L. (1996). Assessing cognitive function. *Geriatric Nursing, 17*(5), 228.

Francis, J., Strong, S., Martin, D. & Kapoor, W. (1988). Delirium in elderly general medical patients: Common but often unrecognized. [abstract]. *Clinical Research,* 36, 711a.

Frankl, V. E. (1984). *Man's search for meaning.* New York: Washington Square Press.

Fraser, D. (1997). Assessing the elderly for infections. *Journal of Gerontological Nursing, 23*(11), 5–10.

Fretwell, M. (1990). Comprehensive Functional assessment (cfa) in everyday practice. In Hazzard, W., Andes, R., Brierman, E. & Blass, J. (Eds). *Principles of geriatric medicine and gerontology,* (2nd ed). New York: McGraw-Hill.

Fretwell, M. D. (1992). Delirium in the elderly patient. In Ferri, F. F. & Fretwell, M. D. *Practical guide to the care of the geriatric patient.* St. Louis: Mosby.

Fretwell, M. D. (1997). Selected functional syndromes. In Ferri, F. & Fretwell, D. (eds). *Practical guide to the care of the geriatric patient,* (2nd ed). St. Louis: Mosby.

Fried, L. P., Storer, D. J. & King, D. E. (1991). Diagnosis of illness presentation in the elderly. *Journal of the American Geriatrics Society,* 39.

Frohlich, E.V. (1995). Hypertension. In Abrams, W.. Beers, M., Berkow, R. (Eds). *The merck manual of geriatrics,* (2nd ed). Whitehouse Station, NY: Merck Research Laboratories.

Fry, P. S. (1990). A factor-analytic investigation of home-bound elderly individuals' concerns about death and dying. *Journal of Clinical Psychology, 46*(6), 737–748.

Gallagher-Allred, C. (1993). Nutrition Screening and Early Intervention: Keys to Preventing Malnutrition. *Journal of Medical Direction,* January, 1993.

Gallager-Alred, C. (1989). *Nutritional care of the terminally ill.* Rockville, MD: Aspen.

Geokas, M. C. (1990). The aging process. *Annals of Internal Medicine, 113*(6), 455–466.

Geringer, E. S. & Stern, T. A. (1986). Coping with medical illness: The impact of personality types. *Psychosomatics, 27,* 251–261.

Greenblatt, D. J., Allen, M. D. & Shader, R. I. (1977). Toxicity of high-dose flurazepam in the elderly. *Clinical Pharmacology and Therapeutics, 21,* 355–361.

Gress, L. M. & Bahr, R. T. (1984). *The aging person: A holistic perspective.* St. Louis: Mosby.

Gross, P. A., Quinnan, G. V. & Weksler, M. E. (1988). Immunization of elderly people with high doses of influenza vaccine. *Journal of the American Geriatrics Society, 36,* 209–212.

Gwyther, L. P. (1985). Care of Alzheimer's patients: A manual for nursing home staff. American Health Care Association and Alzheimer's Disease and Related Disorders Hall, G.R. & Buckwalter, K.C. (1989). Diagnostic clues in the past. *Geriatric Nursing, 10*(4), 202–204.

Hall, G. R. & Buckwalter, K. C. (1987). Progressively lowered stress threshold: A conceptual model for care of adults with Alzheimer's disease. *Archives of Psychiatric Nursing 1*(6), 399–406.

Hall, G. R. (1991). Altered thought processes: Dementia. In Maas, M., Buckwalter, K. C. & Hardy, M. (eds). *Nursing diagnosis and interventions for the elderly.* Redwood City, CA: Addison-Wesley, Nursing.

Hall, N. K. (1997). Health maintenance and promotion. In Ham, R. & Sloane, P. (eds). *Primary care geriatrics,* (3rd ed). St. Louis: Mosby.

Ham, P. (1997). Sexuality. In Ham, R. & Sloane, P. (eds). *Primary Care Geriatrics,* (3rd ed). St. Louis: Mosby.

Ham, R. J. (1992). Confusion, dementia, and delirium. In Ham, R. J. & Sloane, P. D. *Primary care geriatrics,* (2nd ed). St. Louis: Mosby.

Hampton, J. K. (1991). *The biology of human aging.* Dubuque, IA: W. C. Brown.

Harris, S., Casperson, D., DeFriese, G. & Estes, E. H. (1989). Physical activity counseling for healthy adults as a primary preventive intervention in the clinical setting. *Journal of the American Medical Association, 261*(24), 3590–3598.

Hastings Center. (1987). *Guidelines on the termination of life-sustaining treatment and the care of the dying.* Bloomington, IN: Indiana University Press.

Haug, M. R., Breslau, N. & Folmar, S. J. (1989). Coping resources and selective survival in mental health of the elderly. *Research on Aging, 11,* 468–491.

Haynor, P. (1998). Meeting the Challenge of Advanced Directives. *American Journal of Nursing 98*(3): 27–33.

Hayter, J. (1985). To nap or not to nap. *Geriatric Nursing, 6*(2), 104–106.

Health Care Financing Administration. (1992). *State operations manual.* Baltimore: U.S. Department of Health and Human Services.

Heaney, R. P. (1993). Thinking straight about calcium. *New England Journal of Medicine, 328*(7), 503–505.

Heath, J. & Waters, H. (1998). Hearing. In Ham, R. & Sloane, P. (eds). *Primary Care Geriatrics,* (3rd ed). St. Louis: Mosby.

Heinsimer, J. A. & Lefkowitz, R. J. (1985). The impact of aging on adrenergic receptor function: Clinical and biochemical aspects. *Journal of the American Geriatrics Society, 33,* 184–188.

Heitkemper, M. M. & Williams, S. (1985). Present problems caused by enteral feeding. *Journal of Gerontological Nursing,* 11, 25–30.

Hill, L. & Smith, N. (1990). *Self-care nursing: Promotion of health.* Norwalk, CT: Appleton & Lange.

Hoenig, H. M. & Rubenstein, L.Z. (1991). Hospital associated deconditioning and dysfunction. Sexuality and the elderly. In Lewis, C. B. (Ed). *Aging: The health care challenge.* Philadelphia: F. A. Davis.

Hoole, A. J., Greenberg, R. A. & Pickard, C. G. (1988). *Patient care and guidelines for nurse practitioners* (3rd ed). Boston: Little, Brown.

Humphry, D. (1991). *Final exit.* Eugene, OR: The Hemlock Society.

Hurwitz, N. (1969). Admissions to hospital due to drugs. *British Medical Journal,* 1, 539–540.

Hwalek, M., Neale, A., Goodrich, C. & Quinn, K. (1996). The association of elder abuse and substance abuse in the Illinois elder abuse system. *Gerontologist, 36*(5): 694–700.

Inouye, S. K., van Dyck, C. H., Alessi, C. A., Balkin, S., Siegal, A. P. & Horwitz, R. I. (1990). Clarifying confusion: The confusion assessment method, a new method for detection of delirium. *Annals of Internal Medicine, 113*(12), 941–947.

Ives, T. J. (1992). Pharmacotherapeutics. In Ham, R. J. & Sloane, P. D. *Primary care geriatrics,* (2nd ed, chap. 9). St. Louis: Mosby.

Ives, T. J. (1997). Pharmacotherapeutics. In Ham, R. J. & Sloane, P. D. *Primary care geriatrics* (3rd ed, chap. 10). St. Louis: Mosby.

Jackson, J. E. & Ramsdell, J. (1989). *Cognitive impairment: New perspectives in geriatric medicine.* Allen & Hanburys.

Jackson, R. (1997). Geriatric Nutrition. *In The Florida Dietetic Association Handbook of Medical Nutrition Therapy: The Florida Diet Manual,* 1997 Edition. B2.1–B2.20.

Jaffe, M. E. (1987). The clinical investigation of drugs for use by the elderly: Industry initiatives. *Clinical Pharmacology and Therapeutics,* 42, 686–690.

Jahnigen, D. (1997). In Ham, R. & Sloane, P. (eds). *Primary Care Geriatrics,* (3rd ed). St. Louis: Mosby.

Jenike, M. A. (1988). Alzheimer's disease: What the practicing clinician needs to know. *Journal of Geriatric Psychiatry and Neurology,* 1, 37–46.

Jenike, M. A. (1989). *Geriatric psychiatry and psychopharmacology: A clinical approach.* Chicago: YearBook Medical.

Joffrion, L. & Leuszler, L. (1995). The gastrointestinal tract and its problems in the elderly, with nutritional considerations. In Stanley, M. & Beare, P. (eds). *Gerontological nursing.* Philadelphia: FA Davis.

Johnson, M., Haight, B. & Benedict, S. (1998). AIDS in older people: An Integrated literature review for clinical nursing research and practice. *Journal of Gerontological Nursing, 24*(4), 8–13.

Kamath, S. K., Lawler, M. & Smith, A. E. (1986). Hospital malnutrition: A 33-hospital study. *Journal of the American Dietetic Association,* 86, 203–206.

Kane, R. L., Garrard, J. & Buchanan, J. L. (1991). Improving primary care in nursing homes. *Journal of the American Geriatrics Society,* 39, 359–367.

Kaplan, H. & Sadock, B. (1994). *Synopsis of psychiatry,* (6th ed). Baltimore: Williams & Wilkins.

Katz, S., Ford, A. B., Moskowitz, R. W. et al. (1963). Studies of illness in the aged. The index of ADL: A standard measure of biological and psychosocial function. *Journal of the American Medical Association,* 185, 914.

Katzman, R. & Jackson, J. E. (1991). Alzheimer's disease: Basic and clinical advances. *Journal of the American Geriatric Society,* 39, 516–525.

Katzman, R. & Terry, R. (1983). *The neurology of aging.* Philadelphia: F. A. Davis.

Keane, S. M. & Sells, S. (1990). Recognizing depression in the elderly. *Journal of Gerontological Nursing, 16*(1), 21–25.

Kenney, R. A. (1985). Physiology of aging. *Clinical Geriatric Medicine.* 1, 37–40.

Keram, S. & Williams, M. E. (1988). Quantifying the ease or difficulty older persons experience in opening medication containers. *Journal of the American Geriatrics Society,* 36, 198–201.

Kern, S. (1990). The geriatric nurse practitioner in a multipurpose senior center. In Eliopoulos, C. (Ed). *Caring for the elderly in diverse care settings* (pp. 257–265). Philadelphia: Lippincott.

Kerr, H. D. & Byrd, J. C. (1991). Nursing home patients transferred by ambulance to a VA emergency department. *Journal of the American Geriatrics Society,* 39, 132–136.

Kirkpatrick, M. K., Edwards, M. K. & Finch, N. (1991). Assessment and prevention of osteoporosis through use of a client self-supporting tool. *Nurse Practitioner, 16*(7), 16–26.

Knapp, M. T. (1989). A rose is still a rose. *Geriatric nursing, 10*(6), 290–291.

Korn, J. & Poland, G. (1989). Adult immunization. *Primary Care, 16*(1) 177–193.

Kradjan, W. A., Kobayashi, K. A. & Bauer, L. A. (1989). Glipizide pharmacokinetics: Effects of age, diabetes, and multiple dosing. *Journal of Clinical Pharmacology,* 29, 1121–1127.

Kroenke, K. & Pinholt, E. M. (1990). Reducing polypharmacy in the elderly. *Journal of the American Geriatrics Society,* 38, 31–36.

Kubler-Ross, E. (1969). *On death and dying.* New York, McMillan.

Kurrle, S. (1988). Insomnia in the elderly. *Australian Family Physician, 17*(8), 638–639.

LaVoie, A. (1997). *Cold sore virus linked to Alzheimer's disease.* Medical Tribune News Service, Jan. 23.

Leirer, V. O., Morrow, D. G. & Pariante, G. M. (1988). Elders' nonadherence, its assessment, and computer assisted instruction for medication recall training. *Journal of the American Geriatrics Society,* 36, 877–884.

Libow, L. S. & Starer, P. (1989). Care of the nursing home patient. *Medical Intelligence,* 321, 93–96.

Lindsay, R. (1989). Osteoporosis: An updated approach to prevention and management. *Geriatrics, 44*(1), 45–54.

Lipowski, Z. (1989). Delirium in the elderly patient. *New England Journal of Medicine, 320*(9), 578–582.

Lyles, K. (1998). Osteopenia: Osteoporosis and osteomalacia. In Yoshikawa, T., Cobbs, E. & Brummel-Smith, K. (eds). *Practical Care Geriatrics* (2nd ed). St. Louis: Mosby.

Lynch, S. (1997). Elder Abuse: What to look for, how to intervene. *American Journal of Nursing, 97*(1):27-33.

Maas, M., Buckwalter, K. C. & Hardy, M. (1991). *Nursing diagnosis and interventions for the elderly.* Redwood City, CA: Addison-Wesley.

Martin, L. A. & Barkan, H. (1989). Clinical communication strategies of nurse practitioners with patients. *Journal of the American Academy of Nurse Practitioners, 1*(3), 77–83.

Maryland Attorney General's Office. (1990). *Nursing homes: what you need to know,* pp. 17–19.

Master, J. C. (1996). When lithium doesn't help: The use of anticonvulsants and calcium channel blockers in the treatment of bipolar disorder in the older person. *Geriatric nursing, 17*(2), 75.

Matthews, L. E. (1989). Pressure sores: Nutrition care's vital role. *Journal of Nutrition in the Elderly,* 8, 107–113.

Matteson, M. A. & McConnell, E. S. (1988). *Gerontological nursing concepts and practices.* Philadelphia: Saunders.

Mattson, M. & McConnell, E. (1997). Gerontological nursing in acute care settings. In *Gerontological nursing,* (2nd ed). Philadelphia: Saunders.

Matthiesen, V., Lamb, K., McCann, J., Hollinger Smith, L. & Walton, J. (1996). Hospital nurses' views about physical restraint use with older patients. *Journal of Gerontological Nursing,* 22(6):8–16.

Matzo, M. (1997). The search to end meaning: A historical perspective. *Journal of Gerontological Nursing,* 23(3):11–17.

McCelvaney, G., Blackie, S. & Morrison, N. J. (1989). Maximal static respiratory pressures in the normal elderly. *American Review Respiratory Digest,* 139, 277–281.

McCrae, R. R. (1989). Age differences and changes in the use of coping mechanisms. *Journal of Gerontology,* 44(6), 161–169.

Mellick, E., Buckwalter, K.C. & Stolley, J.M. (1992). Suicide in elderly white men: Development of a profile. *Journal of Psychosocial Nursing,* 30(2), 29–34.

Menscer, D. (1997). Hypertension. In Ham, R. & Sloan, P. (eds). *Primary Care Geriatrics* (3rd ed). St. Louis: Mosby.

Meyers, B. S. & Alexopoulas, G.S. (1988). Geriatric depression. *Medical Clinics of North America, 72*(4), 847–863.

Miles, L. E. & Dement, W. C. (1980). Sleep and aging. *Sleep,* 3, 119–120.

Miller, C. (1996). Identifying adverse medication effects when assessing function. *Geriatric Nursing, 17*(6), 295–296.

Miller, C. A. (1990). *Nursing care of older adults.* Glenview, NY: Scott, Foresman.

Miller, I. J. (1988). Human taste bud density across adult age groups. *Journal of Gerontology, 43*(1), 26–30.

Montamat, S. C., Crusack, B. J. & Vestal, R. E. (1989). Management of drug therapy in the elderly. *New England Journal of Medicine, 321*(5), 303–309.

Moody, R. A. (1976). *Life after life.* New York, Bantam Books.

Moon, A. & Williams, O. (1993). Perceptions of elder abuse and help-seeking patterns among African-American, Caucasian-American and Korean-American elderly women. *Gerontologist, 33*(3):386–390.

Moore, M. C. (1988). *Nutrition and diet therapy* (pp. 17-19). St. Louis: Mosby.

Morley, J. (1998). Weight problems. In Yoshikawa, T., Cobbs, E., Brummel-Smith, K. (eds). *Practical Ambulatory Geriatrics* (2nd ed). St. Louis: Mosby.

Morley, J. E., Glick, Z. & Rubenstein, L. (eds). (1990). *Geriatric nutrition: A comprehensive review* (pp. 225–229). New York: Raven.

Morrow, D., Leirer, V. O. & Sheikh, J. (1988). Adherence and medication instructions. *Journal of the American Geriatrics Society,* 36, 1147–1160.

Mosquedo, L. & Brummel-Smith, K. (1997). Stroke. In Ham, R. J. & Sloane, P. D. *Primary care geriatrics,* (3rd ed). St. Louis: Mosby.

Mueller, M. R. (1997). Social barriers to recognizing HIV/AIDS in older adults. *Journal of Gerontological Nursing, 23*(11), 17–21.

Mullan, M., Crawford, F. & Axelman, K. (1992). A pathogenic mutation for probable Alzheimer's disease in the App gene at the N Terminal of b-amyloid. *Nature Genetics,* 1, 2345–2347.

Murphy, D. J., Murray, A. M., Robinson, R. E. & Campion, E. W. (1989). Outcome of cardiopulmonary resuscitation in the elderly. *Annals of Internal Medicine, 111*(3), 199–205.

Murray, R., Huelskoetter, M. & O'Driscoll, D. (1980). *Journal of Gerontology: Medical Sciences, 47*(M), 122–29.

Murray, R. B., Huelskoetter. M. M. W. & O'Driscoll, D. L. (1980). *The nursing process in later maturity.* Englewood Cliffs, NJ: Prentice-Hall.

National Center on Elder Abuse. (1996). Elder abuse in domestic settings. *Elder abuse informational series,* No. 3, Washington D.C.: Author.

Nelson, J., Moxness, K., Jensen, M. & Gastineau, C. (1994). *Mayo Clinic Diet Manual, A Handbook of Nutrition Practices.* Chapter 16, Nutritional Support of Adults. (pp. 385–409), Chapter 7, Cardiovascular Disease (p. 131), and Appendix 2, Interactions between Drugs, Nutrients, and Nutritional Status (pp. 625–646). St. Louis: Mosby.

Nelson, M. & Wernick, S. (1997). *Strong Women Stay Young,* (Chapters 1–4). New York: Bantam Books.

Nelson, R. C. & Franzi, L. R. (1992). Nutrition. In Ham, R. J. & Sloane, P. D. *Primary care geriatrics,* (2nd ed, chap. 9). St. Louis: Mosby.

Neugarten, B. (1973) Adult personality: A developmental view. In Charles, D., & Looft, W., (Eds). *Readings in psychology and development through life* (pp. 356–366). New York: Holt, Rinehart and Winston.

Nolan, L. & O'Malley, K. (1988). Prescribing for the elderly, part II. Prescribing patterns: Differences due to age. *Journal of the American Geriatric Society,* 36, 245–254.

Nolan, L. & O'Malley, K. (1989). Adverse drug reactions in the elderly. *British Journal of Hospital Medicine,* 41, 446–457.

Norton, D., McLaren, R. & Extar-Smith, A. N. (1962). *An investigation of geriatric nursing problems in hospitals.* Edinburgh: Churchill Livingstone.

Nutrition interventions manual for professionals caring for older americans (NIM). (1992). Washington, D.C.: Nutrition Screening Initiative.

O'Malley, K., Crooks, J. & Duke, E. (1971). Effect of age and sex on human drug metabolism. *British Medical Journal,* 3, 607–609.

Oberlink, M., Butler, R., Faye, E., Gauzzo, E. & Kupfer, C. (1997). Keeping an eye on vision: Primary care of age-related ocular disease. *Geriatrics,* (52), 30–41.

Overstall, P. W., Exton-Smith, A. N. & Imms, F. J. (1977). Falls in the elderly related to postural imbalance. *British Medical Journal,* 1, 261–264.

Pannill, F. C., Williams, T. F. & Davis, R. (1988). Evaluation and treatment of urinary incontinence in long-term care. *Journal of the American Geriatrics Society,* 36, 902–910.

Pate, R., Blair, S., Durstine, J., Eddy, D., Hanson, P., Painter, P., Smith, L. & Wolfe, L. (Eds). (1991). *Guidelines for exercise testing and prescription.* Philadelphia: Lea & Febiger.

Payne, B. & Cikovic, R (1996). An empirical examination of the characteristics, consequences and causes of elder abuse in nursing homes. Journal of *Elder Abuse & Neglect, 7*(4): 61–74.

Perrin, K. (1997). Giving voice to the wishes of elders for end-of-life care. *Journal of Gerontological Nursing, 23*(3):18–27.

Perry, P. J., Alexander, B. & Liskow, B. I. (1991). *Psychotropic drug handbook* (6th ed). Cincinnati: Harvey Whitney.

Pillemer, K. & Finkelhof, D. (1988). The prevalence of elder abuse: A random sample survey. *Gerontologist*, 28:51.

Pillemer, K. & Moore, D. (1988). Abuse of patients in nursing homes: Findings from a survey of staff. *Gerontologist, 29*(3):314–326.

Powers, J. S., Krantz, S. B. & Collins, J. C. (1991). Erythropoietin response to anemia as a function of age. *Journal of the American Geriatrics Society,* 39, 30–32.

Quinn, M. & Tomita, S. (1997). *Elder abuse and neglect,* (2nd ed). NY: Springer.

Rader, J. (1995). Use of skillful, creative psychosocial interventions. In Rader, J. & Tornquist, E. (eds). *Individualized Dementia Care.* NY: Springer.

Ray, A., Taylor, J., Meador, K., Lichenstein, M., Griffin, M. Fought, R. & Blazer, D. (1994). Reducing antipsychotic drug use in nursing homes. *Arch Intern Med,* 153:713–721.

Reed, R. (1998). Preventive interventions. In Yoshikawa, T., Cobbs, E. & Brummel-Smith, K. (eds). *Practical ambulatory geriatrics,* (2nd ed). St. Louis: Mosby.

Reddy, U. & Thadepalli, H. (1998). Respiratory infections. In Yoshikawa, T., Cobbs, E. & Brummel-Smith, K. (eds). *Practical Ambulatory Geriatrics,* (2nd ed). St. Louis: Mosby.

Reece, R. D. & Faryna, A. (1990). *Geriatric medicine for the house officer.* Baltimore: Williams & Wilkins.

Reid, I. R., Ames, R. W., Evans, M. C., Gamble, G. D. & Sharpe, S. J. (1993). Effect of calcium supplementation on bone loss in postmenopausal women. *New England Journal of Medicine, 327*(2), 160–164.

Rho, J. & Wong, F. (1998). Principles of prescribing medications. In Yoshikawa, T., Cobbs, E. & Brummel-Smith, K. (eds). *Practical Ambulatory Geriatrics,* (2nd ed). St. Louis: Mosby.

Riggs, B. L. & Melton, L. J. (1992). The prevention and treatment of osteoporosis. *New England Journal of Medicine, 326*(8), 620–627.

Ringsven, M. K. & Bond, D. (1991). *Gerontology and leadership skills for nurses.* Florence: Delmar Publishers, Inc.

Rogers-Seidl, F. F. (1991). *Geriatric nursing care plans.* St. Louis: Mosby-YearBook.

Rosen, W. G., Terry, R. D., Fuld, P. A., et al. (1980). Pathological verification of ischemia score in differentiation of dementia. *Annals of Neurology,* 7, 486–488.

Reuben, D. (1998). Comprehensive assessment in the office. In Yoshikawa, T., Cobbs, E. & Brummel-Smith, K. (eds). *Practical ambulatory geriatrics,* (2nd ed). St. Louis: Mosby.

Rubenstein, L. (1998). Falls. In Yoshikawa, T., Cobbs, E. & Brummel-Smith, K. (eds). *Practical ambulatory geriatrics,* (2nd ed). St. Louis: Mosby.

Rudman, D., Feller, A. G. & Nagraj, H. S. (1990). Effects of human growth hormone in men over 60 years old. *New England Journal of Medicine,* 323, 1–6.

Ryden, M. Pearson, V, Kass, M, Snyder, M., Krichbaum, K., Lee, H., Hagans, E. & Hanscom, J. (1998). Assessment of depression in a population at risk: Newly admitted nursing home residents. *Journal of Gerontological Nursing, 24*(2):21–29.

St. Pierre, J., Craven, R. & Bruno, P. (1986). Late life depression: A guide for assessment. *Journal of Gerontological Nursing, 12*(7), 5–10.

Sarra, K. W. (1988). Audiological assessment program. *Journal of Gerontological Nursing,* 14, 19.

Schafer, R, Bohannon, B., Franz, M., Freeman, J, Holmes, A., McLaughlin, S., Haas, L., Kruger, D., Lorenz, R. & McMahon, M. (1997). Translation of the diabetes nutrition recommendations for health care institutions:technical review. *Journal of the American Dietetic Association, 97*(1), 43–51.

Scharre, D. & Cummings, J. (1998). Dementia. In Yoshikawa, T., Cobb, E. & Brummel-Smith, K. (eds). *Practical Ambulatory Geriatrics,* (2nd ed). St. Louis: Mosby.

Scherer, J. (1985). Nurses drug manual. Philadelphia: Lippincott.

Schneider, L. (1996). Overview of generalized anxiety disorder in the elderly. *J Clin Psychiatry,* 57 (supp 7), 34–45.

Schoene-Sieffert, B. & Childress, J. F. (1986). How much should cancer patients know and decide? *CA-A Journal for Clinicians, 36*(2): 85–94.

Scott, R. B. (1989). Alcohol effects in the elderly. *Comprehensive Therapy, 15*(6), 8–12.

Seghieri, G., Bartolomei, G. C. & De Georgio, L. A. (1989). Serum digoxin and beta-methyldigoxin in elderly patients on hospital admission: Correlation with home compliance and clinical variables. *European Journal of Clinical Pharmacology,* 37, 401–404.

Shea, C., Mahoney, M. & Lacey, J. (1997). Breaking through the barriers to domestic violence intervention. *American Journal of Nursing, 97*(6):26–34.

Singer, C. (1998). Sleep disorders. In Yoshikawa, T., Cobb, E. & Brummel-Smith, K. (eds). *Practical Ambulatory Geriatrics,* (2nd ed). St. Louis: Mosby.

Sloane, P. D. (1997). Normal aging. In Ham, R. J. & Sloane, P. D., (eds). *Primary care geriatrics* (3rd ed). St. Louis: Mosby.

Small, G. (1997). Recognizing and treating anxiety in the elderly. *J Clin Psychiatry,* 58 (supp 3): 41–47.

Smith, N. & Crumpacker, B. (1997). Coronary Artery Disease and Hyperlipidemia. In *The Florida Dietetic Association Handbook of Medical Nutrition Therapy: The Florida Diet Manual.* 1997 Edition. E2.1 – E2.13.

Spagnoli, A., Ostino, G. & Borga, A. D. (1989). Drug compliance and unreported drugs in the elderly. *Journal of the American Geriatrics Society,* 37, 619–624.

Spar, J. E. (1985). Drug treatment. In Chaisson-Stewart, G. M., (Ed). *Depression in the elderly: An interdisciplinary approach* (pp. 193–213). New York: John Wiley and Sons.

Speechley, M. & Tinetti, M. (1991). Falls and injuries in frail and vigorous community elderly persons. *Journal of the American Geriatrics Society,* 39, 46–52.

Staab, A. S. & Lyles, M. K. (1990). *Manual of geriatric nursing.* Philadelphia: Scott, Foresman.

Stanley, M. & Beare, F. (1995). *Gerontological Nursing.* Philadelphia: FA. Davis Co.

Steinke, E. E. (1991). Sexual dysfunction. In Rogers-Seidl, F. F.. *Geriatric nursing care plans.* St. Louis: Mosby-YearBook.

Stolley, J. M. & Buckwalter, K. C. (1991). Iatrogenesis in the elderly: Nosocomial infections. *Journal of Gerontological Nursing, 17*(9), 30–34.

Stolley, J. M., Buckwalter, K. C., Fjordbak, B. & Bush, S. (1991). Iatrogenesis in the elderly: Drug-related problems. *Journal of Gerontological Nursing, 17*(9), 12–17.

Stolley, J. M. & Buckwalter, K. C. (1992). Confusion management. In Bulechek, G. M. & McCloskey, J. C. (eds). *Nursing interventions: Essential nursing treatments* (chap. 9). Philadelphia: Saunders.

Strittmatter, W. J., Saunders, A. M., Schmechel, D., et al. (1993). Apolipoprotein E: High-avidity binding to b-amyloid and increased frequency of type 4-allele in late onset familial Alzheimer's disease. *Proceedings of the National Academy of Sciences of the United States of America, 90*, 1977–1981.

Stromberg, L. (1998). Social and spiritual contributors to independence. In Yoshikawa, T., Cobbs, E & Brummel-Smith, K. (eds). *Practical ambulatory geriatrics,* (2nd ed). St. Louis: Mosby.

Studenski, S. & Laird, R. (1998). Joint problems. In Yoshikawa, T., Cobbs, E., & Brummel-Smith, K. (eds). (1988). *Practical Ambulatory Geriatrics* (2nd ed). St.Louis: Mosby.

Sullivan, R. J. (1989). Respiratory depression requiring ventilatory support following 0.5mg of triazolam. *Journal of the American Geriatrics Society, 37*, 450–452.

Swift, C. G. (1988). Ethical aspects of clinical research in the elderly. *British Journal of Hospital Medicine, 40*, 370–373.

Taggart, H. M. (1988). Do drugs affect the risk of hip fracture in elderly women? *Journal of the American Geriatrics Society, 36*, 1006–1010.

Tatara, T. (1995). *An analysis of state laws addressing elder abuse, neglect and exploitation.* Washington D.C.: National Center on Elder Abuse.

Terry, R. D. (1988). *Aging and the brain.* New York: Raven.

Thun, M. J. (1997). Alcohol consumption and mortality among middle-aged and elderly U.S. adults. *New Eng J of Medicine, 337*(24), 1705–1714.

Tucker, M. A., Andrew, M. F. & Ogle, S. J. (1989). Age-associated change in pain threshold measured by transcutaneous neuronal electrical stimulation. *Age and Ageing, 18*, 241–246.

Tune, L. E. & Lucas-Blaustein, M. J. (1990). Driving and Alzheimer's patients. *San Diego Alzheimer's Association Newsletter, 8*, 2.

U.S. Bureau of the Census. (1996). *Current population reports, (Special Studies, P23-178), Sixty-Five Plus in America.* Washington, DC: U.S. Government Printing Office.

U.S. Preventive Services Task Force (1989). *Guide to clinical preventive services.* Baltimore: William & Wilkins.

U. S. Public Health Service (1990). *Healthy people 2000: national health promotion and disease prevention objectives* (DHHS Publication No. PHS 91-50212). Washington, DC: U.S. Government Printing Office.

Walker, S. N. (1991). Wellness and aging. In Baines, E. M. (Ed). *Perspectives on gerontological nursing.* Newbury Park, CA: Sage.

Weizman, R. & Hart, J. (1987). Sexual behavior in healthy married elderly men. *Archives of Sexual Behavior, 16*, 39–44.

Welch, T. (1998). Liquid Assets: Hydration in the older adult. The Consultant Dietitian. Wellman, N., Weddle, D. & Bates, G. (1997). Nutrition Screening Initiative. In *The Florida Dietetic Association Handbook of Medical Nutrition Therapy: The Florida Diet Manual.* 1997 Edition. B3.1–B3.6.

Whipple, B. & Scura, K. (1996). The overlooked epidemic: HIV in older adults. *American Journal of Nursing, 96*(2), 23–28.

White, J. & Ham, R. (1997). Nutrition. In Ham, R. J. & Sloane, P. D. (eds). *Primary care geriatrics* (3rd ed). St. Louis: Mosby.

Williams, T. F. (1987). Aging or disease? *Clinical Pharmacology and Therapeutics, 42,* 663–665.

Wilson, J. A. & MacLennan, W. J. (1989). Review: Drug-induced parkinsonism in elderly patients. *Age and Ageing,* 18, 208–210.

Wilson, W. (1995). Nose and Throat Disorders in Abrams, W, Beers, M. & Berkow, R. (eds). *The Merck Manual of Geriatrics* (2nd ed). Whitehouse Station, NJ: Merck Research Laboratories.

Windhem, C. T. (1983). Nutrient density of diets in the USDA nationwide food consumption survey: Adequacy of nutrient density consumption practices. *Journal of the American Dietetic Association, 82*(1), 34–43.

Winters, R. K. (1989). Adapting the environment to age-related sensory losses. *Journal of the American Academy of Nurse Practitioners, 1*(4), 106–111.

Wold, S. J. (1990). *Community health nursing.* Norwalk, CT: Appleton & Lange.

Woo, E., Proulx, S. M. & Greenblatt, D. J. (1991). Differential side effect profile of triazolam versus flurazepam in elderly patients undergoing rehabilitation therapy. *Journal of Clinical Pharmacology,* 31, 168–173.

Wood, A. J. J. (1992). The prevention and treatment of osteoporosis. *New England Journal of Medicine, 327*(9), 620–627.

Wooten, P. (1996). Humor: An antidote for stress. *Holistic Nursing Practice, 10*(2), 49–56.

Wynne, H. A., Mutch, E. & Williams, F. M. (1989). The relation of age to the acute effects of ethanol on acetanilide disposition. *Age and Ageing,* 18, 123–126.

Yee, B., Williams, B. J. & O'Hara, N. M. (1990). Medication management and appropriate substance use for elderly persons. In Lewis, C. B. (Ed). *Aging: The health care challenge* (pp. 298–329). Philadelphia: F. A. Davis Co.

Yeomans, A. C. (1991). Assessment and management of gouty arthritis. *Nurse Practitioner, 16*(4).

Yesavage, J. A. & Brink, T. L. (1983). Development and validation of a geriatric depression screening scale: A preliminary report. *Journal of Psychiatric Research, 17*(1), 37–47.

Ying, W. (1996). Deleterious network hypothesis of Alzheimer's disease. *Medical Hypotheses, 46*(5), 421.

Yoshikawa, T., Cobb, E. & Brummel-Smith, K. (1998). *Practical ambulatory geriatrics* (2nd ed). St. Louis: Mosby.

Yuen, G. J. (1990). Altered pharmacokinetics in the elderly. *Clinical Geriatric Medicine, 6*(2), 257–266.

Yura, H. (1978). The need for sleep. In Yura, H. & Walsh, M. B. (eds). *Human needs and the nursing process.* New York: Appleton.

Yurich, A. G., Spier, B. E., Robb, S. S., Elbert, N. J. & Magnussen, M. H. (1989). *The aged person and the nursing process* (3rd ed). Norwalk, CT: Appleton & Lange.

Zatura, A. J., Maxwell, B. M. & Reich, J. W. (1989). Relationships among physical impairment, distress, and well-being in older adults. *Journal of Behavioral Medicine,* 12, 543–557.

Zimberg, S. (1996). Treating alcoholism: An age-specific intervention that works for older patients. *Geriatrics, 51*(10), 45–51.

Zimmer, J. G. & Watson, N. M. (1991). Physician response to notification of acute problems in nursing homes. *Journal of the American Geriatrics Society,* 39, 348–352.

INDEX

PRETEST KEY

1.	C	Chapter 1
2.	B	Chapter 1
3.	C	Chapter 1
4.	D	Chapter 2
5.	D	Chapter 2
6.	A	Chapter 3
7.	B	Chapter 3
8.	D	Chapter 3
9.	A	Chapter 4
10.	D	Chapter 4
11.	D	Chapter 4
12.	B	Chapter 5
13.	C	Chapter 5
14.	C	Chapter 6
15.	B	Chapter 6
16.	B	Chapter 6
17.	B	Chapter 7
18.	B	Chapter 7
19.	B	Chapter 8
20.	A	Chapter 8
21.	A	Chapter 8
22.	D	Chapter 9
23.	D	Chapter 9
24.	B	Chapter 10
25.	B	Chapter 10